Radiation Oncology Primer and Review

Radiation Oncology Primer and Review

Essential Concepts and Protocols

George Rodrigues, MD, FRCPC, MSc
Associate Professor
Departments of Oncology/Epidemiology and Biostatistics
Clinician Scientist, Radiation Oncology
Univeristy of Western Ontario
London Health Sciences Centre
London, Ontario, Canada

Vikram Velker, MD
Radiation Oncology
Department of Oncology
University of Western Ontario
London, Ontario, Canada

Lara Best, MD
Radiation Oncology
Department of Oncology
University of Western Ontario
London, Ontario, Canada

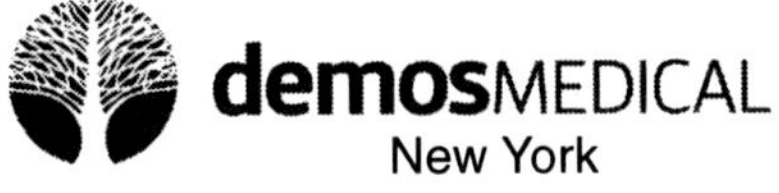

Visit our website at www.demosmedpub.com

ISBN: 9781620700044
e-book ISBN: 9781617051661

Acquisitions Editor: Rich Winters
Compositor: Newgen

Medicine is an ever-changing science. Research and clinical experience are continually expanding our knowledge, in particular our understanding of proper treatment and drug therapy. The authors, editors, and publisher have made every effort to ensure that all information in this book is in accordance with the state of knowledge at the time of production of the book. Nevertheless, the authors, editors, and publisher are not responsible for errors or omissions or for any consequences from application of the information in this book and make no warranty, express or implied, with respect to the contents of the publication. Every reader should examine carefully the package insert accompanying each drug and should carefully check whether the dosage schedules mentioned therein or the contraindications stated by the manufacturer differ from the statements made in this book. Such examination is particularly important with drugs that are either rarely used or have been newly released on the market. Similarly, typical radiation therapy protocols and dosages are stated for reference, but should be carefully examined and confirmed by review of the relevant medical literature prior to any clinical application in order to ensure radiotherapy best practices.

Library of Congress Cataloging-in-Publication Data
Rodrigues, George.
Radiation oncology primer and review : essential concepts and protocols / George Rodrigues, MD FRCPC MSc, associate professor and clinician scientist, Departments of Oncology and Epidemiology/Biostatistics, London Health Sciences Centre and Western University, London, Ontario, Canada, Vikram Velker, MD, resident, Radiation Oncology, Department of Oncology, London Health Sciences Centre and Western University, London, Ontario, Canada, Lara Best, MD, resident, Radiation Oncology, Department of Oncology, London Health Sciences Centre and Western University, London, Ontario, Canada.
p. : cm
Includes bibliographical references and index.
ISBN 978-1-62070-004-4 ; ISBN 978-1-61705-166-1 (E-book)
1. Cancer—Radiotherapy—Textbooks. I. Velker, Vikram. II. Best, Lara. III. Title.
RC271.R3R63 2013
616.99'40642—dc23 2013001188

Cover Image
Illustrated is a Lichtenberg figure: a branching structure formed from an electrical discharge on or inside of an insulator, in this case Perspex®. The structures take their name from Georg Christoph Lichtenberg, the physicist who discovered and studied these entities.

Photograph courtesy of Dr. Marcella Bauman

Special Sales Department
Demos Medical Publishing, LLC
11 West 42nd Street, 15th Floor
New York, NY 10036
Phone: 800–532-8663 or 212-683-0072
Fax: 212–941-7842
E-mail: rsantana@demosmedpub.com

Printed in the United States of America by Gasch Printing.
13 14 15 16 17 / 5 4 3 2 1

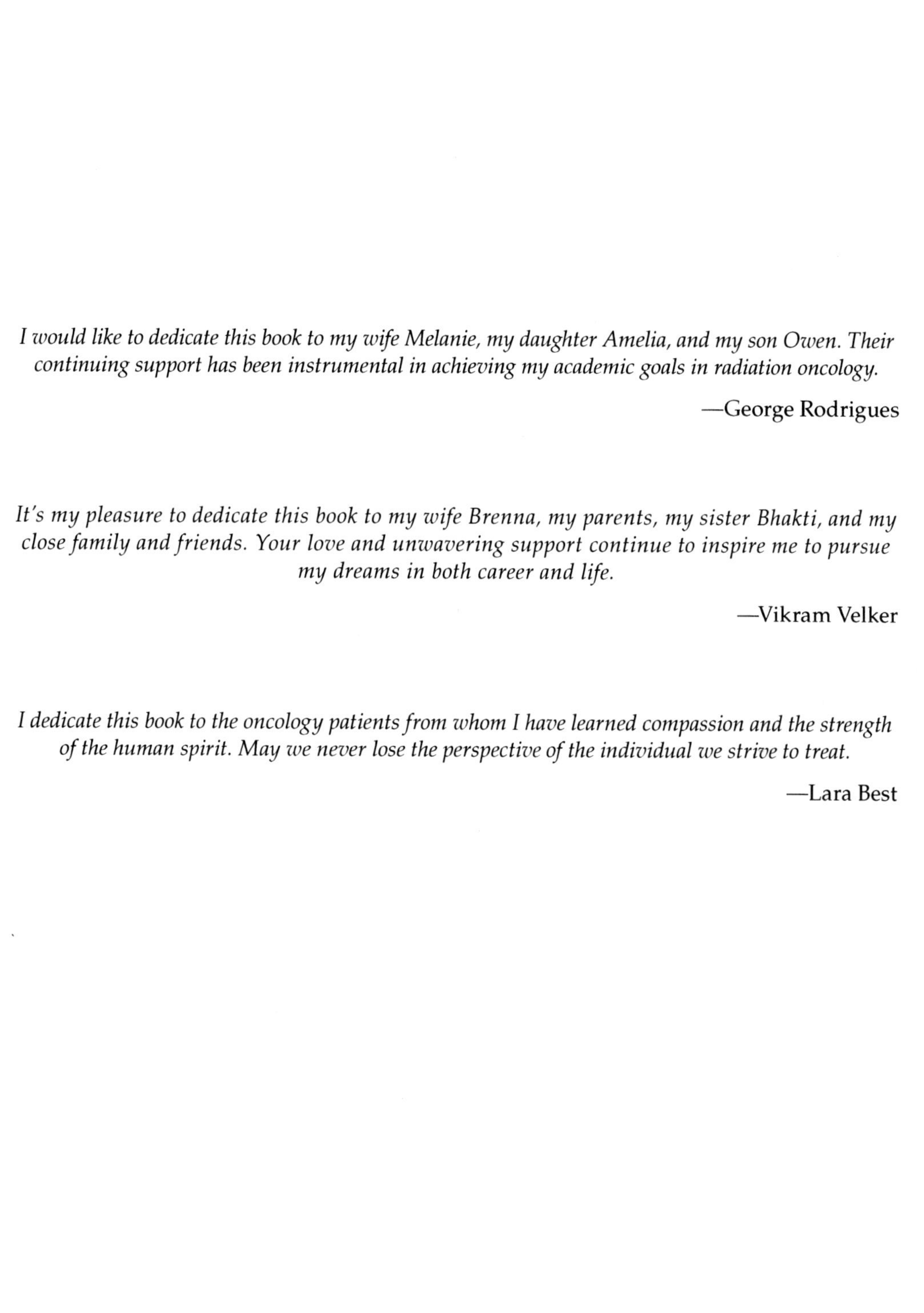

I would like to dedicate this book to my wife Melanie, my daughter Amelia, and my son Owen. Their continuing support has been instrumental in achieving my academic goals in radiation oncology.

—George Rodrigues

It's my pleasure to dedicate this book to my wife Brenna, my parents, my sister Bhakti, and my close family and friends. Your love and unwavering support continue to inspire me to pursue my dreams in both career and life.

—Vikram Velker

I dedicate this book to the oncology patients from whom I have learned compassion and the strength of the human spirit. May we never lose the perspective of the individual we strive to treat.

—Lara Best

Contents

PART III: TREATMENT PLANNING PROTOCOLS AND CONCEPTS

Preface

The practice of radiation oncology requires trainees to integrate a wide range of basic science, clinical science, and treatment planning concepts. This fusion of clinical and technical skills with basic science knowledge attracts many medical trainees to radiation oncology. Many of the concepts relevant to radiation oncology are not routinely integrated in a typical medical school curriculum.

Radiation Oncology Primer and Review was specifically written to efficiently teach high-yield concepts to junior trainees to fill the educational gap not filled by other existing textbooks. The authors of this first edition of *Radiation Oncology Primer and Review* comprise a former program director in radiation oncology, as well as a senior and junior resident in radiation oncology. This editorial team was assembled to provide a relatively consistent presentation of high-yield concepts with high educational relevance to radiation oncology training.

The primary audience for this introductory book in radiation oncology includes junior radiation oncology residents (PGY1–3), senior radiation oncology residents (reviewing for rotations, written examinations, and oral examinations), as well as medical students completing rotations in radiation oncology. Other individuals that would likely benefit from reviewing the concepts and material introduced in this book include: radiation therapist trainees, medical physicist trainees, as well as nursing professionals routinely interacting with radiation oncology professionals and patients.

The first two sections of the book review high-yield basic and clinical science concepts that underlie the practice of radiation oncology. Topics covered in these sections have been cross-referenced to the International Atomic Energy Agency Syllabus for the education and training of radiation oncologists, which has been endorsed by the American Society for Radiation Oncology and the European Society for Therapeutic Radiology and Oncology (report TCS-36). Tables and figures are utilized to clearly illustrate concepts discussed in the text. Many of these tables and figures are specifically designed to be simple in nature to illustrate core information and to maximize the ability of trainees to physically reproduce the information during teaching interactions and examinations.

One common challenge related to treatment planning in radiation oncology is the lack of standardized treatment protocols for training purposes. Textbooks routinely utilize institutional guidelines or expert opinions for the description of treatment planning principles; yet, this approach may not be representative of broader community practice. For this book, we have decided to use control arms from publicly available cooperative group clinical trial protocols and relevant practice guidelines to assist in defining standard best radiotherapy practices. In this way, acceptable radiation treatment planning procedures associated with clinical scenarios commonly seen in radiation oncology practice can be defined. The authors feel that a broader knowledge of community standards of radiotherapy treatment will serve trainees well during examinations, as well as clinical practice. However, the protocols contained within this book should be considered only as a starting point for trainee education in the effective prescription of radiotherapy. While the protocols described in this book are adequate for introductory teaching purposes, interested readers are strongly referred to the source protocols and/or primary medical literature for full details on the implementation of these approaches to direct patient care. Knowledge of local best practice(s) as well as recent innovations in technique, dose-fractionation selection, and treatment planning need to be considered when prescribing radiotherapy to patients.

For radiation oncology trainees, the main objective of this book is that the reader will be able to ultimately tackle other reference textbooks in radiation oncology, as well as return to this book for rapid review of concepts prior to examinations and teaching interactions. We hope all readers of this text successfully and rapidly acquire the essential concepts that radiation oncologists use in practice every day to optimize patient care.

Acknowledgments

The authors would like to thank Abhinay Sathya, Arvand Barghi, and Dr. Alexander Louie for their exhaustive reviews of various early drafts of this textbook.

Abbreviations

2D	Two-Dimensional
3D	Three-Dimensional
3DCRT	Three-Dimensional Conformal Radiation Therapy
4D	Four-Dimensional
5FU	5-Fluorouracil
A	Mass Number, Activity
a	Absolute, Autopsy
ABVD	Adriamycin, Bleomycin, Vinblastine, Dacarbazine
AFP	Alpha-Fetoprotein
AJCC	American Joint Committee on Cancer
AP	Anterior-Posterior
ARR	Absolute Relative Risk
ASCO	American Society of Clinical Oncology
ASCUS	Atypical Squamous Cells of Undetermined Significance
ASIS	Anterior Superior Iliac Spine
ASTRO	American Society of Radiation Oncology
AT	Ataxia-Telangiectasia
B	B Symptoms
BCC	Basal Cell Carcinoma
BED	Biological Equivalent Dose
BID	Twice Daily
BMI	Body Mass Index
Bq	Becquerel
c	Speed of Light, Clinical
C	Cervical
CA	Celiac Axis
CAM	Cell Adhesion Molecules
CAT	Computed Axial Tomography
cc	Cubic Centimeters
CCO	Cancer Care Ontario
cdk	Cyclin Dependent Kinase
cGy	Centigray
Ci	Curie
CI	Conformity Index
cm	Centimeter
CML	Chronic Myeloid Leukemia
CNS	Central Nervous System

CONSORT	Consolidated Standards of Reporting Trials
CR	Complete Response
CT	Computed Tomography
CTV	Clinical Target Volume
d	Distance, Dose
D	Dose, Gastric Resection Level
DCIS	Ductal Carcinoma In Situ
DICOM	Digital Imaging and Communications in Medicine
DNA	Deoxyribonucleic Acid
DRE	Digital Rectal Examination
DRR	Digitally Reconstructed Radiograph
DSB	Double Strand Break
DSMC	Data Safety Monitoring Committee
DVH	Dose Volume Histograms
E	Extranodal
EBM	Evidence-Based Medicine
EBRT	External Beam Radiation Therapy
ECM	Extracellular Matrix
EGF	Epidermal Growth Factor
EMR	Electromagnetic Radiation
EPID	Electronic Portal Imaging Device
ERSPC	European Randomized Study of Screening for Prostate Cancer
eval	Evaluation
F	Female
FAP	Familial Adenomatous Polyposis
FDA	Food and Drug Administration
FDG	Fluorodeoxyglucose
FIGO	Féderation Internationale de Gynécologie et d'Obstétrique
FLAIR	Fluid Attenuated Inversion Recovery
FNA	Fine Needle Aspiration
G	Gap
G-CSF	Granulocyte Colony Simulating Factor
GEJ	Gastroesophageal Junction
GI	Gastrointestinal
GIST	Gastrointestinal Stromal Tumor
GnRH	Gonadotropin-Releasing Hormone
GTV	Gross Tumor Volume
GU	Genitourinary
Gy	Gray
h	Hour
H+E	Hematoxylin and Eosin
HAART	Highly Active Antiretroviral Therapy
Hb	Hemoglobin
HBIG	Hepatitis B Immunoglobulin
HBV	Hepatitis B Virus
HCC	Hepatocellular Carcinoma
hCG	Human Chorionic Gonadotropin
HDR	High-Dose Rate
HIS	Hospital Information System
HIV	Human Immunodeficiency Virus
HPV	Human Papillomavirus
HRQOL	Health-Related Quality of Life
HU	Hounsfield Units

HVL	Half-Value Layer
I	Intensity
ICD	International Classification of Diseases
ICRU	International Commission of Radiation Units and Measurements
IFRT	Involved Field Radiation Therapy
Ig	Immunoglobulin
IGRT	Image-Guided Radiation Therapy
IM	Internal Margin
IMRT	Intensity-Modulated Radiation Therapy
IRB	Institutional Review Board
ITV	Internal Target Volume
IV	Intravenous
J	Joule
K	Kinetic Energy
KERMA	Kinetic Energy Released in the Medium
kg	Kilogram
KPS	Karnofsky Performance Status
kV	Kilovolt
l	Length
L	Lumbar
LDR	Low Dose Rate
LET	Linear Energy Transfer
LHRH	Luteinizing Hormone Releasing Hormone
ln	Natural Logarithm
m	Meters, Multifocal
M	Mitosis, Male, Metastases
max	Maximum
MDR	Medium Dose-Rate
MeV	Million Electron Volts
mg	Milligram
min	Minimum
MLC	Multileaf Collimator
mm	Millimeter
mmHg	Millimeters Mercury
MRI	Magnetic Resonance Imaging
MSK	Musculoskeletal
MV	Megavolt
n	Neutron
N	Number of Particles, Nodes
NCCN	National Comprehensive Cancer Network
NEMA	National Electrical Manufacturers Association
NNH	Number Needed to Harm
NNT	Number Needed to Treat
OAR	Organ at Risk
OD	Daily
p	Proton, Pathological
PA	Posterior-Anterior
PACS	Picture Archiving and Communication System
PD	Progressive Disease
PDR	Pulsed Dose-Rate
PET	Positron Emission Tomography
PGY	Post-Graduate Year
PJ	Pancreaticojejunostomy

PLCO	Prostate, Lung, Colorectal, and Ovarian Cancer
POP	Parallel Opposed Pair
PR	Partial Response
PRV	Planning Organ and Risk Volume
PSA	Prostate Specific Antigen
PTV	Planning Target Volume
PV	Portal Vein
QUANTEC	Quantitative Analyses of Normal Tissue Effects in the Clinic
R	Roentgen, Residual
r	Relative, Retreatment
RBE	Relative Biological Effectiveness
RBG	Red, Blue, and Green
RECIST	Response Evaluation Criteria in Solid Tumors
RILD	Radiation-Induced Liver Disease
RILI	Radiation-Induced Lung Disease
RNA	Ribonucleic Acid
ROI	Region of Interest
RPA	Recursive Partitioning Analysis
RR	Relative Risk
RTOG	Radiation Therapy Oncology Group
s	Second
S	Specific, Synthesis, Surviving Fraction, Sacrum
SABR	Stereotactic Ablative Radiotherapy
SCC	Squamous Cell Carcinoma
SCL	Supraclavicular
SD	Stable Disease
SER	Sensitization Enhancement Ratio
SM	Set-up Margin
SMA	Superior Mesenteric Artery
SNP	Single Nucleotide Polymorphisms
SPECT	Single Photon Emission Computed Tomography
SRS	Stereotactic Radiosurgery
SSB	Single Strand Break
SSD	Source to Skin Distance
STP	Standard Temperature and Pressure
SUV	Standardized Uptake Value
Sv	Sievert
t	Time
T	Mean Lifetime, Time, Tumor, Thoracic
TCP	Tumor Control Probability
TCP/IP	Transmission Control Protocol and Internet Protocol
TCS	Training Course Series
TD	Tolerance Dose
TLD	Thermoluminescent Dosimeter
TNF	Tumor Necrosis Factor
TNM	Tumor, Nodes and Metastases
TPS	Treatment Planning System
TRUS	Transrectal Ultrasound
UICC	International Union Against Cancer
US	Ultrasound
V	Volume
VEGF	Vascular Endothelial Growth Factor

W	Weighting
WBRT	Whole Brain Radiation Therapy
WHO	World Health Organization
x	Unknown Staging
y	Neoadjuvant
Z	Atomic Number

List of Tables

List of Figures

PART I: BASIC SCIENCE CONCEPTS

Chapter 1

Physics

KEY POINTS

- Electromagnetic radiation (EMR, photons) has various important properties including: energy transmission at the speed of light, wave-particle duality, inverse relationship between frequency and wavelength (spectrum), photon energy proportional to wave frequency, energy transfer potential, and wave superposition/refraction/dispersion.
- Atoms consist of positively charged nuclei (proton and neutrons) surrounded by electrons. The physics of atoms are governed by quantum theory with electrons manifesting themselves in statistically constructed electron orbitals. The nucleus is governed by various fundamental forces in nature including the strong nuclear force (attractive), the electromagnetic force (repulsive between protons), and the weak nuclear force (beta decay).
- Radioactive decay is a spontaneous and random process in which atomic nuclei emit particles (usually photons, electrons, or alpha helium particles) in order to achieve lower energy states. Radioactive decay is measured in decays per second (Becquerel—Bq) and is mathematically related to the decay constant of the atomic species of interest and the initial number of atoms present.
- High-energy photons and particles can liberate orbital electrons, creating free radicals in one of two ionization methods [(1) Direct mechanism, where a charged particle liberates orbital electrons directly or (2) Indirect mechanism, where non-charged particles interact with matter to liberate charged particles that subsequently interact under the direct mechanism]. Photon beams are attenuated by matter, which is mathematically related to the initial intensity of the photon beam and the mass attenuation coefficient. Photon interactions with atoms include: coherent scattering, photoelectric absorption, Compton scattering, pair production, and photodisintegration.
- Electrons can interact with atoms in three modes creating bremsstrahlung x-rays, characteristic x-rays, and Auger electrons. These interactions can be utilized to create radiation that can be clinically useful in terms of x-ray tubes, kilovoltage x-ray units, and linear accelerators.
- Radiation exposure in air is measured in units of total charge per mass of air (R—Roentgen). Kinetic energy released in the medium (KERMA) and absorbed dose (deposited radiation) are related concepts both measured in units of J/kg (Gray—Gy).
- Radiation dosimetry in humans can be visually depicted in multiple ways including: depth dose curves, isodose charts, and isodose distributions. Single and/or multiple electron/photon beams can be utilized to deliver radiation therapy to a wide variety of clinical situations.

1.1. ELECTROMAGNETIC RADIATION

Properties of EMR

The existence and nature of EMR was theorized by James Maxwell and experimentally confirmed by Henrick Hertz. Properties of EMR include the following:

1. EMR consists of sinusoidally varying symmetric electric and magnetic fields, which are perpendicular to each other and both perpendicular to the direction of motion. This motion of EMR allows for the transmission of energy from one location to another (Figure 1.1).
2. The speed of EMR waves is equal to the speed of light (c = 299,792,458 m/s), which is confirmatory evidence that light consists of EMR.
3. According to the physics of electromagnetism, changes in electric fields induce changes in local magnetic fields (principle of electromagnetic induction). The opposite relationship is true as well (a changing magnetic field will induce changes in electric field). This reciprocal relationship of induction of electric and magnetic fields in EMR leads to wave propagation (i.e., motion).
4. EMR have properties consistent with both waves and particles, otherwise known as the wave-particle duality of EMR. Wave-like properties of EMR are usually manifested in large distances (macroscopic scale), whereas, particle properties usually occur in small distances (microscopic scale).
5. The wave properties of EMR were developed in relation with the deBroglie hypothesis, which related the velocity of waves to the product of the frequency and wavelength of the wave. In the case of EMR, velocity is equal to the speed of light; therefore, the following relationship is appropriate to EMR:

$$\text{speed of light} = \text{frequency} \times \text{wavelength}$$

6. Einstein hypothesized the particle nature of EMR by describing the existence of photons (discrete packets of energy or quanta) in the physical explanation of the photoelectric

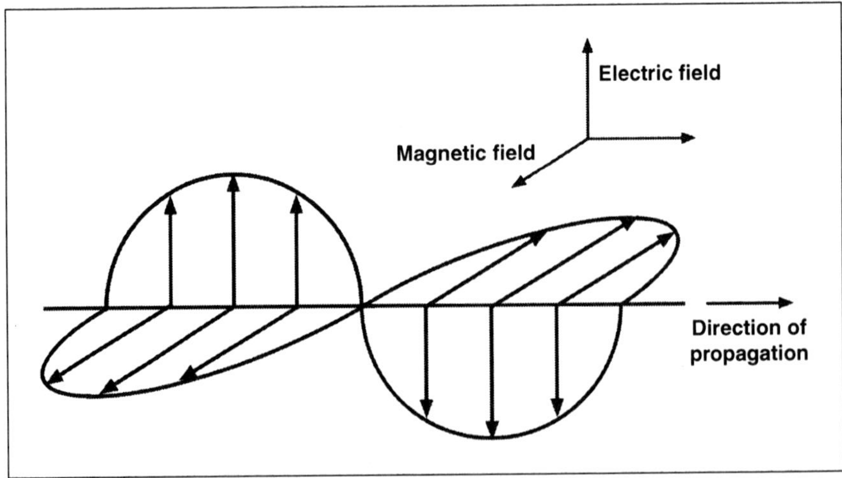

FIGURE 1.1 Electromagnetic radiation

effect (see section 1.4). Photon energy is related to photon frequency and Planck's constant by the following mathematical relationship:

$$\text{photon energy} = \text{frequency} \times 6.626 \times 10^{-34}\ \text{Js}$$

7. Combining the wave and particle equations together leads to the relationship that photon energy is directly related to frequency and inversely proportional to wavelength. For example, high-energy photons (such as those used in radiotherapy) consist of high frequency and low wavelength forms of EMR.
8. Due to the wave nature of EMR, various general wave and optical properties apply to EMR. These include superposition (destructive and constructive interference), refraction (alteration of EMR direction based on medium density), and dispersion (separation of EMR into component parts).
9. EMR can interact with various forms of matter to transfer energy. These interactions can include several photo-electron interactions (see section 1.4), as well as interactions with atomic nuclei (photodisintegration).

The EMR Spectrum

The EMR spectrum is defined as the entire range of all possible frequencies and wavelengths of EMR (Figure 1.2). In terms of wavelength, EMR can typically range from 1 km (radio waves) to 10^{-12} m (gamma rays). X-rays, with wavelengths of ~10^{-10} m, usually arise from the release of energy from electron-atomic transitions, whereas gamma rays are created from nuclear transitions from high to low-energy states. X-rays are capable of various interactions with matter including electron ejection and photon scattering. Gamma rays are also able to exhibit these interactions, as well as additional interactions including electron–positron pair production and nuclear excitation/dissociation, due to the higher energies involved.

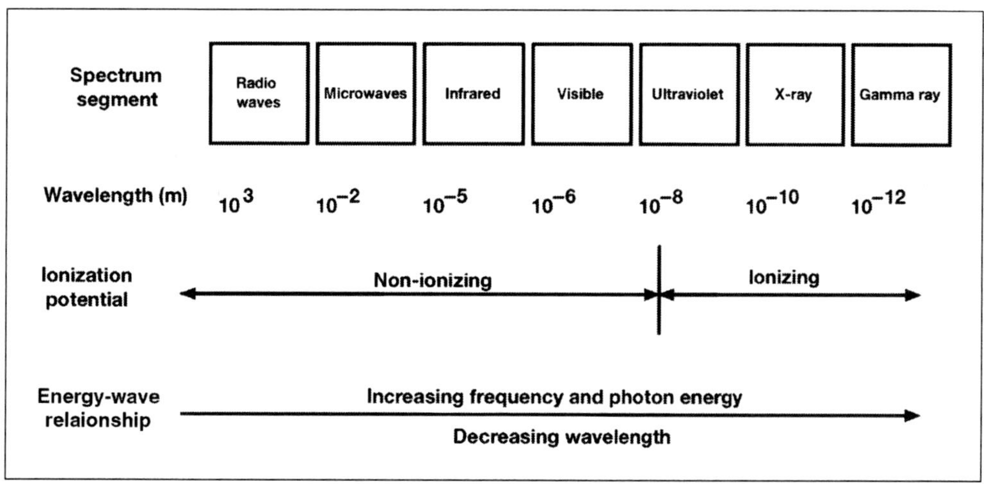

FIGURE 1.2 Electromagnetic spectrum

1.2. STRUCTURE OF MATTER

Atomic Structure

The atom is a basic unit of matter that has a substructure of a core nucleus and a cloud of electrons surrounding the nucleus. The nucleus contains the vast majority of atomic mass in a very small volume (radius on the order of 10^{-14} m), and the electron cloud occupies a substantially larger volume (radius on the order of 10^{-10} m). The nucleus contains two particles, the positively charged proton and the neutron (no charge). Atoms are specified by the shorthand notation $^{A}X_{Z}$ where X is the chemical symbol for the element in question, A is the mass number representing the total number of nucleons (protons and neutrons) in the atom, and Z is the atomic number reflecting the number of protons in the nucleus (as well as the number of electrons orbiting the atom in a neutrally charged atom). One can calculate the number of neutrons in the atom by subtracting Z from the total number of nucleons A (therefore, #neutrons = A − Z).

Atoms are commonly classified according to the relative content of nucleons contained within the nucleus of the atom:

1. *Isotope.* Two atoms with the same Z but different A (e.g., $^{12}C_6$ and $^{13}C_6$).
2. *Isotone.* Two atoms with different A and Z but the same number of neutrons, that is, the same A − Z value (e.g., $^{12}B_5$ and $^{13}C_6$).
3. *Isobar.* Two atoms with same A but different Z (e.g., $^{40}S_{16}$, $^{40}K_{19}$, and $^{40}Ca_{20}$).
4. *Isomer.* Two atoms with the same A and Z but different energy states (e.g., $^{99m}Tc_{43}$ and $^{99}Tc_{43}$).

Models of the Atom

There are four successively more complicated mathematical and conceptual models of the atom that evolved in conjunction with both theoretical and observational scientific investigation (Figure 1.3).

1. *The Thomson model.* Otherwise known as the "plum and pudding" model of the atom, electrons were considered to be residing within an area of positive charge but free to travel within this positive charge area. As the electron would naturally stray away from the center of the positively charged zone, the electron would be subject to increasingly intense electrostatic attractive forces, which would prevent the electron from leaving the positively charged zone.
2. *The Rutherford model.* This model introduced the concept of a central, dense, positively charged nucleus with electrons orbiting this nucleus in a manner similar to planetary motion. This model explained experimental observations of alpha particles ($^{4}He_2$) being deflected by a thin gold leaf; however, other observations were not explained by this model (sharp absorption spectra observed with atoms, and the lack of expected EMR emissions due to electrons rotating around a fixed point in space).
3. *The Bohr model.* This model built on aspects of the Rutherford model but added the new complexity of electron quantum orbits. For any specific atom, electrons were required to exist in very specific quantum orbits with correspondingly specific energy states. Electrons moving from one quantum energy state to another would either release or absorb a discrete amount of energy. Although this model explained the two limitations of the Rutherford model, the Bohr model could only be applied to a simple system such

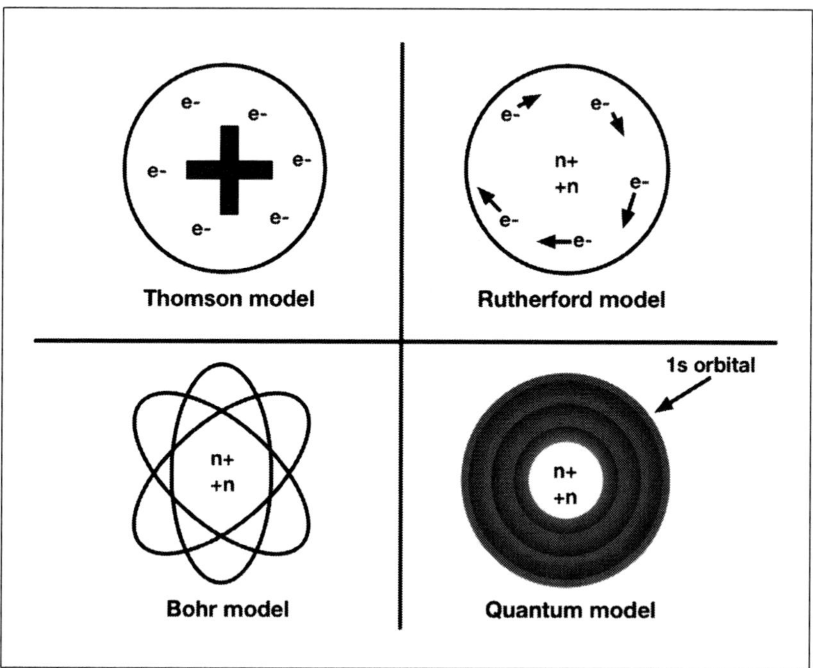

FIGURE 1.3 Atomic models

as a hydrogen atom. The Bohr model could not predict the properties and characteristics of more complex atoms.

4. *The Quantum (orbital) model.* This model of the atom builds upon the existence of the wave-particle duality of matter. Schrodinger demonstrated that electrons have wave-like properties that manifest themselves in statistically-based electron probability clouds (also known as electron orbitals) when they are part of an atom. Orbitals consist of various shapes (spherical, dumbbell, and torus) based on harmonic values explained by the Schrodinger equations. This fusion of atomic theory and quantum mechanics was able to explain the properties of more complex atoms, as well as chemical interactions between atoms to form molecular bonds.

Nuclear Stability

There are four known fundamental forces in nature, which include the gravitational force (attractive force between two masses over long distances), electromagnetic forces (attractive and repulsive forces related to charge and magnetism), the weak nuclear force (a nuclear disruptive force related to beta decay), as well as the strong nuclear force (attractive force between two nucleons to keep neutrons and protons together, mediated by a gluon particle over extremely small distances). The nucleus is held together by nuclear binding energy, which is a manifestation of the collective strong nuclear force between nucleons overcoming the collective electromagnetic repulsive forces between protons contained within a nucleus. Neutrons tend to stabilize the nucleus as they are subject to the strong nuclear force but not the repulsive electromagnetic force. For atoms with Z numbers of up to 20, an equal number of neutrons are able to associate with an equal number of protons to form stable nuclei (i.e., an n/p ratio of 1). However for larger atoms, a larger n/p ratio is required to facilitate nuclear stability. Of the known 300 or so stable nuclei observed in nature, over 50% have even proton and even neutron numbers. Stable atoms with odd proton and odd neutron numbers occur rarely in nature (e.g., $^{2}H_{1}$, $^{6}Li_{3}$,$^{10}B_{5}$, and $^{14}N_{7}$).

1.3. RADIOACTIVE DECAY AND RADIONUCLIDES

Radioactivity

Radioactive decay is the process by which unstable nuclei emit charged particles (e.g., alpha $^{4}He_2$ or beta electrons) or gamma photons in order to achieve lower energy states (that tend to be more stable). This process is both stochastic (random) and spontaneous (does not require any interactions with other particles to initiate the process) in nature. Radioactive decay is mediated by interactions between various fundamental forces in nature including the strong nuclear force (which tends to stabilize the nucleus by attracting nucleons together), electrostatic forces (which tend to disrupt the nucleus by repulsing protons from each other) as well as the weak nuclear force (responsible for beta decay). Random energy exchange between nucleons and the surrounding quantum vacuum (empty space in the universe with underlying energy) can provide sufficient energy to allow for spontaneous and stochastic radioactive decay.

Given the random nature of the radioactive decay process, it is not possible to predict when a particular nucleus will undergo this process; yet, if the number of nuclei involved is large, then prediction is possible using statistical computation. The rate of radioactive decay is known as the activity and is measured in Becquerel (Bq). One Bq is defined as one radioactive decay per second. Historically, another unit of radioactivity was the Curie (Ci), which was defined as the rate of decay of 1 g of Radium-226 (equal to 3.7×10^{10} Bq). In the process of radioactive decay, an initial radionuclide (the parent) decays to a lower energy nuclide (daughter) with the same chemical element (with gamma decay) or a different chemical element (with alpha or beta decay).

Modes of Radioactive Decay

Three major modes of radioactive decay exist in nature and are classified as nucleon emission, beta decay, and nuclear transitions.

1. *Nucleon emission:*
   - Alpha decay—Alpha particle emitted with daughter nucleus $^{A-4}X_{Z-2}$.
   - Proton emission—Proton ejection with daughter nucleus $^{A-1}X_{Z-1}$.
   - Neutron emission—Neutron ejection with daughter nucleus $^{A-1}X_{Z}$.
2. *Beta decay:*
   - Beta decay—Electron ejection from nucleus with daughter nucleus $^{A}X_{Z+1}$.
   - Positron emission—Positron (positive electron antiparticle) ejection from nucleus with daughter nucleus $^{A}X_{Z-1}$.
   - Electron capture—Nucleus captures orbital electron (functionally equivalent to positron emission) with daughter nucleus $^{A}X_{Z-1}$.
3. *Nuclear transitions:*
   - Isomeric transition—Nucleus releases high energy photon (gamma-ray) with daughter nucleus $^{A}X_{Z}$ at a lower energy state.

- Internal conversion—Nucleus transfers energy to orbital electron with an electron ejected from the atom. Daughter nucleus $^{A}X_{Z}$ at a lower energy state is created. Vacant electron orbital is created, which will lead to emission of electrons (Auger electrons) and photons (characteristic x-rays) in order for the atom to reach a lower energy state.

Mathematics of Radioactive Decay

The mathematical construct to describe the process of radioactive decay involves various constants and relationships. The following definitions apply to radioactive decay:

- Half-life ($t_{1/2}$)—Time to reach 50% of original radioactivity level.
- Mean lifetime (T)—Average lifetime of a radionuclide prior to decay.
- Decay constant (λ)—Inverse of mean lifetime.
- Total activity (A)—Number of decays per second (A_0 = initial activity at time zero, A_t = activity at time t).
- Number of particles (N)—Total number of radionuclide atoms in a sample of interest (N_0 = initial number and time zero, N_t = number at time t).
- Specific Activity (S_A)—Number of decays per second per amount (mass or volume).

Given the fact that radioactive decay has been observed to be a logarithmic process, the following mathematical relationships exist between the various definitions listed above.

$$t_{1/2} = \ln 2/\lambda = T \ln 2, \text{ where } \ln 2 = 0.693$$

(relationship between half-life, mean lifetime, and the decay constant)

$$A = \lambda N = -dN/dt$$

(relationship demonstrating direct relationship between activity and radionuclide number and decay constant)

$$N_t = N_0 e^{-\lambda t} \text{ and } A_t = A_0 e^{-\lambda t}$$

(exponential decay equations relating initial vs. time = t radionuclide number and activity).

Radioactive Decay Schema and Series

A radioactive decay schema is a graphical representation of the process of radioactive decay that plots the transition of a parent to daughter radionuclide, as well as the production of any radioactive particles (e.g., alpha, beta, gamma). Energy is plotted on the *y*-axis and the atomic number (number of protons) is plotted on the *x*-axis. The specific energy and the maximum energy associated with any photons and particles are reported on the graph, respectively.

A radioactive decay series is sometimes otherwise known in the literature as a decay chain. This series/chain is a collection of various successive radioactive transitions starting with an unstable radionuclide and eventually leading to a stable nuclide. A series of parent to daughter transitions occurs with various daughter radionuclides becoming parent radionuclides within the sequence of radionuclide transitions. This process can be visually demonstrated by plotting a series of connected radioactive decay schema in a two-dimensional plot. The uranium (^{238}U), actinium (^{235}U), and the thorium (^{232}Th) radioactive series are well known examples of this process found in nature.

Nuclear Reactions

Various nuclear reactions are known to occur, where radionuclides can transition from one species to another. These reactions can be written in a shorthand notation, where parent(x,y) daughter refers to the "x" particle or photon reacting with the parent nucleus to create a daughter nucleus with the production of a new "y" particle or photon. For example, an early nuclear reaction experiment conducted by Rutherford converted nitrogen to oxygen:

$$^{14}N_7 + {}^4He_2 \rightarrow {}^1H_1 + {}^{17}O_8 + \text{energy}$$

which, in nuclear shorthand, can be written as

$$^{14}N_7(\alpha,p)^{17}O_8$$

Other reaction classes with nuclear shorthand notation are described in Table 1.1.

Important Radionuclides in Radiation Oncology

Radionuclides have various applications in diagnostic medicine and therapy. Commonly used radionuclides are summarized in Table 1.2.

TABLE 1.1 Nuclear Reaction Classes and Shorthand

Reaction Class	Nuclear Shorthand
Alpha particle reactions	(α, p) and (α, n)
Proton-based	(p, γ), (p, n), (p, d), and (p, α)
Neutron-based	(n, α), (n, p), and (n, γ)
Deuteron-based	(d, n) and (d, p)
Photodisintegration	(γ, n), (γ, p), (γ, d), (γ, t), and (γ, α)
Other	Fission (neutron bombardment of nuclei to create smaller nuclei with neutron and energy release) and fusion (combination of two or more nuclei to create heavier nuclei with release of neutrons and energy)

α, alpha particle; n, neutron; p, proton, d, deuteron ($^2H_1$); t, tritium ($^3H_1$); γ, gamma photon.

TABLE 1.2 Common Radionuclides in Radiation Oncology

Application	Radionuclide	Specific Application
External-beam	^{60}Co	Radiation units (i.e., cobalt unit)
	^{137}Cs (historical)	
	^{226}Ra (historical)	
Brachytherapy	^{60}Co	Pellets
	^{137}Cs	Interstitial needles, tubes, and pellets
	^{192}Ir	High dose rate source, seeds, and pellets
	^{125}I	Seeds
	^{103}Pd	Seeds
	^{198}Au	Seeds
	^{226}Ra (historical)	Needles
Systemic therapy	^{89}Sr and ^{153}Sa	Systemic bone metastases treatment
	^{131}I	Radioactive iodine thyroid treatment
Diagnostic	^{99m}Tc	Bone scanning
	^{67}Ga and ^{201}Th	Thyroid imaging
	^{18}F	Positron emission tomography imaging

1.4. IONIZING RADIATION

Direct and Indirect Ionizing Radiation

Photons and particles with sufficient energy have the ability to liberate orbital electrons from atoms and their corresponding molecules. When this process occurs, highly reactive free radicals are formed by the creation of unpaired electrons. This leads to highly reactive atomic and molecular species that can interact with other atoms and molecules. In biological systems, free radicals can interact with DNA and cause either repairable or non-repairable damage with important downstream effects (e.g., cell death). Interactions between photons/particles and atoms/molecules are classified as either directly or indirectly ionizing (Figure 1.4).

1. *Direct ionization.* This process occurs when charged particles such as electrons (e^-) or alpha particles ($^4He_2^{2+}$) with sufficient kinetic energy interact with atoms and molecules to liberate electrons and create free radicals. This process is known as direct due to the fact that no intermediary step is required (i.e., the interaction occurs directly between the particle and the atom/molecule). The charged particle can interact with several atoms/molecules, in turn, losing kinetic energy with each successive interaction until all energy has been absorbed by the material/medium.
2. *Indirect ionization.* This process occurs when non-charged particles such as photons and neutrons interact with atoms and molecules. These interactions result in the release of charged particles (such as electrons) that then go on to interact with atoms and molecules by the direct mechanism explained above. The term "indirect" refers to the fact that the uncharged particles themselves do not create the free radicals that ultimately cause biological damage. This effect requires the intermediate step of the creation of charged particles.

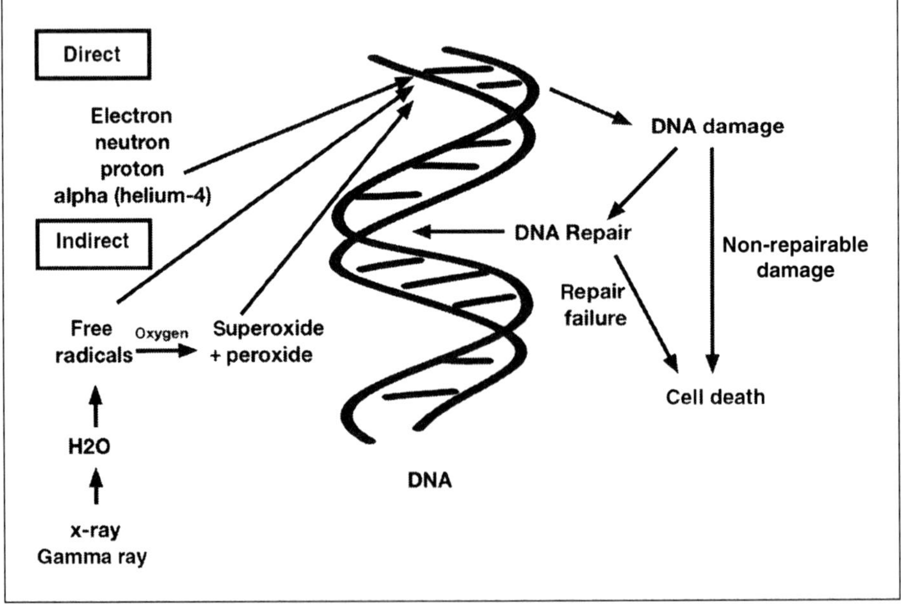

FIGURE 1.4 Direct and indirect DNA damage

Photon Beam Attenuation and Characterization

As a photon beam travels through a medium (such as water, human tissue, etc.), various possible interactions can take place. Any individual photon may not interact at all and pass through the medium unchanged. Alternatively, a photon–atom/molecule interaction can occur and can result in either absorption (photon does not leave the medium) or scattering (photon direction and/or energy is altered) of the photon. This collective process of photon absorption and scattering is known as attenuation. The process of attenuation is highly dependent on both the physical characteristics of the medium/material in question, as well as the photon beam energy spectrum (the relative proportions of various photon energies contained within the photon beam).

Photon beams can be characterized by several concepts related to the number of photons and total energy per cross-sectional area (fluence and energy fluence, respectively, see Table 1.3). In addition, photon beams can be characterized by the amount of a pre-specified material that will halve the beam's initial intensity (the half-value layer [HVL]).

In terms of the HVL, this can be mathematically described as a logarithmic process (similar to radioactive decay) in monoenergetic photon beams (i.e., a pure radiation beam of a solitary energy). The concept of a linear attenuation coefficient is defined as:

$$\mu = \ln 2/\text{HVL} = 0.693/\text{HVL}$$

This linear attenuation coefficient can be used in conjunction with the thickness of the medium (x) to define the reduction in beam intensity with the following equation:

$$I_x = I_0 e^{-\mu x}$$

where I_0 is the initial intensity prior to attenuation and I_x is the intensity after passing through x thickness of medium.

An additional concept related to the linear attenuation coefficient is the mass attenuation coefficient, which is defined as μ/ρ where ρ is the density of the medium in question. This coefficient is a more fundamental constant as it is independent of the density of the medium and is directly proportional to the probability of photon-atomic interactions.

In the context of a polyenergetic photon beam, a process known as beam hardening can occur whereby lower energy photons are disproportionately more likely to be attenuated than higher energy photons. This process will change the distribution of energies within the photon beam as the photons progress through the medium in question. The end result is that the first HVL (attenuation from 100% to 50% intensity) will be smaller than the second HVL (attenuation from 50% to 25% intensity).

TABLE 1.3 Photon Beam Fluence Concepts

Concept	Definition
Fluence	The number of photons within a cross sectional area in space at an instant in time
Energy fluence	The sum of energy of all photons within a cross sectional area in space at an instant in time
HVL	The thickness (usually in centimeters) of material required to attenuate a photon beam to one-half intensity (or fluence)

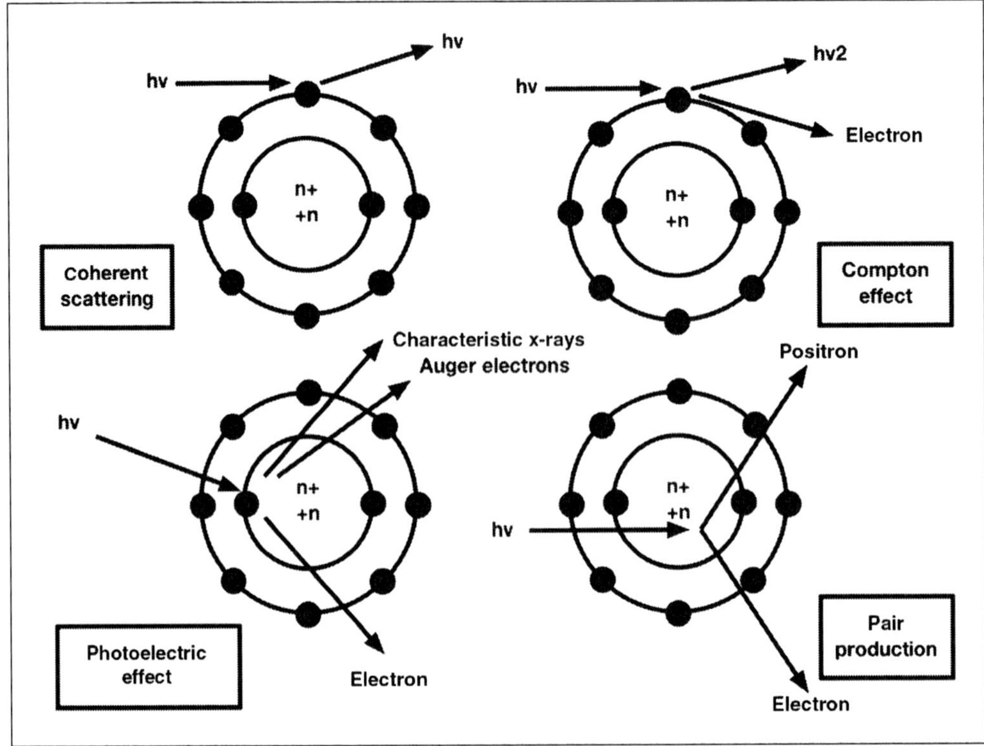

FIGURE 1.5 Photon-atomic interactions

Photon Interactions at the Atomic Level

There are five main methods by which photons can interact with atoms (Figure 1.5). Depending on which processes dominate in specific photon beam situations, important consequences with regards to the characteristics of photon beam radiation deposition can occur.

1. *Coherent scattering.* This process, which is also known as Rayleigh scattering, essentially absorbs and releases a photon from an atom with the same energy, although the direction of the photon has changed. No energy is gained or lost in this process. The photon energy, wavelength, and frequency are identical. The atom itself is also unchanged. This interaction is significant in situations with low photon energies and/or high Z (atomic number) materials.
2. *Photoelectric absorption effect.* In this photon-atomic interaction, the photon is completely absorbed by the atom with the release of an electron (usually an inner orbital electron) with kinetic energy equal to the photon energy minus the binding electron energy (potential energy to be overcome to release the electron). Therefore, the minimum energy for the photoelectric effect to occur is directly related to the binding energies of the various electrons in a particular atom. After the photoelectric interaction is complete, an electron vacancy is created within the atom that leads to outer electrons filling the vacancy with the release of energy (in the form of characteristic x-rays and/or Auger electrons, see

section 1.4). The probability of photoelectric interaction is related to the photoelectric mass attenuation coefficient, which is also related to both the cube of the atomic number and the inverse cube of the photon energy.

$$\text{Probability of photoelectric interaction} = \text{photoelectric } \mu/\rho \propto (Z^3/E^3)$$

Therefore, the probability of photoelectric interaction is higher for high Z materials (bone > air) and lower for higher energy photon beams (where other types of interactions dominate). It is this relative atomic number difference in photoelectric effect probability that is utilized in x-ray imaging, computed tomography, as well as in the use of high Z contrast agents (e.g., oral/rectal barium contrast and intravenous iodine contrast).

3. *Compton scattering effect.* In this interaction scenario, an incident photon will lose a portion of its energy, usually to an outer orbital electron which will result in the release of that electron with some kinetic energy (equal to transferred energy minus binding energy) and the creation of a new photon with reduced energy (and reduced frequency/increased wavelength) and a new direction (up to maximum 180° change in direction from incident direction, the 180° situation is commonly known as photon backscatter). The probability of interaction is related to the Compton mass attenuation coefficient, which in this case is independent on atomic number and photon energy. However, this value is directly related to the electron density of the medium/tissue of interest. Conveniently, the intensities obtained from computed tomography (otherwise known as the Hounsfield unit) are directly related to the Compton mass attenuation coefficient. A significant proportion of photon interactions given as part of external-beam radiation therapy is in the Compton range; therefore, all modern treatment planning systems (TPS) utilize CT-based information to provide predictions of photon dose deposition related to radiation treatment.
4. *Pair production.* In this scenario, the incident photon disappears after interaction with the atom and the sum of the energy is converted into an electron and positron (electron antiparticle) pair. Any remaining energy after this interaction is apportioned equally between the particles in the form of kinetic energy. A minimum threshold energy applies to this form of interaction, which is equal to the energy equivalent of the pair mass (2 × 0.511 MeV = 1.022 MeV). The probability of this interaction is related to the pair production mass attenuation coefficient, which in turn is directly proportional to the square of the atomic number (Z^2) per atom, and directly proportional to the atomic number (Z) per electron and per gram.
5. *Photodisintegration.* This concept was introduced in section 1.3 and relates to the absorption of a high-energy photon by an atomic nucleus with the release of a subatomic particle (e.g., proton or neutron) and potential disruption of the nucleus itself.

The Relationship Between Photon Energy and Photon-Matter Interactions

There is a dependence of photoelectric effect, Compton, and pair production mass attenuation coefficient (and hence interaction probability) on photon energy (Figure 1.6). It is important to note that at 0.026 MV, an equal contribution to total attenuation between photoelectric effect (50%) and Compton scattering (50%) exists. Similarly, at 24 MV an equal proportion of attenuation from Compton (50%) and pair production (50%) exists. At 4 MV, 94% of attenuation is from Compton effect and at 10 MV 77% of attenuation is Compton based (with the remainder from pair production).

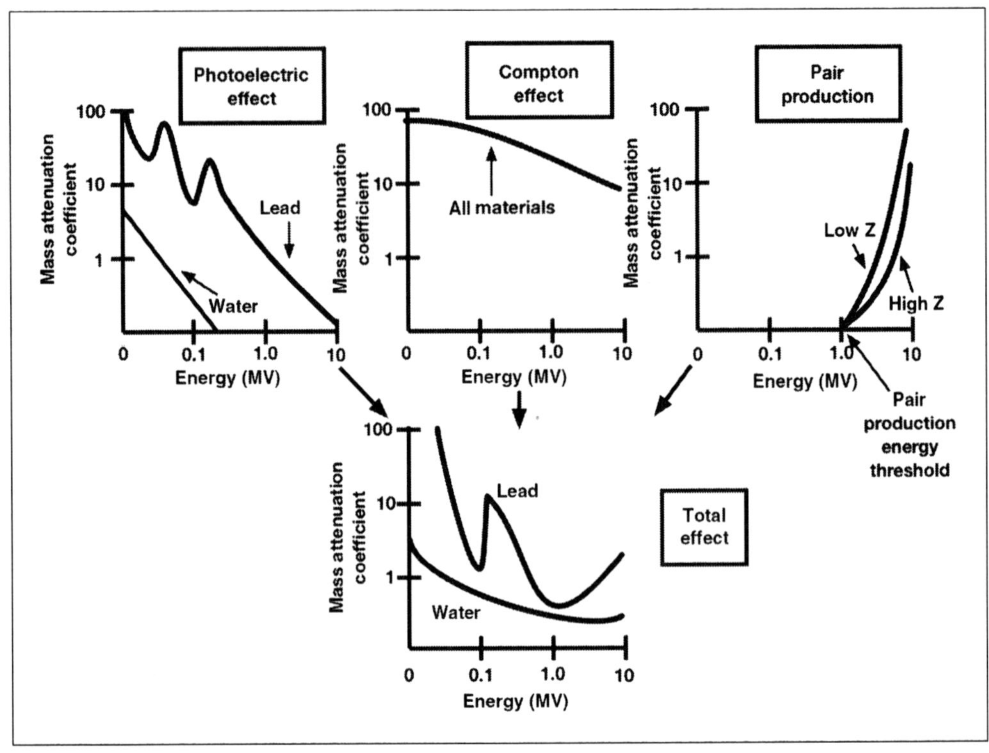

FIGURE 1.6 Photon attenuation

1.5. X-RAY PRODUCTION

X-Ray Production at the Atomic Level

X-ray radiation can be created by the interactions between electrons and atoms in two distinct modes (Figure 1.7). These x-ray production methods are capitalized upon to generate radiation for both diagnostic and therapeutic purposes.

1. *Bremsstrahlung x-rays.* One method by which electrons can interact with atoms to create x-ray radiation is by travelling near to the atomic nucleus. The positive charge of the nucleus will cause the trajectory of the travelling electron track to detect towards the nucleus. The electron will lose energy (and speed) in the process; however, the total amount of energy will be conserved by the creation of an x-ray photon. It is important to note that a single electron can interact with several atomic nuclei in sequence with the production of multiple bremsstahlung (braking radiation) x-ray photons. This interaction occurs frequently in high Z materials. Additionally, the angle of x-ray production is related to the electron energy (perpendicular to electron track for low-energy and parallel and forward for high-energy situations).
2. *Characteristic x-rays.* As opposed to the Bremsstrahlung process, characteristic x-rays are created by the interaction between a free electron and an orbital electron (as opposed to an

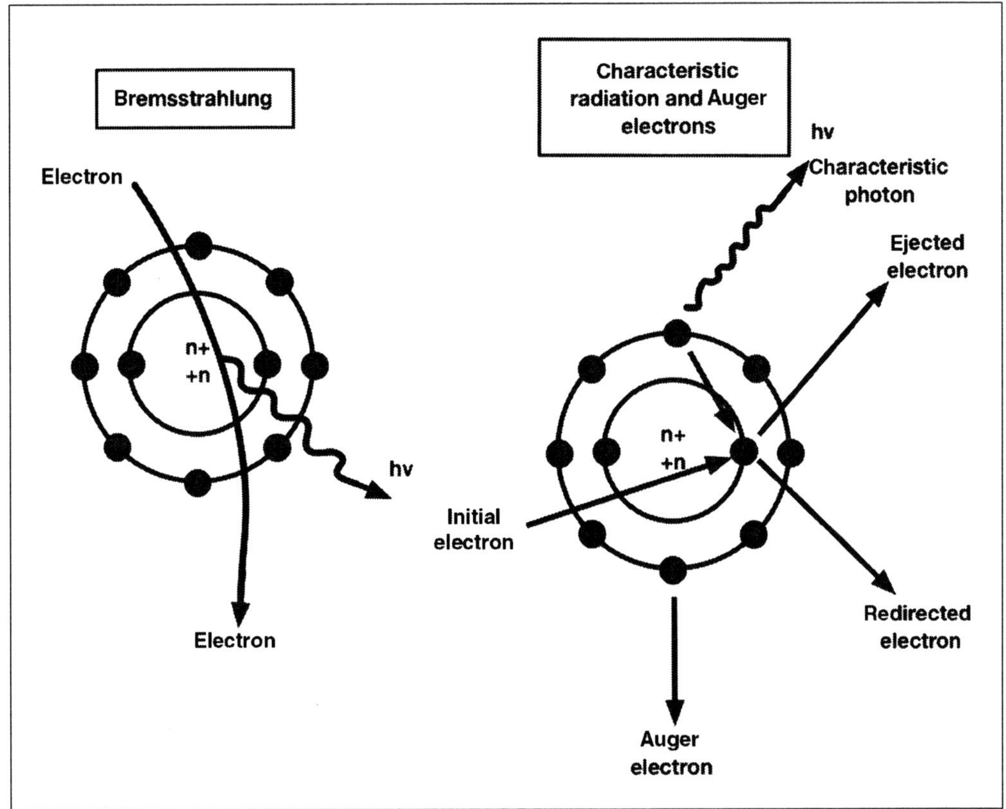

FIGURE 1.7 X-ray production

atomic nucleus). In this interaction, the free moving electron imparts energy to the orbital electron, freeing the orbital electron from the atom. The resultant empty orbital is filled either by another free electron or from another orbital electron. Whatever the method, this process of filling the empty electron orbital releases very specific (i.e., characteristic) amounts of energy (by the creation of x-ray photons) related to the difference in orbital energies. Similar to the bremsstrahlung process, the initial free electron (now with lower energy) can still interact with other atomic nuclei and atomic electron orbitals to create new bremsstrahlung and characteristic interactions, respectively. Of note, Auger electrons can be created in a related process. Instead of the production of a characteristic x-ray photon, occasionally the atom can release energy by ejecting an additional electron. This is equivalent to an internal photoelectric effect, in which the characteristic x-ray does not leave the atom but is absorbed by another electron within the atom, leading to electron ejection.

The X-Ray Tube

The x-ray tube is utilized for multiple purposes including radiography, fluoroscopy, computed tomography, kilovoltage imaging (on-board cone-beam imaging systems), as well as orthovoltage treatment systems (Figure 1.8). The main components of the x-ray tube are listed in Table 1.4.

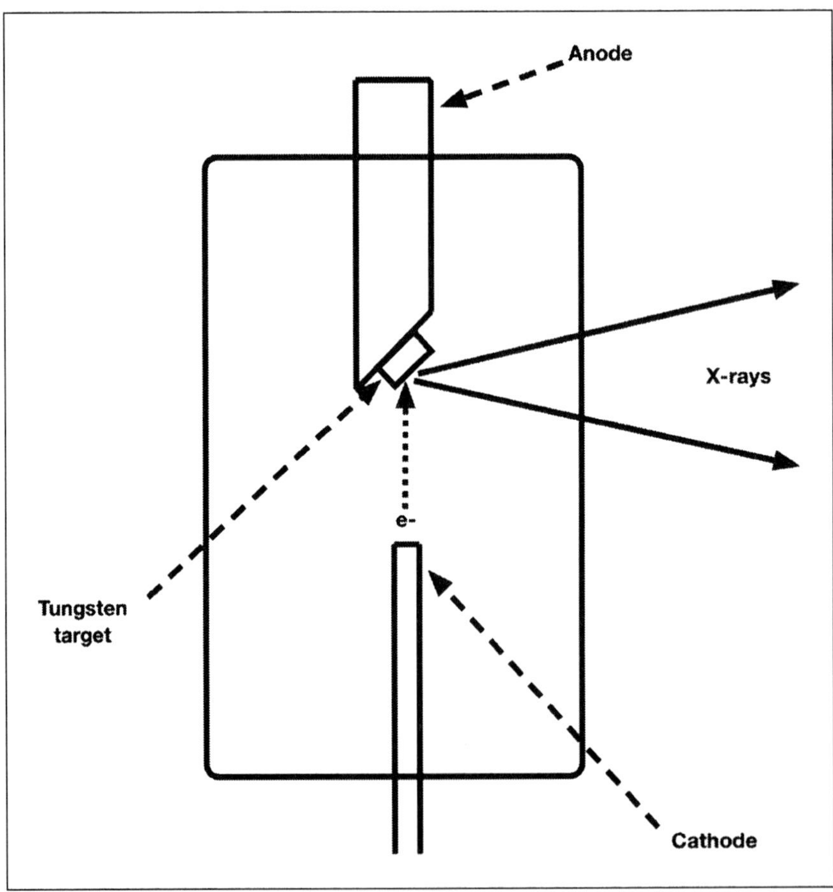

FIGURE 1.8 X-ray tube

TABLE 1.4 X-Ray Tube Components

Component	Description
Cathode	Negative electrode used to generate and repel electron beam towards anode target
Filament	Material within cathode that can release electrons upon addition of heat (thermonic emission)
Focusing cup	On cathode, shaped to focus electron beam created from filament onto the target
Anode	Positive electrode to attract electron beam and dissipate heat generated in x-ray process
Target	Required to be a high Z material with high melting point to facilitate x-ray production
Glass window	To allow x-ray radiation to leave the tube but also must maintain the vacuum of the system
Vacuum (cathode–anode gap)	A vacuum is required between the cathode (focusing cup) and the anode (target) in order to generate a high-speed electron beam to facilitate electron-atomic interactions
Glass housing	To create vacuum within the x-ray tube

TABLE 1.5 Kilovoltage Therapy Machine Options

Therapy Unit	Description
Contact	40–50 kV, 1–2 mm aluminum HVL, SSD of 2 cm, in contact with skin, maximum treatment depth of 2 cm
Superficial	50–150 kV, 1–8 mm aluminum HVL, SSD 15–20 cm, skin in contact with end of glass/steel cone
Orthovoltage	200–350 kV, SSD of 50 cm, use of cones or collimation system, maximum dose about 2 cm

Kilovoltage X-Ray Units

Prior to the advent of modern megavoltage (>1000 kV) machines, various kilovoltage (kV) systems were utilized to treat various cancers. Treatment would consist of multiple beam treatments until skin tolerance was reached. Kilovoltage therapy still is utilized in the treatment of superficial skin lesions, as well as other specialized treatment indications (e.g., endorectal therapy) with various therapy options depicted in Table 1.5.

Radionuclide-based Gamma-Ray Unit

The best known example of a radionuclide-based gamma-ray radiation machine is the cobalt-60 unit. This type of radiation unit has provided reliable and low-cost megavoltage range radiotherapy since its development in 1951. Cobalt-60 is created by the neutron-based nuclear reaction $^{59}Co(n,\gamma)^{60}Co$, with ^{60}Co subsequently undergoing beta decay to ^{60}Ni. Cobalt-60 pellets, cylinders, and/or discs are stored within a 1–2 cm sealed steel container containing ~10,000 Ci of activity.

The Linear Accelerator

A medical linear accelerator (linac) is a medical device that generates electron and/or photon beams usually for cancer treatment purposes. Linacs have various components that work together to produce therapeutic beams of radiation (Figure 1.9).

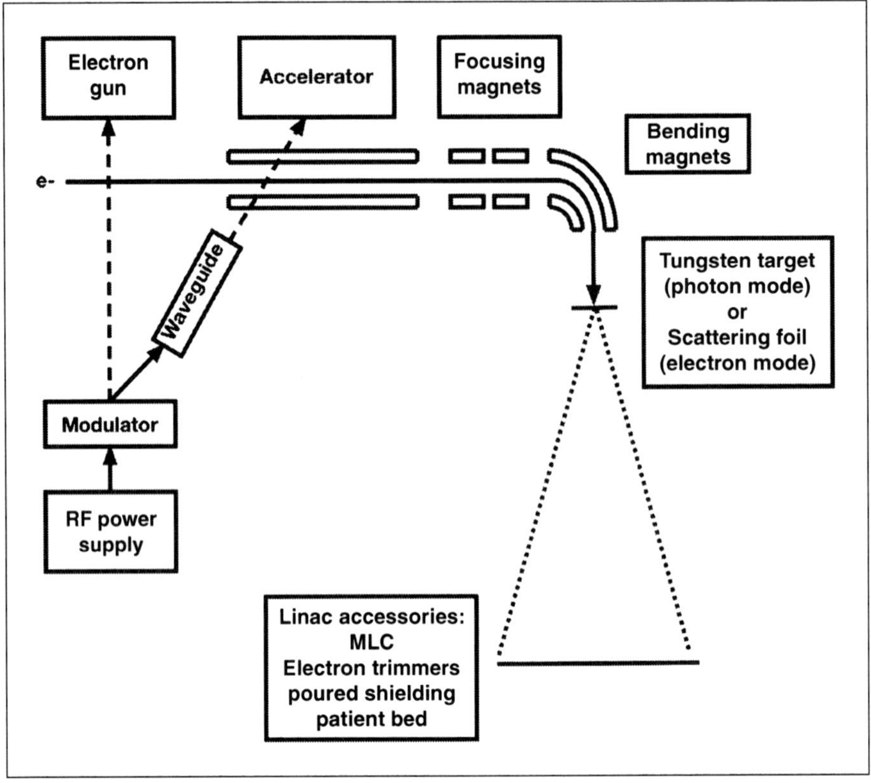

FIGURE 1.9 Linear accelerator

1. *Electron source.* These can be created by a variety of methods including a photocathode, cold/hot cathode, or radio-frequency ion source.
2. *Injection device.* High voltage device to inject electrons into the vacuum chamber for acceleration.
3. *Accelerator guide.* A vacuum chamber is used to serve as a conduit for the electrons to move to their ultimate destination (the target). The chamber contains cylindrical electrodes, which are charged with radiofrequency energy to accelerate the electrons towards the target using standing waves. Bending magnets are used in higher energy linacs, in order to direct the beam towards the patient (treatment bed).
4. *Target.* A high-density target (with high melting point, usually tungsten) is used to convert incoming electrons into a photon beam by the bremsstrahlung mechanism. If the linac is in electron beam mode, the tungsten target is removed and replaced by an electron scattering foil in order to convert an electron pencil beam (small non-clinical beam) into a beam that can be used clinically.
5. *Treatment head.* Various devices are placed within the treatment head to support clinical treatment delivery. These devices include primary beam collimators/jaws (to define beam size), ionization monitors (for beam quality assurance), flattening filter (to homogenize photon beams), multileaf collimators (to support computer-controlled shielding and intensity-modulated radiation therapy), and treatment head trays (for wedges or electron trimmers).

1.7. ISODOSE CURVES

Graphical Methods

Various graphical methods exist for the depiction of radiotherapy beam dose deposition (Figure 1.11).

1. *Depth dose distribution.* This approach can characterize the change in dose along a one-dimensional line, usually along the center path of a radiotherapy beam, otherwise known as the central axis. The percentage depth dose curve is usually normalized on the *y*-axis as a percentage of the maximum dose (which is usually referred to as the d_{max}). Depth dose distribution profiles can vary according to various parameters including: radiation type, radiation energy, density (or density changes) in the medium, field size, field shape (shielding), and source to skin distance (SSD).

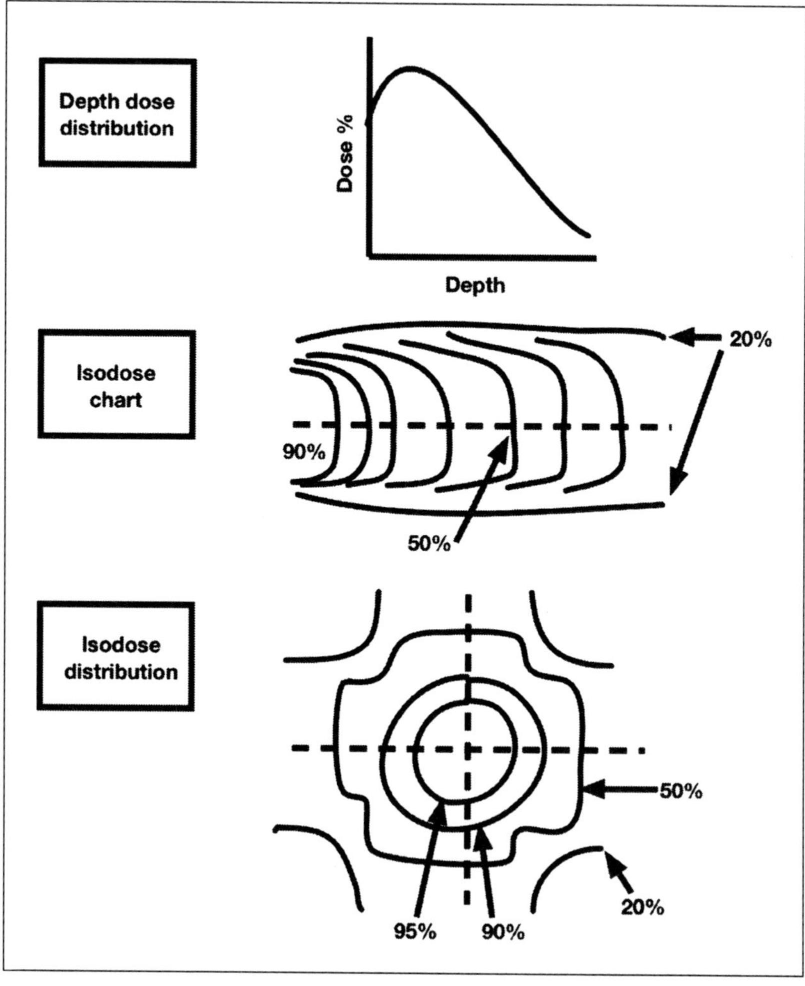

FIGURE 1.11 Dose depiction graphical methods

2. *Isodose chart.* This is a two-dimensional representation of isodose curves (a line connecting points in space receiving the same dose of radiotherapy) assessing the relationship between dose, depth from the surface, and distance from the central axis (usually for a single photon or election field). At any given depth, a depth dose beam profile can be generated to demonstrate the relationship between relative dose and distance from the central axis.
3. *Isodose distribution.* A two-dimensional representation of isodose lines relating to a three-dimensional (3D) radiotherapy plan. Although commonly visualized in axial planes, coronal and sagittal isodose distributions can also be generated for review by radiotherapy personnel. With the advent of modern TPS, 3D isodose distributions can also be generated using various 3D visualization methods.

Single Beam Considerations

1. *Single field electron beam.* Electron beams exhibit rapid fall-off with depth for most clinical energies. The rapid reduction in delivered radiation dose is clinically utilized for the treatment of superficial tumors including those of the skin, head and neck, and rib metastases. Additionally, electron isodose lines bow outward from the initial treatment beam due to lateral scatter of electrons as they interact with matter (Figure 1.12). There are several rules of thumb to describe the depth dose characteristics of an electron beam including:

$$\text{surface dose} = 70 + \text{electron beam energy (in percent)}$$

$$90\% \text{ isodose line} = \text{electron energy (in MeV)}/4 \text{ (in cm)}$$

$$80\% \text{ isodose line} = \text{electron energy (in MeV)}/3 \text{ (in cm)}$$

$$\text{electron range} = \text{electron energy (in MeV)}/2 \text{ (in cm)}$$

2. *Single field photon beam.* Photon beams can be generated by orthovoltage (<1 MeV), radionuclides (^{60}Co), or by linear accelerator (≥4 MV). The beam profile and depth of maximum dose (d_{max}) of single field photon beams depend on the beam energy, field size/shape, source to skin distance, and direction/angle of the incident beam to the surface. As the photon energy increases, d_{max} and the effective range of radiotherapy will increase, while the surface dose will decrease. These properties of megavoltage radiation are exploited to treat deep tumors of the human body with a significant skin-sparing (and hence toxicity-sparing) effect (Figure 1.12). Conversely, as tangential beams of radiation (glancing along the surface) are used (e.g., breast cancer tangent fields), the d_{max} is reduced and the surface dose increases, which may lead to more superficial skin toxicity.

Other Radiation Beam Considerations

Clinically, single photon or electron beams are used in palliative situations involving the spine or superficial ribs. More commonly, one or more beams are used in concert to treat various target volumes. Some common field arrangement scenarios are listed below (Figure 1.13).

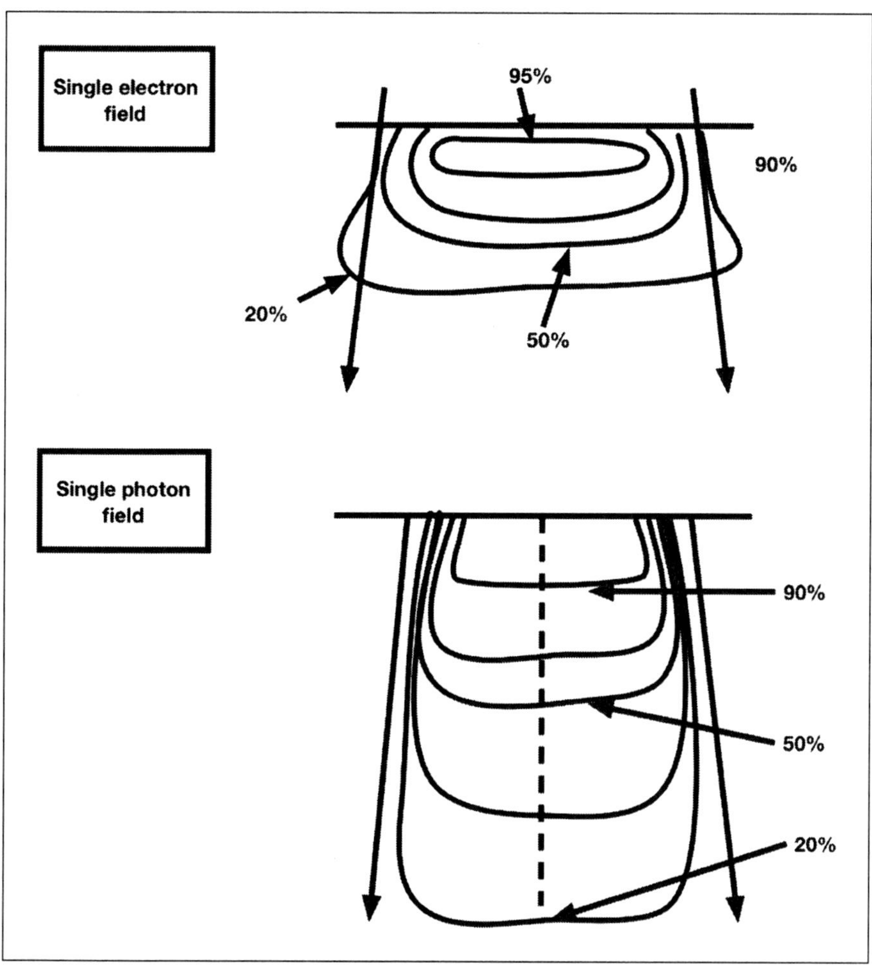

FIGURE 1.12 Single photon/electron radiation beams

1. *Single field wedged photon beam.* Modification of a single photon beam by a wedge filter (of high Z material) in order to change the central axis of the radiation beam to a value other than 90°. The wedge angle is the angle between the central axis of the radiation beam and the isodose lines that cross it. It is important to note that the physical angle of the wedge filter to create the wedge angle and the wedge angle itself are not the same (the physical angle is smaller than the wedge angle).
2. *Parallel opposed pair photon beam.* When two radiation beams oppose each other, a more uniform radiation dose is delivered. Some heterogeneity of delivered dose still occurs at the superficial surfaces (both anterior and posterior) due to buildup; however, when compared to a single beam of radiation, the build-up region is smaller given the exit dose of the opposite beam.
3. *Wedged-pair photon beam.* Wedged-pair beams can be used to treat relatively superficial tumors, while sparing the contralateral volume of interest. This technique has been historically used to treat the ipsilateral neck and neck tumors (e.g., parotid), while sparing the contralateral parotid gland (to spare salivary function). Two important concepts that are associated with this technique are the wedge angle (see above) and the hinge angle (the angle between the two central axes as defined by both wedged beams). A mathematical relationship exists between these two concepts:

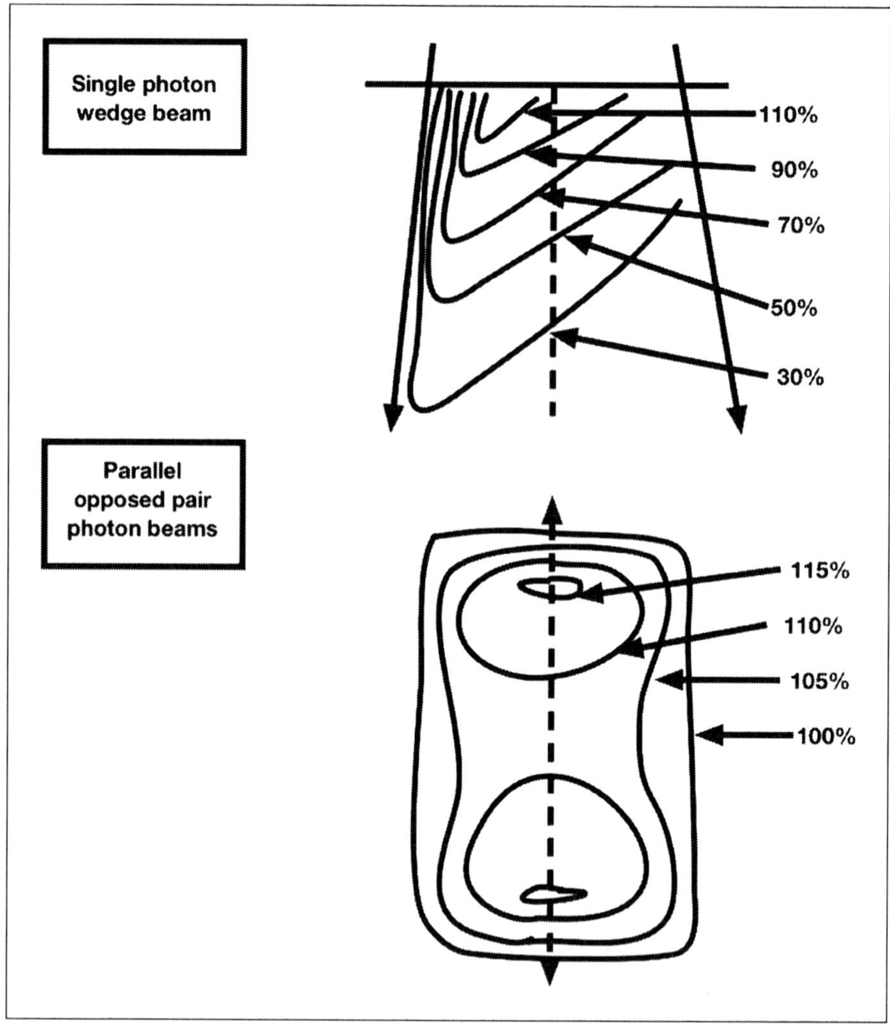

FIGURE 1.13 Other radiation beam considerations

$$\text{wedge angle} = 90 - (\text{hinge angle}/2)$$

or

$$\text{hinge angle} = 2 \times (90 - \text{wedge angle})$$

4. *Multiple photon beams.* Modern treatment of patients with radiotherapy routinely utilizes multiple fields (three or more). Isodose distributions that result from such beam arrangements depend on the number of beams, location/angle of beams, beam energy, beam weighting, use of overlapping or non-overlapping beams, use of non-coplanar beams (beams not aligned in the same axis), and the use of devices that may modulate the beam (shielding, wedges, tissue equivalent compensation/bolus, multileaf collimation).

Chapter 2

Biology

KEY POINTS

- The hallmarks of cancer include: evading apoptosis, self-sufficiency in growth signals, insensitivity to antigrowth signals, tissue invasion and metastasis, limitless replication potential, and sustained angiogenesis.
- The cell cycle consists of mitosis, first gap, synthesis, second gap, and a return to mitosis (with gap zero for nondividing cells). The cycle is highly regulated by multiple proteins including: cyclin-dependent kinase, myc transcription factor, and ras signaling.
- Cell death can occur through necrosis and apoptosis (programmed cell death). Cell lifespan is regulated by chromosomal shortening and telomeres.
- Tumor populations consist of clonal cell populations that can exhibit phenotypic and genotypic heterogeneity. This can lead to sequential mutations that change the nature of the tumor over time.
- Angiogenesis is a mechanism by which new blood vessels are formed. In cancer cells, various angiogenesis factors (vascular endothelial growth factor [VEGF] and epidermal growth factor [EGF]) are utilized to secure blood supply for growing tumors.
- The tumor microenvironment can have a profound impact on tumor growth and spread. Degradation of the extracellular matrix (ECM) surrounding tumors by endogenous factors (such as altered cell adhesion molecules [CAMs]) can lead to metastatic cancer potential.
- Cancer cells can often have hypoxic regions either with inadequate or tenuous blood supply. These areas are clinically important due to potential increased radiation resistance as well as possible genetic alterations, which can lead to further invasion and metastases.
- Modes of cancer spread include local invasion and distant metastases (lymphatic and hematogenous). Invasive tumors are thought to develop metastases through a sequence of events including: primary tumor development, localized invasion, detachment and intravasation, arrest, extravasation, micrometastasis formation, and macrometastasis formation.
- Genetic mechanisms/mutation that can lead to cancer potential can be classified by the following: oncogenes, tumor suppressor genes, gene amplification, viral interactions, and epigenetic phenomena.
- The majority of cancer is sporadic in nature; however, familial cancer syndromes and inheritable risks are known to exist.

2.1. WHAT IS CANCER?

The growth of cells in the human body is governed through an interconnected system of checks and feedback loops. These processes are coded for by the DNA of a cell, collectively termed the *genome*. Alterations and mutations of the genetic code can disrupt these processes, culminating in errors that may lead to cancer, which is essentially the uncontrolled division of cells in the body. Given this vague definition, a common misconception is that cancer is a singular disease, when it is actually a broad term that encompasses a vastly heterogeneous group of diseases, with numerous factors and variations determining the severity and potential lethality of each individual diagnosis.

Carcinogenesis

The process by which normal cells undergo transformation to cancer cells is termed *carcinogenesis*. This vastly complex process can be thought of as a cell that undergoes a series of genetic alterations and mutations, through inherited, environmental, and acquired causes, which eventually leads to the cell's inability to control its proliferation, differentiation, and ultimately death.

This process of carcinogenesis, the development of malignant cells, has been proposed to be the product of six characteristic hallmarks of cancer (Figure 2.1):

1. Evading apoptosis
2. Self-sufficiency in growth signals
3. Insensitivity to antigrowth signals
4. Tissue invasion and metastasis
5. Limitless replication potential
6. Sustained angiogenesis

These hallmarks describe the biology of cancer (Hanahan and Weinberg, 2000), and will be further discussed in this chapter.

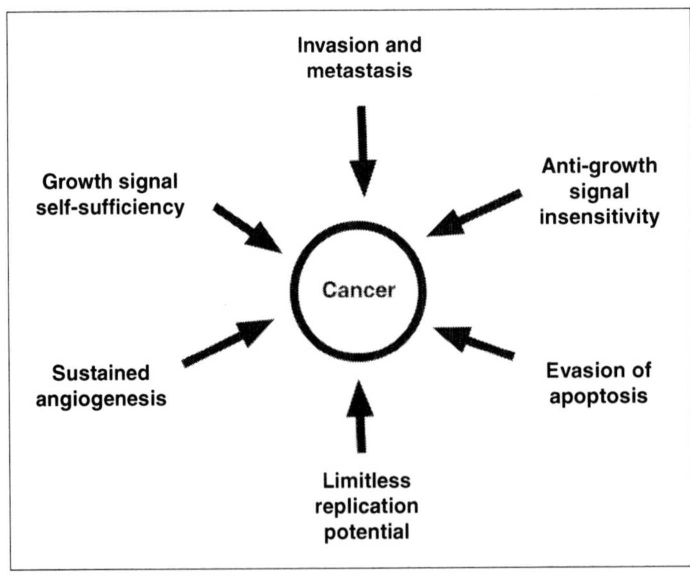

FIGURE 2.1 Hallmarks of cancer

2.2. CELL CYCLE AND PROLIFERATION

Phases of the Cell Cycle

The growth and propagation of mammalian cell populations occur through mitotic division, a process by which a single cell duplicates its chromosomes and divides to form two daughter cells with identical DNA to the parent cell. The main events in the cell cycle of actively growing cells are the period of duplication of chromosomal material (synthesis) and the period of active division (mitosis), which are separated by two time gaps (Figure 2.2). The cell cycle of actively growing cells can be broken down into four sequential phases defined as M (mitosis), G_1 (the first gap phase preceding synthesis during which growth occurs), S (synthesis), and G_2 (the second gap phase preceding mitosis during which chromosomes condense and prepare for separation), and then M again. Cells that are not actively dividing are said to be in G_0, or interphase. Mitosis can be further broken down into the following subphases: prophase, metaphase, anaphase, telophase, and cytokinesis.

Cell Cycle Regulation

The cell cycle is under the regulation of multiple molecules and proteins with some examples provided below.

1. *Cyclin-dependent kinase (Cdk).* One of the most important groups of cell cycle regulators in mammalian cells are the Cdk family of proteins. Cdk proteins bind to molecules known

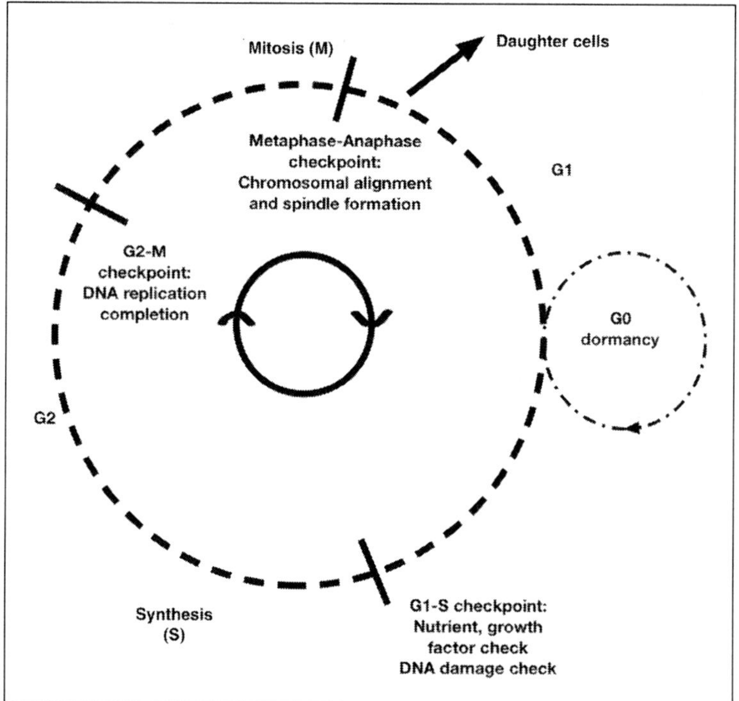

FIGURE 2.2 Cell cycle

as cyclins, which cause the activation of the Cdk protein complex. Activated Cdk-cyclin complexes act at the various phases of the cell cycle to regulate progression. Therefore, the activation and deactivation of Cdk are regulated in response to environmental signals to the cell Cdk inhibitor molecules, including the kinase inhibitory protein (KIP) and inhibitor of Cdk4 (INK4) family of proteins.

2. *Myc transcription factor.* The Myc gene codes for a protein transcription factor that regulates cell proliferation. Expression of Myc causes a cell to enter the active phases of the cell cycle, even in the absence of growth factors. Therefore, Myc expression is controlled by growth inhibition and differentiation signals. Activation of Myc is a common feature of many human tumor cells.
3. *Ras signaling.* The Ras signaling pathways are crucial for the interpretation of extracellular signals that trigger intracellular changes and ultimately lead to cell cycle progression. Extracellular signals are received by cell membrane-bound tyrosine kinase receptors, which in turn lead to a cascade that increases Ras activation. This activation is carried through a variety of pathways to trigger changes in the nucleus that play a critical role in transition through the cell cycle, and thus promote proliferation.

Regulation of Differentiation and Senescence

Normal cells will not proliferate indefinitely, and typically terminal differentiation will lead to the arrest of proliferation. This is a precisely timed and regulated process to ensure appropriate numbers of differentiated cells. Similarly, cells that have undergone a determined number of doublings arrest their proliferative potential and will enter senescence. Senescence is a mechanism to reduce the formation of malignant cells by limiting the number of cellular divisions, and, therefore, limiting the number of genetic errors that might accumulate in a given cell. Tumor cells are cells that gain unlimited proliferative potential through genetic and environmental factors that lead to an ability to block normal differentiation, insensitivity to growth inhibitory signals, and avoidance of cellular senescence.

2.3. CELL IMMORTALITY AND DEATH

Cell death is an integral process of mammalian cells, and it is estimated that humans have approximately 10 billion cells that undergo death on a daily basis. Therefore, it is vital that the human body be able to regulate the balance between cell proliferation and cell death in its various body systems. Normal human cells generally have a finite lifespan as they are programmed to limit their own replication. Cancer cells typically display a limitless potential for replication, known as cell immortality (Figure 2.3).

Cell death occurs through the two processes of necrosis and programmed cellular death (apoptosis). While necrosis is a passive process that serves to remove damaged cells from the organism, apoptosis is a genetically regulated and active natural process which is disrupted in the cancer cell.

Programmed Cell Death (Apoptosis)

Apoptosis, programmed cellular death, consists of a highly intricate regulatory process governed by a complex interplay of multiple genes and their protein products. It can be triggered by endogenous factors, such as DNA damage and growth factor deprivation, and

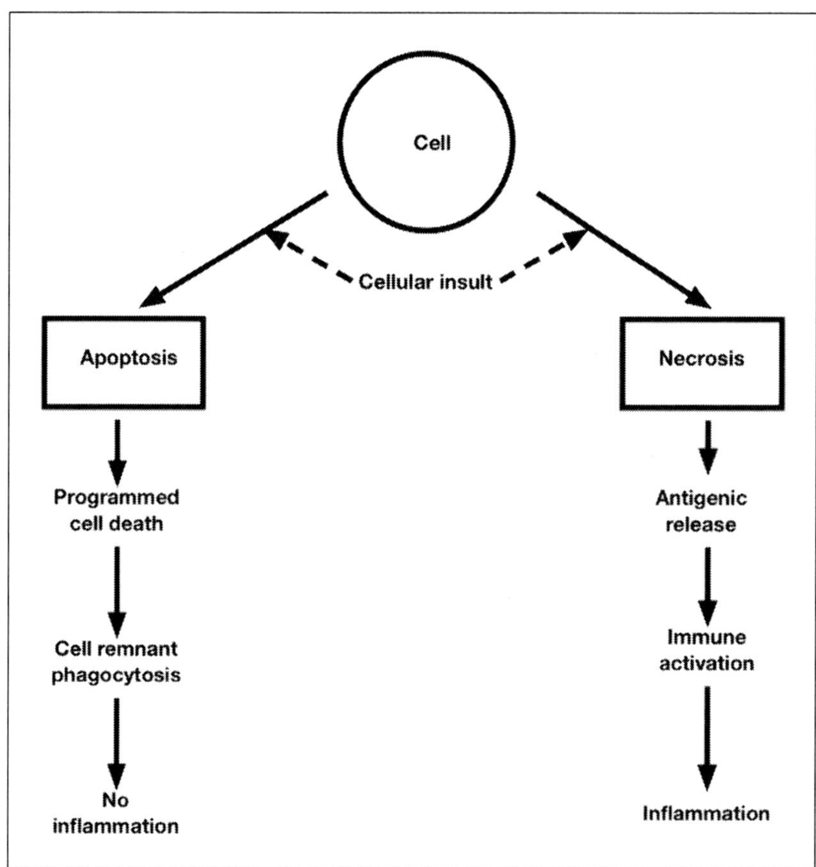

FIGURE 2.3 Cell mortality

exogenous factors such as radiation and chemotherapeutic agents. The integrity of the apoptotic machinery ensures that cells with irreparable DNA damage that could progress to cancer will be eliminated from the population. Loss of integrity of the apoptotic pathways and regulators can allow cells to evade apoptosis and continue growth, a key mechanism of cancer development. An example of one of the most important and frequently disrupted apoptotic regulators is the p53 tumor suppressor gene. The p53 protein is a transcription factor that plays a key role in apoptosis, and mutations of the p53 gene are found with increased frequency in a variety of human tumors.

Cell Immortality

The finite lifespan of normal human cells is related to the phenomena of chromosomal shortening and telomeres. With each successive replication of a cell, the DNA at the end of its chromosomes cannot be properly replicated. To protect cells from the degradation of these chromosomal ends, cells evolved protective repeated sequences of DNA called telomeres, which form a nucleoprotein structure that link to the chromosomal ends and prevent loss of vital DNA. Telomeres can be maintained by a special protein called telomerase, which is normally suppressed in most human cells. Therefore, normal human cells exhibit the phenomena of progressively shortening telomeric ends with each successive doubling. It has been demonstrated that after cells typically undergo between 50 and 80 doublings (known as the Hayflick limit), their telomeric protection will have been expended and this is associated with loss of cell proliferative capacity. Eventually, the cell will undergo critical DNA damage to its chromosome ends and loss of stability that will lead to cell death, often mediated by tumor suppressor genes such as p53. Tumor cells often exhibit rare mutations that can lead to the activation of telomerase, which allows the cell to prevent telomere shortening and to achieve cell immortality.

2.4. TUMOR HETEROGENEITY

Tumor Heterogeneity

Although cancer is a clonal disease characterized by recurrent cellular division, tumor populations consist of a heterogeneous and evolving population of tumor cells. The model of Darwinian evolution and concept of "survival of the fittest" can be loosely applied to a growing cancer cell population. The process begins with the transformation of a normal cell to a malignant precursor cell, a mutation which gives this cell some proliferative and possibly survival advantage over the surrounding cells. This cell divides to form the first clonal expansion, a population of cells with the mutation significant enough to displace the cells that lack the mutation and survival advantage. Subsequently, a few of the cells in the first clonal expansion population may acquire a mutation that gives them an advantage, ultimately leading to a second clonal expansion of cells that can displace the first generation. Through the repetition of this process, greater genetic instability is propagated and more aggressive colonies of cells are generated (Figure 2.4).

Tumor Progression

Tumor progression is the evolution of cells within a tumor to give it greater capacity for autonomous growth and leads to cancerous cells with the ability to invade and metastasize.

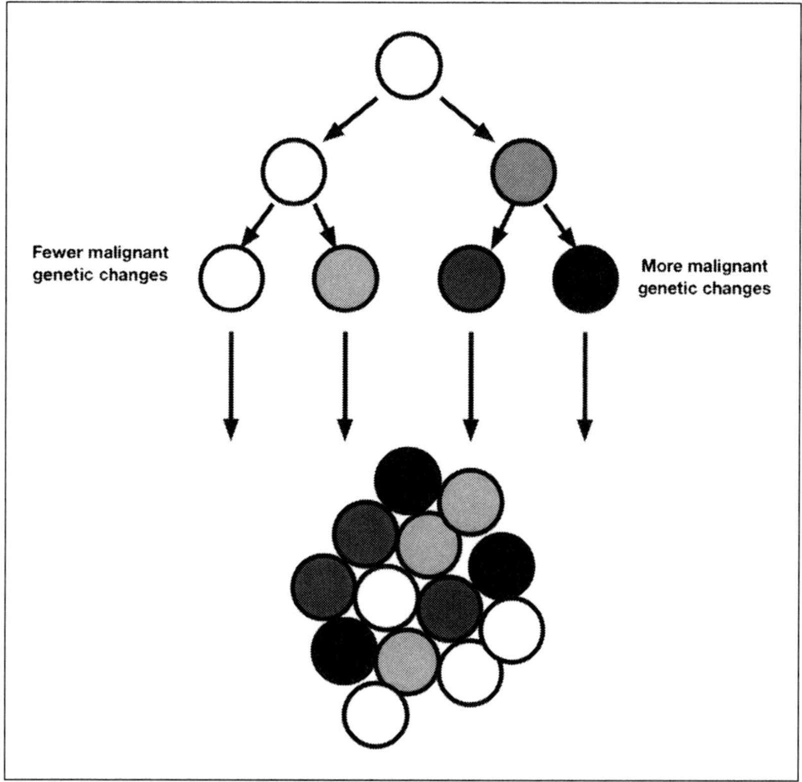

FIGURE 2.4 Tumor heterogeneity

2.5. ANGIOGENESIS

Normal Angiogenesis

The formation of new blood vessels from preexisting larger vessels is termed *angiogenesis*. It is a naturally occurring process to ensure that oxygen and nutrients are provided to cells, which occurs in limited instances in adults. In adults, normal angiogenesis occurs in the female reproductive system in the lining of the uterus, and also in damaged tissues as a part of wound healing. In the embryo and children, it occurs as a normal part of development and growth.

Regulation of Angiogenesis and Vascular Endothelial Growth Factor (VEGF)

Angiogenesis requires a cascade of events beginning with vasodilation and an increase in vascular permeability. Vasodilation is mediated primarily by the molecule nitric oxide. An increase in nitric oxide signals an increase of VEGF, which permits vessel leakiness. This increased permeability allows for extravasation and sprouting of new endothelial cells, ultimately leading to new blood vessel formation. Multiple inducers and inhibitors of VEGF and angiogenesis have been described, including epidermal growth factor (EGF) and tumor necrosis factor alpha that contribute to the tumor's complex regulation of this process.

Tumor Angiogenesis

Cancerous cells require oxygen and nutrients to grow and divide, which requires close proximity to capillary blood vessels (Figure 2.5). Without the ability to induce the sprouting of new vessels, growing tumors would quickly outstrip their own blood supply. However, in tumors, it has been observed that these cancerous cells are able to affect the regulation of angiogenesis through the release of multiple signaling factors that induce angiogenesis and downregulate the inhibiting factors. This activates an angiogenic switch that results in the enhanced angiogenesis displayed by tumors. Recent cancer therapies have focused on the inhibition of angiogenesis by blocking the action of factors such as VEGF and EGF.

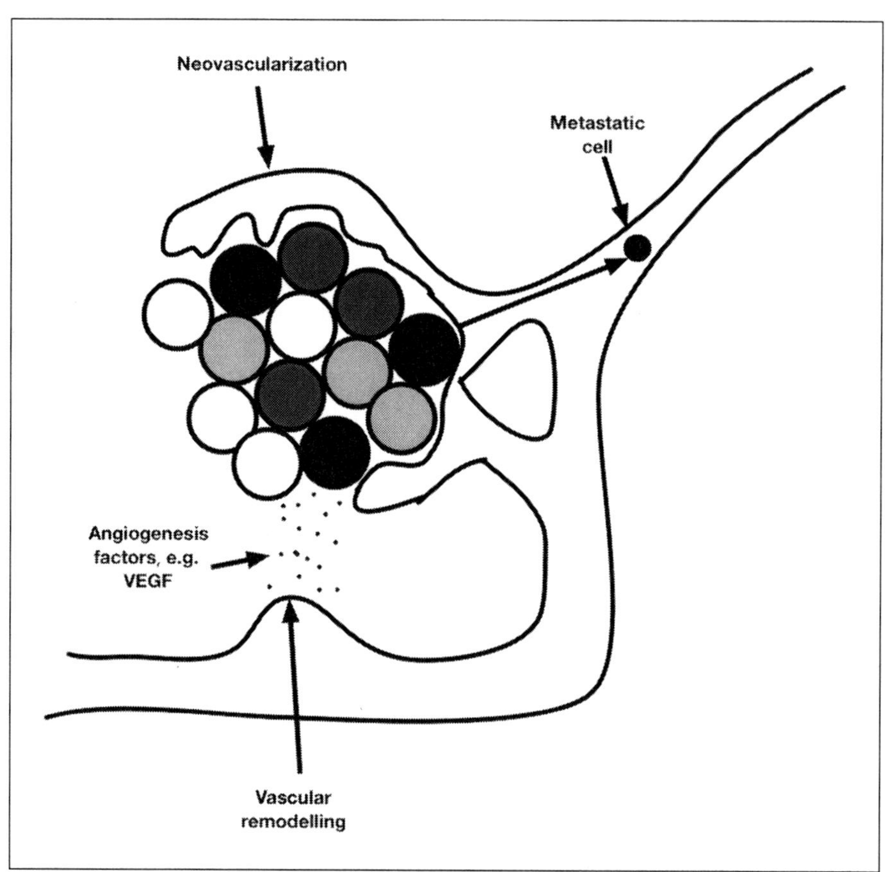

FIGURE 2.5 Tumor angiogenesis

2.6. TUMOR MICROENVIRONMENT

Extracellular Matrix and Cell Microenvironment

The ECM varies according to the type of cells, location, and developmental stage. These differences in the connective tissue, proteins, and proteoglycans surrounding different types of cells provide specialized three-dimensional environments. The ECM serves to provide adhesive structure, facilitate communication between adjacent cells, and harbor molecules such as growth factors and proteinases. The matrix also contributes to cell signaling by bringing signaling molecules, such as growth factors, into close proximity.

Tumor Microenvironment

In tumor cell populations, a disruption in the balance of proteolysis, adhesion, and signaling in the ECM is observed. Aberrant proteolysis can lead to a cascade that causes cleavage of the ECM. This, in turn, releases normally sequestered growth factors into the matrix, which can lead to increased proliferation of the cells. Degradation of the ECM removes some of the physical barriers to cell migration, while modification of the CAMs allows increased motility. Fragments of the ECM can also initiate a number of tumor-promoting processes, including angiogenesis.

Cell Adhesion Molecules

Cell adhesion molecules (CAMs) are specialized transmembrane proteins that facilitate cell–cell and cell–ECM interactions. Examples of the types of CAMs include integrins, cadherins, and selectins. CAMs allow signaling between cell and environment, and function prominently in tumor cell proliferation, invasion, and metastases. Alteration of the CAMs and signaling within a tumor between adjacent cells may allow the cell to migrate away from its primary site of development to form distant metastases. Similarly, this may explain why certain tumor types are more likely to metastasize to various organs.

Gap Junctions

Gap junctions are clusters of connexin proteins which form communication "tunnels" between adjacent cells. This allows the sharing of signaling molecules and metabolites. Increased gap junction formation has been associated with greater metastatic potential of tumor cells.

2.7. TUMOR HYPOXIA AND REOXYGENATION

Tumor Hypoxia

The metabolism of cells is influenced by numerous environmental factors, including oxygen concentration of the surrounding environment (Figure 2.6). Tumors tend to have regions of hypoxic environments, with oxygen concentrations < 5 mmHg. Normal tissue oxygen concentration typically ranges between 10 and 80 mmHg. These observed pockets of tumor hypoxia are secondary to the irregular vascular architecture caused by the abnormal angiogenesis within tumor tissues. The models used to describe tumor hypoxia typically focus on the distance of hypoxic cells from the blood vessel and on abnormal blood flow. Cells further away from the blood vessel can experience increasing hypoxia as they reach the diffusion limit, typically between 70 and 150 µM. However, recent studies have also shown that there are regions of both acute and chronic hypoxia within a tumor owing to acute changes in blood flow.

Effect of Oxygen Concentration on Tumor Cells

Oxygen plays a vital role in radiation treatment as a potent radiosensitizer, and hypoxic tumors have been shown to be less responsive to treatment. The modified behavior of tumor cells in hypoxic environments is thought to be due to alterations in gene expression. Increases in the gene expression of various factors allows the cell to compensate for

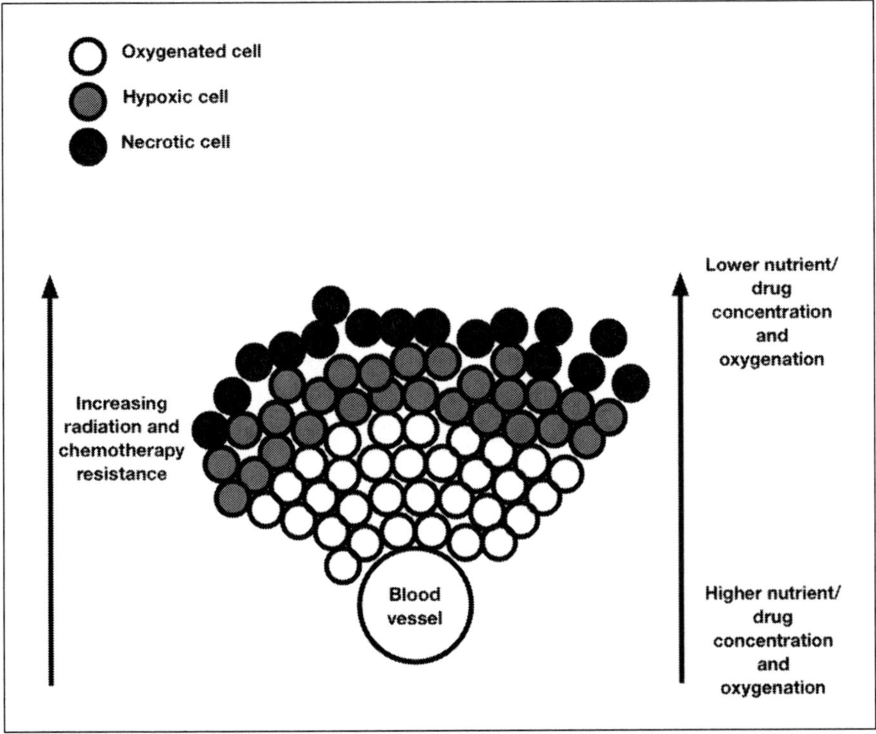

FIGURE 2.6 Tumor hypoxia

its environmental changes, including switching to anaerobic metabolism. Coupled with an increase in the expression of angiogenesis promoters, there is also an increase in factors, which lead to greater propensity for invasion and metastatic spread. Although prolonged hypoxia will typically lead to apoptosis, studies have revealed that tumor cells with mutated p53 demonstrate hypoxia resistance, and that hypoxic environments can lead to deficient DNA repair mechanisms. By selecting for p53 mutations and allowing increased genetic variability to mutations, selective hypoxia appears to be an important mechanism by which tumors progress.

Methods of Tumor Reoxygenation

To overcome the radioresistance of hypoxic tumor cells, various mechanisms of reoxygenating tumor cells have been explored. Oncology patients often experience anemia secondary to their disease or other concomitant treatments, such as chemotherapy. These lower concentrations of hemoglobin, and therefore oxygen delivery, have been demonstrated to lead to poorer outcomes of radiotherapy, provoking the use of blood transfusions and erythropoietin injections during treatment to obtain normal red blood cell levels. Another method that has been explored to increase oxygenation is the use of hyperbaric oxygen environments during radiation, which has been shown to have some improvement in treatment response for head and neck and cervical cancers. Literature has also suggested an interest in the use of antiangiogenesis drugs, such as VEGF inhibitors, concurrently with radiation, to paradoxically improve tumor oxygenation by the manipulation of the vascular architecture.

2.8. INVASION AND METASTASES

Metastasis

Metastasis, the spread of cancer from the area of primary tumor development to distant organs, is responsible for the majority of cancer deaths. As mentioned earlier in this chapter, tumor progression is marked by the selection for more aggressive populations of cells within a tumor. Coupled with changes in environment, including change of the CAMs, these cells will potentially have the ability to leave the primary tumor site.

Modes of Cancer Spread

The two typical methods of spread are through the lymphatic drainage system and the vasculature (hematogenous). A common first site of lymphatic spread is the regional lymph nodes, although it is not unusual for malignant cells to be absent in the lymph nodes and still ultimately be found in more distant organ sites. Clinically, it has been observed that certain cancers are more likely to spread to certain organ systems than others (i.e., prostate cancer most commonly to bone, lung cancer most commonly to brain). Although this may be partially a function of its pattern of spread, experiments using rodent model systems have concluded that this "homing in" of certain cancer cells to various organs is a function of cell signaling. This includes cancer cells overexpressing receptors for signaling molecules, called chemokines, which are normally used by white blood cells to target specific organs, but can also function to allow the cancer cell to preferentially spread to an organ with greater expression of the chemokine ligand.

Invasion to Metastasis Cascade

The process of metastasis formation from a primary tumor can be described in a series of sequential steps (Figure 2.7):

1. *Primary tumor development.* An initial premalignant cell undergoes transformation to a malignant cell, and through a series of successive proliferations generates a malignant tumor growth.
2. *Localized invasion.* The primary tumor gains access to the vasculature either through direct invasion or through the formation of microvascular channels.
3. *Detachment and intravasation.* Decreased expression of cellular adhesion molecules, increased expression of proteases, and leaky vasculature allow tumor cells to enter the circulation and be transported to different sites through the body.
4. *Arrest.* Initially, tumor cells in the circulation will typically become physically arrested, due to their relative size, in the first capillary bed they encounter, often the liver or lung. Through physical deformation, some may continue to pass through the capillary eventually to lodge in other areas. Many cells will die following arrest, but some will extravasate through the capillary bed and enter adjacent tissue.
5. *Extravasation.* Arrested tumor cells may extravasate into the tissue parenchyma through complex interactions between the tumor cells, endothelial cells of the capillary, and the basement membrane. The tumor cells may extend projections known as invadopodia between the endothelial cell junctions, which facilitates proteolytic penetrance and

allows access to the basement membrane. The tumor cell then interacts with the ECM and basement membrane through CAMs and binding molecules, releasing proteases to lyse the matrix proteins and enter the tissue parenchyma.

6. *Micrometastasis formation.* Following extravasation of a tumor cell into the parenchyma, it will often find itself in a microenvironment that differs from its normally associated tissue. Therefore, in order for the cell to survive and grow to form a micrometastasis, it must be able to respond to growth factors found within its new environment, or be independent in producing its own growth factor (a hallmark of most tumor cells). Both during and after extravasation, the tumor is also susceptible to normal tissue defense mechanisms against foreign cells, which includes both immune system–mediated cytotoxic killing and the normal tissue's ability to attempt to signal apoptosis in the new foreign cell. These defenses must be overcome for the cell to take hold and form a metastatic deposit.
7. *Macrometastasis formation.* Progression from micrometastasis to a larger, clinically detectable growth requires continued proliferative capacity and the ability to induce angiogenesis in the surrounding tissue to maintain blood supply. Many tumor deposits will not progress beyond the micrometastasis stage, because they either undergo eventual cell death through apoptosis and necrosis or enter a prolonged period of dormancy. The pathways and triggers affecting the reactivation of dormant micrometastases after prolonged periods of time, a frequent occurrence in certain cancers such as breast cancer, is the subject of ongoing research into the environmental stresses and changes that affect this switch.

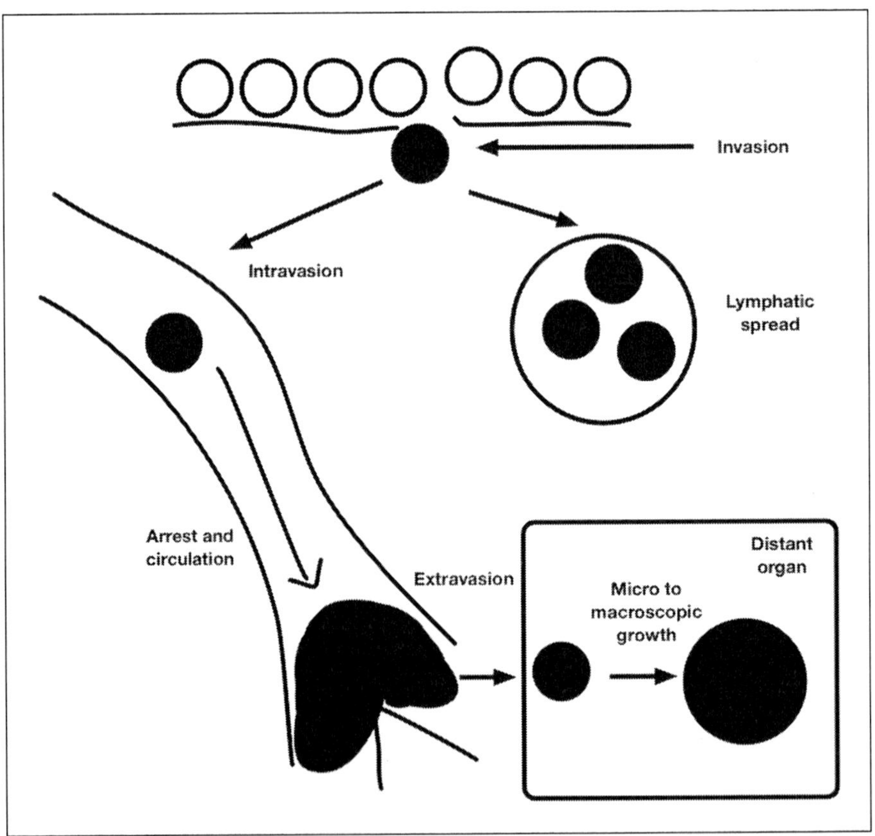

FIGURE 2.7 Invasion to metastases pathway

2.9. CANCER GENETICS

Genomic Mutations Predispose to Cancer

The majority of malignant disease is caused by mutations that result in genetic instability (Figure 2.8). These changes can occur at the germline stage, in which case they are propagated into every cell in the body and can be potentially inherited, or through a mutation in a single cell. Mutations typically occur in response to carcinogens, environmental molecules, and factors that cause DNA damage, which can predispose one to the development of malignant disease. Most often, damage is repaired by DNA repair mechanisms, but inherited or new mutations causing faulty DNA repair mechanisms can result in increased predisposition to cancer development. These genes that encode critical processes, which if altered can lead to tumor formation, can be classified as oncogenes and tumor suppressor genes.

Oncogenes

Genes that code for a protein product that could lead to cancer development and progression are termed proto-oncogenes. Normally, each cell has two alleles (copies) of DNA coding for a specific gene. A mutation to a single allele can lead to activation of the proto-oncogene to an oncogene, which, in this activated form, may contribute to carcinogenesis. Oncogenes

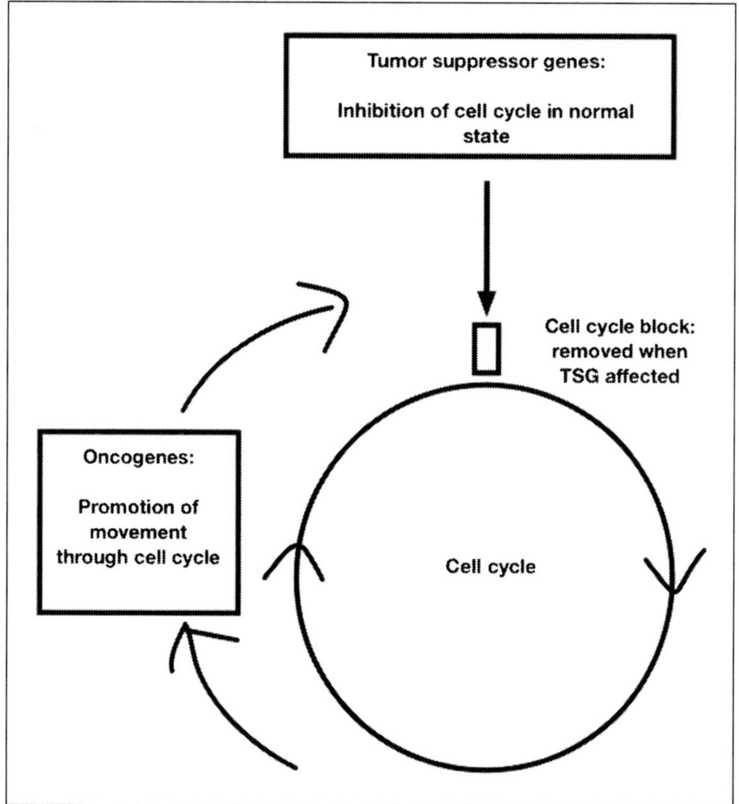

FIGURE 2.8 Cancer genetics

typically code for growth factors, cytoplasmic kinases, transcription factors, and antiapoptotic proteins. Their activation through various pathways results in a gain of function to support tumor development. A few examples of the numerous oncogenes, some of which were described previously in this chapter, are VEGF, EGFR, Ras, c-Myc, and HER2/neu.

Tumor Suppressor Genes

As suggested by their name, tumor suppressor genes act to inhibit the proliferation of malignant cells, and thus alterations resulting in a loss of their function can lead to tumor development. Unlike oncogenes, they require both copies to be mutated to lead to carcinogenesis. Tumor suppressors can be broadly classified as gatekeepers or caretakers. Gatekeepers work to limit tumor cell proliferation and promote cell death, whereas caretakers work to maintain genomic stability, often facilitating DNA repair functions. Examples of commonly mutated tumor suppressor gatekeeper genes are *p53*, *RB*, *PTEN*, and *BRCA* genes.

p53 acts in numerous capacities to control progression through the cell cycle and apoptosis, and is mutated in over half of human cancers. A rare autosomal-dominant mutation of *p53* is found in Li-Fraumeni syndrome, which predisposes the carrier to early onset of a variety of malignancies. PTEN (phosphatase and tensin homolog deleted on chromosome 10) is a negative regulator of cellular pathways, and mutations are often found in many glioblastomas, prostate, thyroid, breast, and skin malignancies. *RB* is the retinoblastoma gene, and although first described in its namesake eye tumor, alterations are often found in osteosarcoma, small-cell lung carcinoma, prostate, and breast cancers. Familial breast cancer is often associated with autosomal-dominant mutations of *BRCA* tumor suppressor genes, with *BRCA1* also associated with increased ovarian and prostate cancers, whereas *BRCA2* mutations are associated with ovarian, male breast, prostate, pancreatic, bile duct, and gastric cancers.

Gene Amplification

Genetic mutations and instability may lead to an increased number of copies of a specific gene, known as gene amplification. The enhanced number of copies typically leads to enhanced expression of the gene and its coded phenotype. Gene amplification of oncogenes can lead to enhanced cellular proliferation and transformation. Furthermore, gene amplification of drug-resistant genes has been associated with increased resistance of certain tumors to chemotherapeutic agents.

Epigenetics

Epigenetics refers to the process by which cells modify the structure and activity of chromatin, thereby controlling the transcription of various genes. This process is primarily mediated through DNA methylation, which acts as an effective "on/off" switch, allowing the cell to access and transcribe a particular gene or not. Disruption of normal epigenetic patterns can lead to abnormal silencing or activation of genes that control tumor suppression, DNA repair, cell cycle control, and cell signaling. DNA methylation patterns are normally inherited from the maternal and paternal contributions to DNA in a process known as genomic imprinting. Loss of imprinting has been recently implicated in a number of human cancers, including colorectal cancer.

Viruses and Cancer

Viruses may induce malignant transformation by inhibiting the normal control of cellular growth through actions on tumor suppressor genes, direct insertion or activation of oncogenes, alteration of cellular signal transduction, or immune system modification. Viruses containing DNA or RNA sequences are thought to be involved in up to 15%–20% of human cancers. Numerous human tumor viruses have been identified, examples of which are summarized in Table 2.1.

TABLE 2.1 Examples of Human Tumor Viruses

Virus	Name	Cancer Association	Notes
HPV	Human papilloma virus	Cervical, oropharyngeal, anal, vulvar, penile, nonmelanoma skin cancers	HPV 16, 18 most common high-risk subtypes (also 31, 33, and 45)
EBV	Epstein-Barr virus	Burkitt's lymphoma, nasopharyngeal carcinoma, lymphomas, posttransplant	90% of population by age 20 infected; NPC most common in Southeast Asians
HBV	Hepatitis B virus	Hepatocellular carcinoma	Widespread in Asia, Africa, and South America
KSHV	Kaposi sarcoma–associated herpesvirus	Kaposi sarcoma, primary effusion lymphoma, multicentric Castleman's disease	Kaposi sarcoma endemic in Mediterranean and African elderly men
HTLV-1	Human T-cell leukemia virus	Adult T-cell leukemia	Only retroviruses known to lead directly to cancer in humans
HCV	Hepatitis C virus	Hepatocellular carcinoma	Blood-borne infection

2.10. HERITABLE CANCER

Inherited Cancer Risk

The majority of human cancers are thought to be of a sporadic nature, with inherited cancer syndromes thought to be responsible for approximately 1–15 out of every 100 human cancer cases, depending on the study. Studies of monozygotic twins (twins who share nearly identical genes) reveal that environmental factors and somatic factors are the main determinants of cancer development. Concordance rates for cancer observed amongst twins vary widely depending on disease site, and are typically < 0.10. However, for colorectal, prostate, and breast, rates of concordant cancer development were reported to be 35%, 42%, and 27%, respectively, in monozygotic twins in a Scandinavian study (Lichtenstein et al., 2000). This suggests that certain cancers have increased genetic risk factors, whereas others are largely sporadic events. Some of this discordance may be explained by increased understanding of epigenetics and the inheritance of DNA methylation patterns, known as genomic imprinting. Further research is required to understand the overall contribution of inheritance to cancer risk.

Familial Cancer Syndromes

Most familial cancer syndromes are linked to mutations in the tumor suppressor genes of germline cells. These are typically similar to the mutations that can occur in somatic cells, but they can be propagated through generations given their presence in germline cells. These syndromes are most commonly associated with a loss of function mutation of a single allele of a tumor suppressor gene often leading to deficient DNA repair. Given that a single allele is typically affected, these mutations generally act in a recessive manner, requiring inactivation of the remaining wild-type allele to promote cancer development. Common heritable human cancer syndromes related to tumor suppressor genes are summarized in Table 2.2.

TABLE 2.2 Heritable Human Syndromes of DNA Repair

Syndrome	Repair Pathway Affected	Defective Protein	Cancer Predisposition
Xeroderma pigmentosum	Excision repair	XP	UV-induced skin cancer
		CS	
Ataxia telangiectasia	DNA DSB response	ATM	Lymphomas
AT-like disorder (ATLD)	DNA DSB response	MRE11	Lymphomas
Nijmegen breakage syndrome (NBS)	DNA DSB response	NBS1	Lymphomas
BRCA1/BRCA2	Homologous recombination	BRCA1	Breast (ovarian) cancer
		BRCA2	
Werner syndrome	Homologous recombination	WRN helicase	Various cancers
Bloom syndrome	Homologous recombination	BLM helicase	Leukemia, lymphoma, others
Hereditary nonpolyposis colorectal cancer (HNPCC)	Mismatch repair	MLH 1	Colorectal cancer
		MLH 2	
Fanconi's anemia	DNA cross-link repair	FANC-D2	Leukemia, others

Chapter 3

Radiobiology

KEY POINTS

- Ionizing radiation interacts with matter to create charged particles that can cause DNA damage by the creation of intermediate free radical species (created by the breakdown of water).
- Cell survival curves relate the proportion of surviving cells on the y-axis (usually on a logarithmic scale) versus the radiation dose on the x-axis. Creation of cell survival curves, based on experimental data of cell populations before and after a known radiation exposure, can be used to investigate the impact of different radiation modalities, oxygenation, and drug exposure.
- The preeminent model to explain cell survival curves is the linear quadratic equation:

$$S(D) = e^{(-\alpha D - \beta D2)}$$

- Radiobiologically, cells in various points of the cell cycle have variable radiosensitivities (most sensitive at G2-M checkpoint of successful DNA replication).
- DNA damage can be expressed as: single-strand breaks, double-strand breaks, and base damage. Double-strand breaks are the most difficult to repair.
- Cell radiosensitivity is directly related to the rate of cell division and level of differentiation. Various drugs (radiosensitizers and radioprotectors) and oxygen level can modify cell radiosensitivity.
- The four Rs of radiobiology are: repair, reassortment, repopulation, and reoxygenation. Repair and repopulation tend to result in lower cell kill and normal tissue effects, whereas reassortment and reoxygenation can result in greater cell kill and normal tissue effects.
- Early normal tissue effects (days to weeks) of radiotherapy are usually seen in tissues with high cell turnover (e.g., skin and mucosa), whereas late normal tissue effects (months to years) are usually seen in slowly proliferating tissues (e.g., lung and heart).
- Radiation dose rate is defined as the amount of radiation delivered per unit of time. Lower dose rates are generally associated with higher DNA repair although an inverse dose rate effect is known to exist with very low dose rates. Radiation is usually delivered in fractions to capitalize on tumor cell reoxygenation and reassortment and normal

tissue repair and repopulation. Fractionated radiation of different fraction sizes can be compared using the biological equivalent dose equation:

$$BED = nd\ (1 + d/(\alpha/\beta))\ [\text{in units } Gy_{(\alpha/\beta)}]$$

- Biological effects of radiotherapy can be deterministic (with a threshold dose and increasing risk as dose increases) or stochastic (random risk with no known threshold). Radiation exposure can lead to known acute and late radiotherapy syndromes.

3.1. RADIATION INTERACTIONS AT THE MOLECULAR LEVEL

Ionizing Radiation

The study of the effect of ionizing radiation on living processes is termed *radiobiology*. A basic understanding of the core principles of radiobiology is integral in the practice of radiation therapy. Ionizing radiation occurs indirectly through the release of charged particles. These charged particles cause a complex series of biochemical events that cause DNA damage to cells and organ tissues. Ionizing radiation damage can only be mediated through charged particles. However, radiation is not delivered in a homogeneous manner through tissue, and the amount of absorbed dose depends on a quantity known as linear energy transfer (Figure 3.1).

Linear Energy Transfer

As a charged particle travels through a tissue (absorber), energy is lost unevenly across the path. Linear energy transfer is defined as:

$$LET = dE/dl$$

where dE is the change in kinetic energy and dl is the change in length.

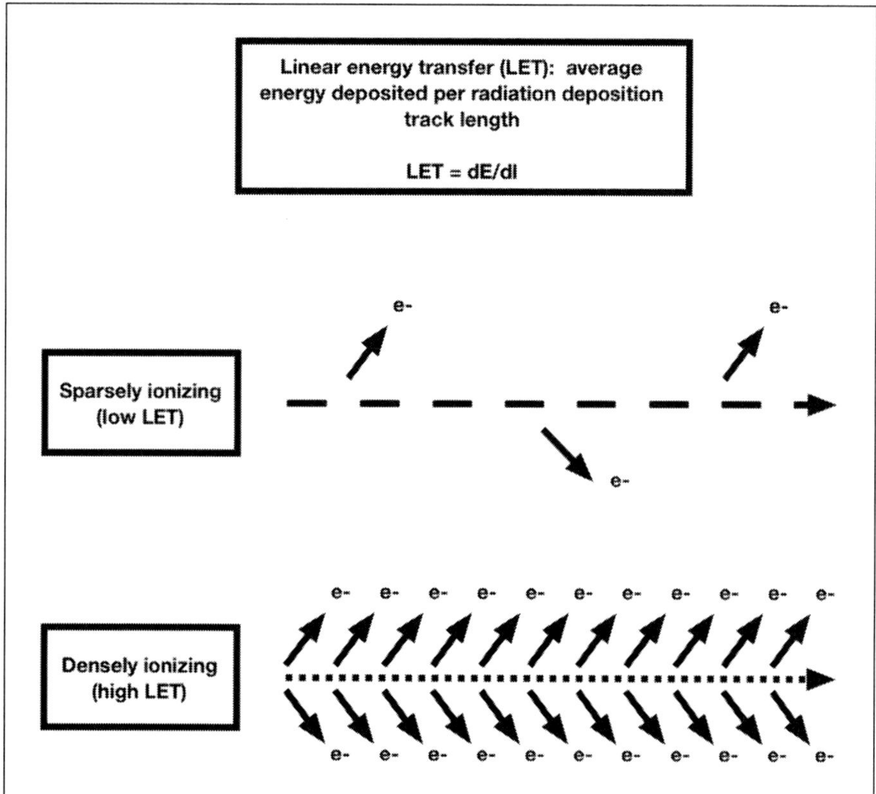

FIGURE 3.1 Radiation deposition and linear energy transfer

Therefore, linear energy transfer (LET) is commonly expressed in units of KeV/µm. The LET depends on the particle charge, energy (speed), absorbed (tissue) type, and its density. Heavier particles, such as protons and neutrons, tend to be much higher LET particles compared to electrons. Most therapeutic particles deposit all their energy within a range of centimeters within tissue. Lower LET particles will travel a longer range in tissue and deposit their energy exponentially along the path. Higher LET particles will travel within a lesser range and have a sharper drop-off of their dose, resulting in more focal energy deposition.

H_2O Radiolysis

The majority of DNA damage is mediated through the indirect action of directly ionizing radiation. This means that a charged particle (as it passes through tissue) will cause the breakdown (radiolysis) of water to form free radicals in close proximity to the DNA of cells. H_2O radiolysis is a relatively quick process that occurs on a time scale of 10^{-12} to 10^{-6} seconds following radiation exposure along the track of the charged particle (Figure 3.2). Reactive species formed by the radiolysis of water include OH^-, H_3O^+, e^-_{aq}, and H. These species can then interact with oxygen and are thought to form more potent radical species, such as superoxide radical O_2^- and toxic peroxides, that can cause more effective DNA damage.

Free Radicals

Free radicals are highly reactive species that are characterized by an unpaired electron in the outer shell of their structures. These are unstable species, typically short-lived, that will attempt to sequester the electron of a nearby molecule. Radicals react with nearby molecules

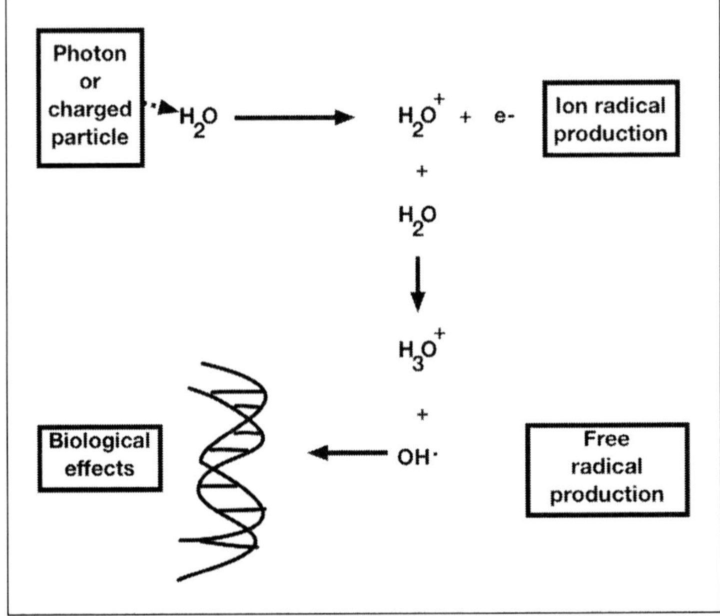

FIGURE 3.2 Hydrolysis and free radical production

to neutralize themselves, including other free radicals, solutes such as oxygen, and molecules such as DNA. Free radicals are the mediators of DNA damage by reacting with and oxidizing the sugar–phosphate bonds and bases that comprise a DNA molecule.

LET affects the balance between the direct and indirect actions of DNA damage. As the LET increases, a lesser dependence on indirect DNA damage and more pronounced direct damage is noted. As the LET increases, more energy is deposited along the path of radiation. This results in a significantly increased amount of water hydrolysis and causes free radical formation. First, as the density of free radicals increases, there is increased likelihood of these particles recombining and neutralizing themselves prior to mediating DNA damage. Second, as the density of energy deposition increases, the likelihood of directly damaging the molecules within the DNA backbone increases. As a result, there is a reduced dependence on indirect DNA damage and a reduced dependence on the presence of oxygen with higher LET.

3.2. CELL SURVIVAL CURVES

Cell Survival

DNA damage caused by the application of radiation can result in cell transformation, mutation, or death. In order to quantify the effect of radiation on a population of cells, one should plot the survival of a population of cells against a given dose of radiation. In the context of radiobiology, mammalian cell survival is typically defined as a cell retaining its ability to proliferate and thus "reproduce."

Plotting Survival Curves

A typical mammalian cell survival curve is represented by a graph assessing the relationship between fractions of surviving cells versus radiation dose (Figure 3.3). The fraction of surviving cells (S) is represented logarithmically on the x-axis. The dose of radiation (D) is represented linearly on the y-axis. The advantage of plotting cell survival on a logarithmic scale is that differences in very small surviving fractions can be adequately highlighted and compared.

Comparisons Using Survival Curves

The survival curves of multiple cell populations can be plotted on a single graph to allow comparison of the amount of radiation exposure required to produce the same biological outcome (i.e., cell survival of 50%). These curve comparisons can be used to determine the relative biological effectiveness (RBE) or the sensitization enhancement ratio (SER). RBE is the comparison of effects of different radiation types on similar cell populations or conditions. SER is the comparison of the same radiation on variations of cell populations or conditions. Both the RBE and SER are calculated by the ratio of the dose required to population B (D_b) to that required to achieve the same surviving cell fraction in population A (D_a).

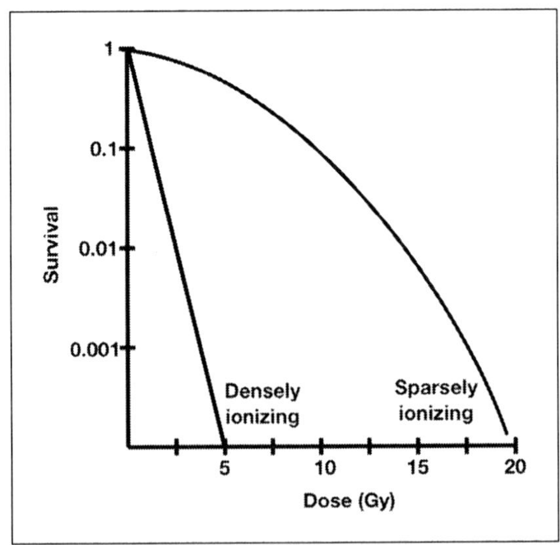

FIGURE 3.3 Cell survival curves

3.3. CELL KILLING MODELS

Linear Quadratic Model

The linear quadratic model is the most widely accepted model to represent tumor cell survival following exposure to ionizing radiation (Figure 3.4). This model is a curve fit that most closely approximates the observed cell survival for a given amount of x-ray radiation exposure. It is expressed by the equation:

$$S\,(D) = e^{(-\alpha D - \beta D2)}$$

where S is the surviving fraction, D is the dose exposed, α is the initial slope of the curve at low dose, which represents the susceptibility to single-track damage, and β is the slope at larger doses, which represents the susceptibility to dual-track damage.

Two chromosome breaks are required to cause DNA damage that results in cell death. At lower doses of radiation, this is more probably the result of a single electron that damages two chromosomal strands. This leads to the dominant effect in the linear portion of the curve represented by the α term. At higher doses of radiation, the probability of two separate electron tracks cooperating to produce two chromosome breaks is increased, leading to the quadratic portion of the observed curve, represented by the β term.

α/β Ratio

The α and β terms differ for various tumor cells in the body. The α/β ratio is the dose at which the killing effect of single-track damage is equal to that caused by dual-track damage,

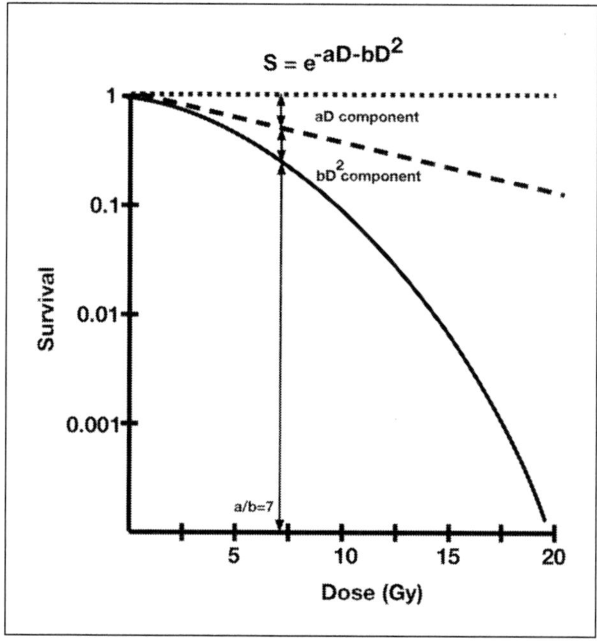

FIGURE 3.4 Linear quadratic model

and is expressed in Gy. It is used to compare different tissue susceptibilities to radiation damage. The α/β ratio is typically higher (approximately 10) for tumors and early reacting normal tissues such as skin, gut, and oral mucosa. The curves for normal and late reacting tissue, such as spinal cord, brain, and lung, have a higher β value and more dominant quadratic component, and a typically lower α/β ratio of approximately 3. The higher the α/β ratio, the more insensitive the tissue to the fractionation of radiotherapy dose (see dose fractionation considerations, Chapter 3.9).

Tumor Control Probability

An idealized model is used to illustrate the amount of radiation required to sterilize a given population of tumor cells (N_o) by reducing the population of cells to less than one cell.

$$TCP = e^{-N_o S}$$

$$\text{where } S(D) = e^{-N_o (e \wedge (-\alpha D - \beta D^2))}.$$

Tumor control probability (TCP) is plotted against radiation dose and usually results in a sigmoidal curve. Increases in tumor size will typically shift the curve to the right, as an increased radiation dose would be required to achieve the same tumor control. Increased sensitivity of the tumor to radiation (increased α) will shift the curve to the left, requiring less radiation dose to achieve the same tumor control.

3.4. MITOTIC CELL CYCLE

Phases of the Cell Cycle

To review, the cell cycle of actively growing cells can be broken down into four sequential phases defined as: M (mitosis), G_1 (the first gap phase preceding synthesis during which growth occurs), S (synthesis), and G_2 (the second gap phase preceding mitosis during which chromosomes condense and prepare for separation), and then M again. Cells that are not actively dividing are said to be in G_0, or interphase. Mitosis can be further broken down into subphases such as prophase, metaphase, anaphase, telophase, and cytokinesis.

Cell Cycle Time and Distribution

The cell cycle time (T_c) is defined as the total time between each mitotic event. The human cell cycle time varies by the type of cell, environmental changes, and a complex interplay of molecular signaling events. These events are governed by protein kinases and are activated by a family of cyclin proteins. G_1 has the most variable duration of time, whereas mitosis has a relatively consistent duration of 1 hour for most cells. Individual cells in a given population will be found in different phases of the cell cycle simultaneously, and are said to be asynchronously distributed through the cell cycle. The greatest percentage of cells will be found in the G_1 phase, since the population has doubled in number following mitosis. Cells are most radiosensitive during the G_2-M phases of the cell cycle as the chromosomal material is condensed and duplicated, increasing the likelihood of radiation-induced DNA damage.

Cell Cycle Checkpoints

Checkpoints exist throughout the mitotic cell cycle to ensure fidelity of the chromosome and DNA duplication process. An error in this process, either occurring randomly or as a result of deliberate therapeutic intervention (such as radiotherapy or chemotherapy), should be sensed at a checkpoint and will often trigger cell death. Once a cell crosses from G_0 interphase into G_1, it is committed to proceed through the cell cycle to division, or be arrested during a checkpoint in the cycle and relegated to apoptosis and cell death. A cell that has entered the mitotic cycle may not cross back into G_0 interphase. Major cell cycle checkpoints occur during G_1/S, G_2/M (check for successful DNA replication), and M (check for correct spindle attachment) phases.

3.5. DNA DAMAGE AND REPAIR

Types of DNA Damage

Recall that DNA damage is mediated by the direct and indirect effects of ionizing radiation. These DNA-induced changes can lead either to cell transformation, mutation, or cellular death. DNA is a double-stranded molecule of coding bases linked together by a sugar–phosphate backbone. There are three important types of DNA damage: single-strand breaks, double-strand breaks, and base damage (Figure 3.5).

1. *Single-Strand Break (SSB).* Formed by the deposition of energy directly into the sugar–phosphate backbone structure.
2. *Double-Strand Break (DSB).* Formed when two SSBs occur on opposite strands of DNA at a distance of < 10 base pairs apart.
3. *Base Damage.* Energy deposition changes the chemical structure of the base and the faulty coding of the DNA.

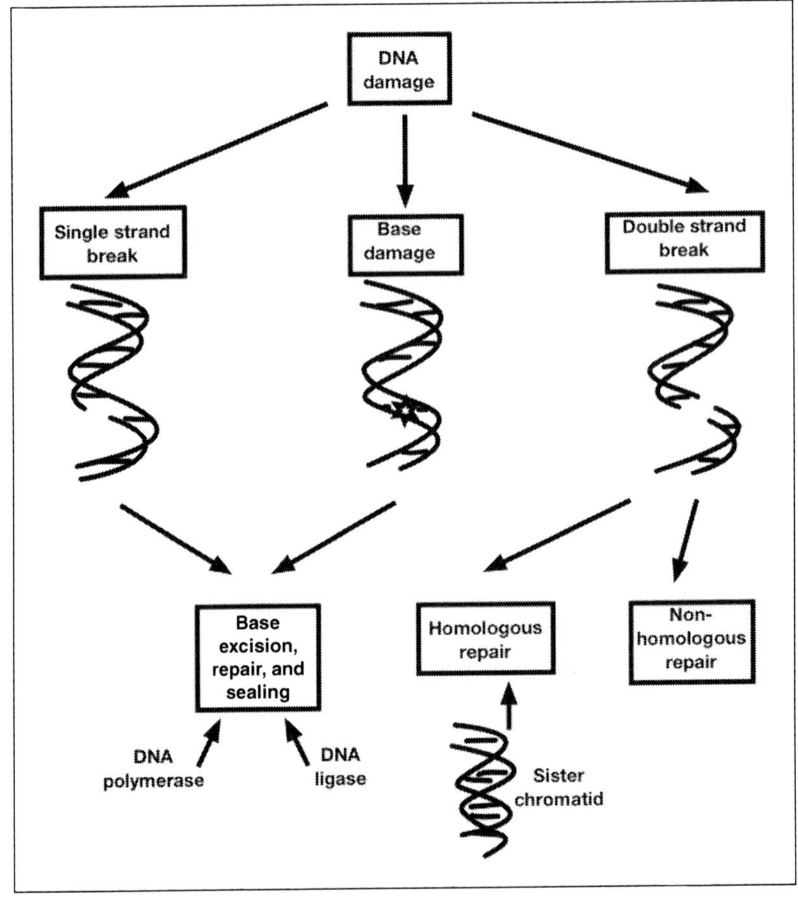

FIGURE 3.5 DNA damage and repair

Chromosomal Damage/Aberrations

To affect cellular damage, individual DNA damage must add up to an insult that causes a chromosomal aberration. The majority of DNA damage is repaired by the cell through mechanisms of DNA repair. DNA damage that is incorrectly repaired or not repaired can lead to chromosomal aberrations, which can be classified as stable or unstable.

Unstable chromosomal aberrations interfere with cell division and cause cell death. These typically occur in metaphase when the faulty chromosome affects the cell's ability to evenly distribute its DNA to daughter cells. The ability of a dose of radiation to cause unstable chromosomal aberrations is proportional to its ability to be lethal to cells. Stable chromosomal aberrations are changes that do not affect the cell's ability to proliferate, and thus will be propagated into future generations of cells (how mutations are passed down through generations). These are usually translocations and deletions.

Repair Mechanisms

Studies have revealed that every 100 cGy of radiation delivered is expected to yield between 25 and 60 double-strand breaks per cell, but we observe only one chromosomal aberration. This is because the majority of DNA damage is sensed by the cell through a continuous system of checks and is repaired very efficiently. Cells have a complex set of pathways to sense DNA damage, excise damaged components, and then repair the deficits with significant fidelity. Defects in DNA repair mechanisms can lead to familial syndromes, which predispose individuals to higher rates of cancer. Examples of cancer syndromes linked to defective repair mechanisms include hereditary nonpolyposis colorectal cancer, *BRCA*-linked breast cancer, and ataxia-telangiectasia.

Single-strand breaks are typically repaired by the cell sensing DNA damage and excising the damaged portion. Single-base codon damage can be readily repaired through the excision of the damaged base. DNA polymerase then acts to replace the excised portion, using the opposite intact strand as a template. DNA ligase then seals the break in the sugar–phosphate backbone.

Double-stranded DNA repair can occur through either homologous or nonhomologous repair methods. In homologous repair, this typically occurs during the cell cycle when there are two sister chromatids (two copies of identical chromosomes), and the cell can use the sister chromatid as a template to repair the damaged one. Nonhomologous repair is required when the cell has not yet replicated its DNA, and there is no template to guide the repair. Therefore, errors are more likely to occur during nonhomologous DSB repair.

3.6. RADIOSENSITIVITY AND RADIORESISTANCE

Radiosensitivity

Radiosensitivity refers to the relative ability to cause cell killing by exposure to ionizing radiation (Figure 3.6). Cells of differing populations vary in their sensitivity to radiation. The radiosensitivity of tumor cells is primarily mediated by both the intrinsic properties of the cell and the cell's in vivo environment.

The intrinsic radiosensitivity of a tumor cell population is governed by the *Law of Bergonie and Tribondeau,* which states that sensitivity to radiation is directly proportional to the rate of cell division, and inversely proportional to the cell's degree of differentiation. Therefore, aggressively dividing, poorly differentiated malignancies tend to be intrinsically more radiosensitive than indolent, slow-growing tumor cell populations.

The presence of certain molecules in the tumor environment can increase sensitivity to radiation (radiosensitizers) or decrease the effects on normal tissue (radioprotectors). Some radiosensitizers can enhance radiation effects by directly increasing the amount of DNA damage, while others attempt to increase the sensitivity of cells in low oxygen environments. The most clinically relevant radiosensitizer in radiobiology is oxygen.

Oxygen as a Radiosensitizer

Recall that the majority of radiation damage to DNA is mediated through indirect effects through the hydrolysis of water and formation of free radicals. These reactions are facilitated and enhanced in the presence of oxygen. Therefore, hypoxic (low oxygen tension) environments are associated with lower tumor cell kill. Hypoxia is specifically an issue with tumors that tend to grow spherically away from blood supply, and thus demonstrate reduced oxygen tension as cells grow further from the nearest blood capillary. One method of overcoming these low oxygen environments to increase tumor cell kill is to use higher LET radiation, which is more dependent on the direct effect of DNA damage, and thus less dependent on the presence of oxygen. Radioprotectors are typically molecules that interfere with the action of free radicals (such as antioxidants) or reduce oxygenation of tumors (such as vasoconstrictors).

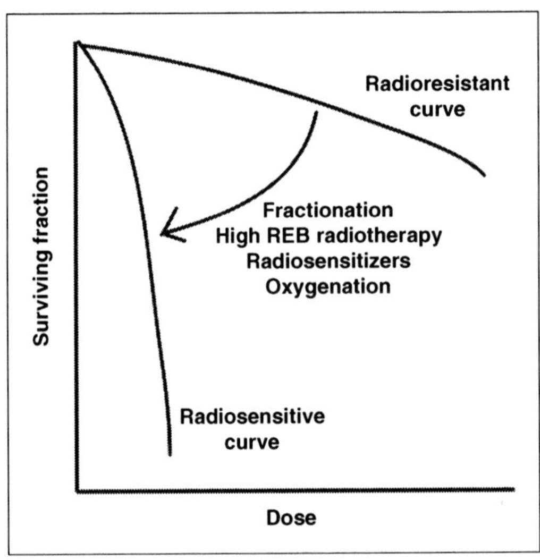

FIGURE 3.6 Radiosensitivity and radioresistance

3.7. TUMOR RESPONSE

The observed response of a biological population of tumor cells to an increasing dose of ionization radiation exposure is different from the linear response that would be predicted in an ideal system. In vivo behavior of tumor cells in response to radiation is mediated through a complex interplay of four key mechanisms, known as the four Rs of radiobiology: Repair, Reassortment, Repopulation, and Reoxygenation (Figure 3.7).

1. *Repair.* DNA repair of sublethal damage (such as single-strand breaks) decreases the ultimate number of chromosomal aberrations and reduces cell kill. Since DNA repair takes time, it would make sense that the lower the rate at which radiation dose is delivered, the more cellular repair can take place. This concept is exploited during radiation therapy delivery through fractionation schemes in order to protect normal tissues, while maintaining tumor cell kill (see Chapter 3.9).
2. *Reassortment (also known as Redistribution).* Although lowering the dose rate initially results in increased repair and thus reduced cell kill, a paradoxical increase in tumor kill is noted at very low dose rates. This is called the inverse dose rate effect. Cells are most sensitive to radiation during the G_2-M cell cycle phase. In a tumor cell population, the

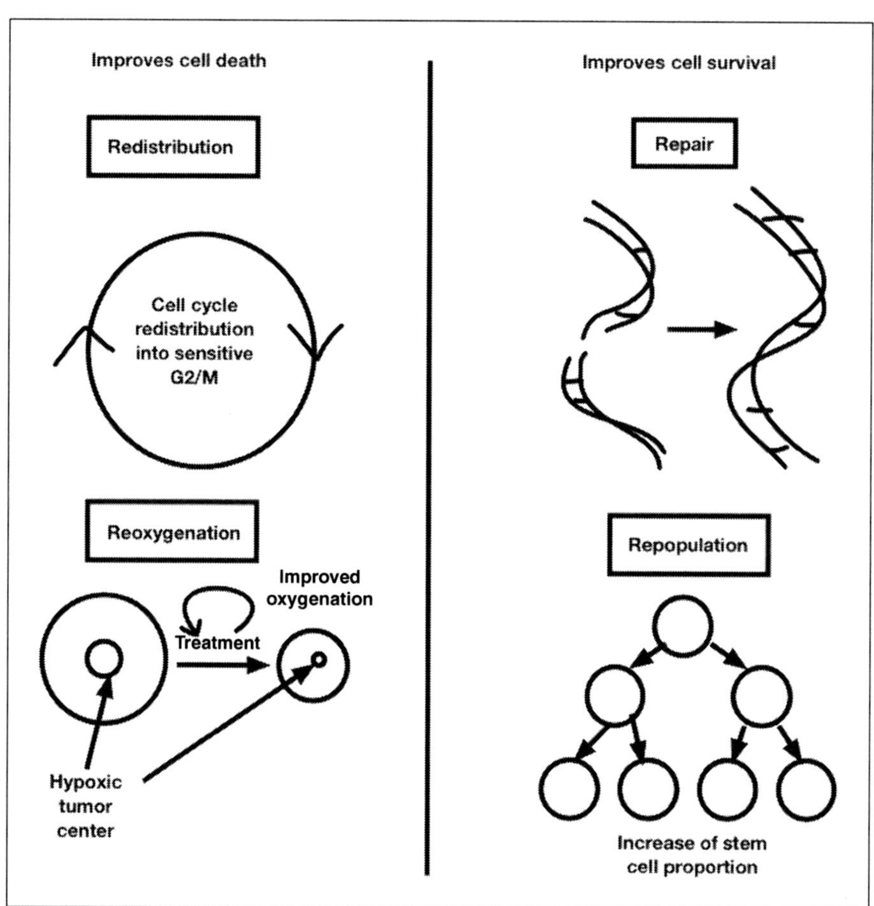

FIGURE 3.7 Four Rs of radiobiology

cells are asynchronously distributed in various phases of the cell cycle, and only a portion is in the radiosensitive phase at a given time. Exposure to continuous low-dose radiation causes cells to become blocked or frozen at G_2-M. Therefore, cells become bunched or redistributed into G_2-M, which increases tumor cell kill.

3. *Repopulation.* The population of tumor cells undergoing radiation is mediated by a balance of the degree of cell killing effects versus the amount of cellular replication by the remaining cells. If the given dose rate of radiation is not kept ahead of the remaining cells' ability to replicate, then the tumor will repopulate.
4. *Reoxygenation.* Recall that the presence of oxygen increases the radiosensitivity of tumors. According to the spheroid tumor model of cell growth, an enlarging tumor will outgrow its blood supply, which results in a shell of well-aerated cells surrounding a hypoxic core. Fractionating radiation doses allows one fraction of radiation to be delivered, which will be much more effective against the aerated cells. These damaged cells are then sloughed off and cleared, resulting in reoxygenation of the deeper cells, in time for the next fraction of radiation to be delivered. Therefore, reoxygenation increases tumor cell kill and is exploited by radiation dose fractionation.

Tumor and normal tissues have differential responses to radiation; thus, the four Rs of radiobiology are exploited to maintain the balance between antitumor and normal tissue preserving effects. In general, repair and repopulation result in lower tumor cell kill, but increased normal tissue recovery. Conversely, reassortment and reoxygenation are associated with improved tumor cell kill, but likely more normal tissue effects.

3.8. ACUTE AND LATE NORMAL TISSUE RESPONSES

Effects of radiation on normal tissue can be divided into early/acute and late effects.

Early/Acute Effects

Early/acute effects manifest within a few days to weeks, caused by the death of a large number of cells. This is typically seen in tissues with rapid rates of turnover, such as the gastrointestinal epithelium, skin epidermis, and hematopoietic system. These effects are rapid and typically reversible. Early/acute effects that lead to permanent dysfunction are termed *consequential late effects* and are likely due to stem cell depletion or irreversible damage to underlying tissue structure(s).

Late Effects

Late effects manifest within months to years, and are caused by damage to slowly proliferating tissues, such as the lung, kidney, heart, liver, and central nervous system. While early effects tend to be reversible, late effects are often marked by incomplete repair and can lead to chronic deficits.

Normal Tissue Complication Probability

Various models have been proposed to estimate the probability of causing a normal tissue complication. Most models are based on the variables of dose delivered and volume exposed (Figure 3.8). The TD_{50} is the dose that, if delivered uniformly to a given volume, would result in 50% of a population of patients having a specific complication. The amount of volume needed to be exposed to increase the likelihood of complication depends on the type of organ being irradiated. For simplicity sake, organs are thought of as being serial or parallel. A serial organ is one where dysfunction at any given part of the organ would result in downstream dysfunction (e.g., spinal cord). Parallel organs have redundant anatomical structure that can withstand the dysfunction of part of the organ (e.g., lung and kidney). The serial versus parallel nature of the organ can have a significant impact on TD_{50} and hence the susceptibility of the organ to radiobiological damage.

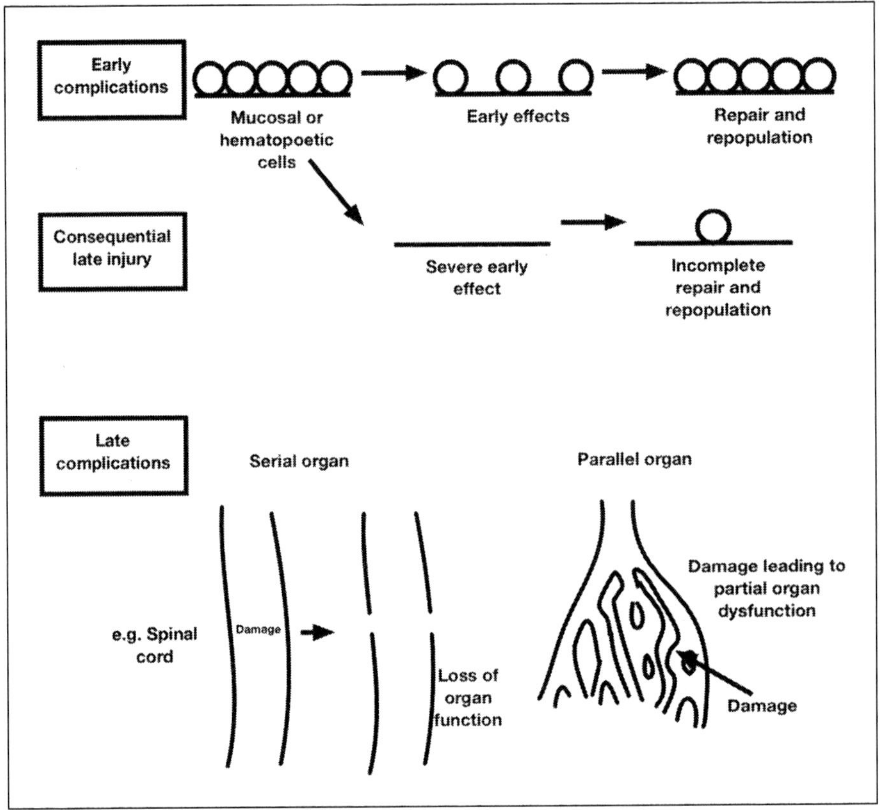

FIGURE 3.8 Normal tissue complications

3.9. TIME, DOSE, AND FRACTIONATION CONSIDERATIONS

The delivery of radiotherapy is dependent on the exploitation of the four Rs of radiobiology to balance the efficiency of tumor cell killing with the effects on normal tissue. Two important concepts in radiation therapy delivery are that of dose rate and dose fractionation (Figure 3.9).

Dose Rate

Radiation dose rate is defined as the amount of radiation delivered to a volume of interest per unit of time. Within the therapeutic realm of radiation, external beam radiation is delivered at higher dose rates than interstitial and intracavitary brachytherapy. Lower dose rates can be associated with increased DNA repair. As previously mentioned, at very low doses, the inverse dose rate effect is noted, and tumor cell kill can be enhanced. This is the basis of low-dose rate brachytherapy.

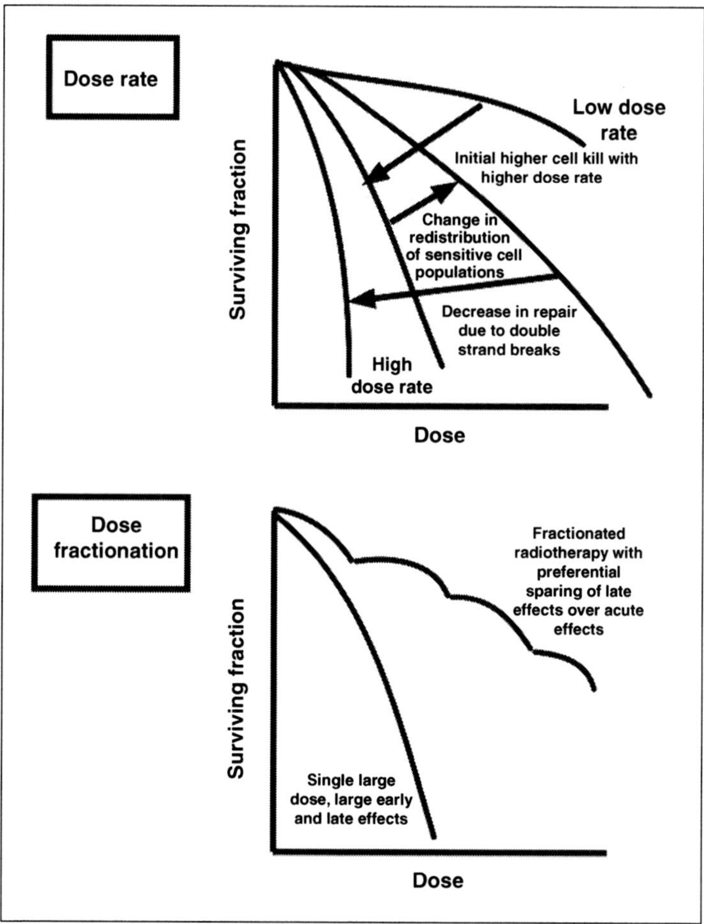

FIGURE 3.9 Effect of dose rate and dose fractionation

Dose Fractionation

Breaking a large dose of radiation into smaller packets or fractions of radiation over a period of time is a strategy used to improve tumor kill through reoxygenation, while reducing normal tissue effects. Fractionation exploits the differential radiosensitivity of tumor cells compared to normal tissues. Recall that the alpha/beta ratio is higher for tumor and early responding tissues compared to normal and late-responding tissue cells. The cell survival curves for tumor cells are more linear, while normal cells' survival curves have an initial curved shoulder. Giving a single fraction of high-dose radiation would have a significant tumor effect, but would also grossly impact the surrounding normal tissues. Fractionating the dose allows divergence of the two cell survival curves, as the normal tissue curve continues to re-express the shoulder of the curve sparing more normal tissues. Therefore, the alpha/beta ratio is a measure of the insensitivity to dose fractionation schemes. In summary, dividing dose into a number of fractions spares normal tissue (repair, repopulation) and increases damage to tumor cells (reoxygenation, reassortment).

Isoeffect and BED Calculations

The therapeutic use of different doses and fractionation schemes requires the ability to compare the effectiveness of these different treatment regimens. Whole treatment regimens with different dose per fraction will require a change in total dose to yield the same effect. This can be calculated using the isoeffect equation:

$$D_2/D_1 = (d_1 + \alpha/\beta)/(d_2 + \alpha/\beta)$$

where D is the total dose, d is the dose per fraction for each fractionation regimen, and alpha/beta refers to the tissue of interest.

The ability to define a common reference value for the comparison of biological effects is important in radiotherapy. This quantity is known as the biologically equivalent dose (BED). The following calculation defines the BED:

$$BED = nd\,(1 + d/(\alpha/\beta))\ [\text{in units } Gy_{(\alpha/\beta)}]$$

where n is the number of fractions and d is the dose per fraction.

The BED calculation is a useful quantity as different exposures can be added for cumulative biological effect when they are converted to this common reference value. Furthermore, BED allows comparison and correction for radiotherapy treatments that are interrupted or split either intentionally or unintentionally. The BED calculation noted above is a simplification and ignores correction factors for repair and repopulation. Other BED equations are available that can adjust for the overall time frame of treatment.

3.10. ISSUES IN HUMAN RADIATION EXPOSURE

Radiation exposure will ultimately result in biochemical changes that can alter cell metabolism, causing both acute and late biological side effects. These effects can be classified as either deterministic or stochastic, and are dependent on the effective dose of exposure.

Effective Dose Concept

As radiosensitivity varies by tissue type and as certain organs are more crucial to survival than others, one can crudely quantify the effect of partial body exposures with a calculation of effective dose. Effective dose is the product of cumulative dose to each organ or tissue with a weighting factor for that tissue type.

$$\text{Effective dose} = \text{Sum of } (D_{Ti} \times W_{Ti})$$

where D_{Ti} is the total dose to each organ and W_{Ti} is the tissue weighting factors. Similar to equivalent dose, the effective dose is expressed in Sieverts (Sv).

Deterministic Effects

Deterministic biological effects are guaranteed when radiation exposure crosses a given threshold dose, and will increase in severity with dose given beyond that threshold (Figure 3.10). These include nuisance side effects seen in many types of therapeutic radiation such as skin erythema and hair loss, but can also result in a more serious and possibly fatal acute radiation syndrome. A whole body dose of 4 Gy is lethal in 50% of humans at 60 days. No one has ever been known to have survived an acute whole body exposure of > 10 Gy.

Acute Radiation Syndrome

Acute radiation syndrome encompasses the signs and symptoms of whole body radiation exposure, and the manifestation is dependent on the total dose received. It can be classified as cerebrovascular, gastrointestinal, and hematopoietic syndrome, as shown in Table 3.1.

TABLE 3.1 Acute Radiation Syndromes

	Cerebrovascular	Gastrointestinal	Hematopoeitic
Dose range	> 100 Gy	10 Gy < D < 100 Gy	2.5 Gy < D < 10 Gy
Time to death	24–48 hr	3–10 d	< 60 d if no intervention
Symptoms	Disorientation, muscular movement, respiratory distress, nausea, convulsive seizures, coma, death	Nausea, vomiting, diarrhea, anorexia, lethargy, weight loss, emaciation, exhaustion	Fevers, chills, hemorrhages, infections, ulceration, epilation
Remediation	None	None	If < 8 Gy -> antibiotics If 8–10 Gy -> bone marrow transplantation

Stochastic Effects

Stochastic effects are nonguaranteed effects typically associated with lower dose exposures that are variable and are not associated with a threshold dose, but become more likely with increasing dose (Figure 3.10). The severity of these effects is not proportional to the exposure. Long-term and delayed effects of radiation, such as inherited genetic mutations and cancer are examples of stochastic (random) effects.

Secondary Malignancies

Radiation exposure is associated with the risk of development of secondary radiation-induced malignancy. They are typically seen as delayed effects associated with long latency periods with hematologic malignancies, such as leukemia, occurring 10 years after exposure and solid tumors, such as thyroid and breast cancers, occurring 25 years after exposure.

Hereditary Effects

Data on the hereditary effects of radiation exposure has been studied extensively in Japanese survivors of the atomic bombs and survivors from Chernobyl. Radiation does not cause new or bizarre mutations in cells that it affects, but instead results in a greater frequency of mutations that occur spontaneously.

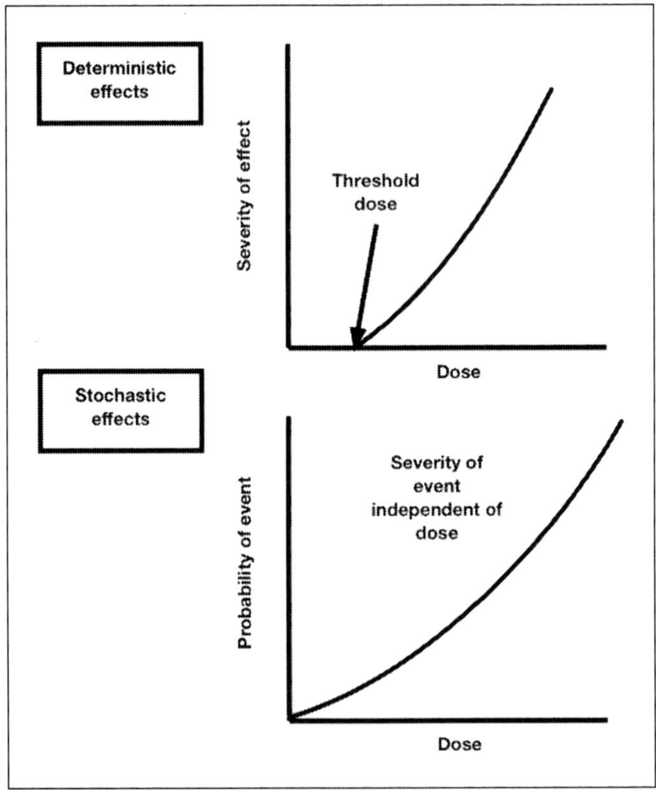

FIGURE 3.10 Deterministic and stochastic effects

Chapter 4

Pathology

KEY POINTS

- Pathology is the study of the etiology, pathogenesis, morphological properties, and clinical significance of various disease processes including cancer. In the context of cancer, pathological diagnosis and classification underpin clinical decision making from staging to treatment.
- The acquisition of adequate specimen(s) to confirm malignancies can include a variety of procedures ranging from relatively noninvasive fine-needle aspirations/punch biopsies to invasive excisional biopsies.
- Pathological examination of samples usually begins with a macroscopic evaluation including: various specimen phenotypic features, margin status, and preliminary diagnostic impression(s).
- Microscopic evaluation of specimens usually involves a multistep process including: fixation, embedding, sectioning, staining, and light microscopy. Frozen section techniques are available to support decision making during surgical procedures.
- Cytological evaluations are used to assess cellular material as opposed to full tissues and have clinical application in gynecological, thoracic, and hematological malignancies as well as the assessment of fine-needle aspiration materials.
- Immunohistochemistry generally utilizes labeled antibodies to known tumor antigens to assist in the diagnosis of cancer specimens. These techniques are particularly useful in tumors of unknown primary and/or poorly differentiated cancers. Another specialized technique occasionally used for pathological diagnosis is electron microscopy.
- Abnormal cell growth is usually classified by various terms in the following subcategories: change in cell number, change in cell size, and change in cell maturity.
- Tumors are typically classified as benign or malignant usually depending on various pathological features such as: invasion, encapsulation, differentiation, and mitotic activity.

4.1. INTRODUCTION

Pathology is the branch of medicine that is devoted to the study of the changes in the function and structure of cells and cellular tissues in the body secondary to disease processes. Etymologically, pathology is derived from the Greek roots of *logia* (the study of) and *pathos* (suffering). The aim of pathology is to study the etiology, pathogenesis, morphologic changes, and clinical significance of the disease process. Pathological study and diagnosis are critical to the field of oncology in order to differentiate between benign and malignant disease processes, and because the subsequent investigation and management of cancer patients hinge on the pathological tissue diagnosis. Furthermore, correct interpretation of pathological reports is crucial to clinical decision making. In this chapter, we will discuss the basic techniques and terminology relevant to oncological pathology.

4.2. SPECIMEN ACQUISITION

Tissue specimens are obtained in the practice of oncology, termed *biopsy*, for the purpose of diagnostic evaluation of abnormally appearing tissue and for the evaluation of the adequacy of treatment (usually following definitive surgical, chemotherapeutic, and/or radiotherapeutic management). Specimens obtained can range in size from a small sampling of cells to entire organs and their surrounding tissue.

Types of Biopsies

A *biopsy* refers to an examination of a sample of tissue that is obtained from an individual for the purpose of diagnosing a disease. It can be obtained from nearly any tissue in the body, using a variety of techniques. Types of biopsies include:

1. *Excisional.* A whole organ or lump is removed. Most commonly used for suspected lymphomas, where evaluation of the whole lymph node is essential for diagnosis. Also occasionally used for highly suspicious breast lumps.
2. *Incisional.* A portion of a mass, most commonly soft tissue, is sampled surgically for diagnosis.
3. *Core needle.* A small core of tissue is obtained, often percutaneously, using a specialized hollow needle. Most commonly used for breast masses.
4. *Punch.* A small circular 2- to 5-mm-diameter area of epidermis and dermis is punched out using a specialized biopsy tool. Used for dermal changes suspicious for skin cancer.
5. *Endoscopic.* A fiberoptic scope is used to evaluate an area of concern and a small tissue sample can be obtained through the scope with the use of forceps and cautery. Examples include the diagnosis of gastrointestinal tumors (esophagogastroduodenoscopy, colonoscopy), urological tumors (cystoscopy, ureteroscopy), and intra-abdominal tumors (laparoscopy), as well as the sampling of mediastinal lymph nodes (mediastinoscopy).
6. *Panendoscopy.* Used in the evaluation of suspected head and neck cancers; involves the insertion of a rigid laryngoscope under general anesthesia for direct visual evaluation of the pharynx, larynx, and hypopharynx, and biopsies of suspicious areas.
7. *Colposcopy.* A specialized procedure for evaluating areas of cervical dysplasia, where a focused telescope is used to guide core biopsies of the cervix.
8. *Ultrasound/computed tomography (CT)-guided/stereotactic biopsy.* Ultrasound and CT-guided biopsies utilize radiologic imaging to guide the precise placement of the biopsy needle into the tissue to be sampled. CT-guided techniques are commonly used for intrathoracic (i.e., lung) and intraabdominal (i.e., liver) biopsies. Stereotactic biopsy implies that the tumor is localized in three-dimensional space using an x-y-z coordinate system and possible immobilization to reduce tissue motion. It is employed when accurate targeting is required (i.e., brain biopsy).
9. *Bone marrow.* A core and aspirate sample of bone marrow is acquired by inserting a specialized needle into the pelvic bone under local anesthesia, typically into the posterior superior iliac spine. Rarely, aspirate samples are obtained from the sternum. Used for suspected hematological malignancies.
10. *Fine-needle aspiration.* A small needle is inserted into a mass, and a syringe is used to draw up a sample of cells for cytological evaluation (see Section 4.5). Commonly employed for thyroid nodules, masses of the breast, pancreatic cysts, and enlarged peripheral lymph nodes.

4.3. MACROSCOPIC EVALUATION

Macroscopic, or gross, evaluation is the qualitative and quantitative assessment of each specimen received by the pathologist prior to more detailed microscopic evaluation of cellular details. The pathologist examines the submitted specimen commenting on its labeled identification, appearance, texture, shape, composition, completeness, and gross findings suggestive of abnormal pathology. The specimen is oriented using anatomical cues, as well as information provided by the individual obtaining the specimen, often in the form of differentially inked or sutured edges by the surgeon at the time of resection. Quantitative measurements including size and weight are recorded, as well as the appearance of margins for tumors. The pathologist will often section larger specimens, so that the extent of tumor involvement can be accurately described. Preliminary diagnoses and impressions are made based on the gross macroscopic evaluation. Furthermore, for large resected specimens, these impressions will guide the pathologist as to which areas of the specimen should be prepared for microscopic evaluation.

4.4. MICROSCOPIC EVALUATION

The study of cells and their extracellular matrix is termed histology. Histologic evaluation requires the use of light microscopes to examine tissue specimens. Within oncology, microscopic tissue evaluation not only provides diagnosis but also allows for tumor grading based on the degree of differentiation, nuclear features, and mitotic rate. Preparation of the tissue specimen for microscopic evaluation requires that they be sectioned into thin fragments, preserved to avoid breakdown (fixation), impregnated to maintain tissue rigidity (embedding), and stained for evaluation. The steps to light microscopic evaluation are:

1. *Fixation.* Tissue degradation secondary to enzymes within the tissue and bacteria is prevented by preservation of the tissue—termed fixation. Specimens are usually chemically fixed by submerging them in an agent that will stabilize the tissue, often by creating cross-links within the tissue's proteins. Formaldehyde and glutaraldehyde are examples of commonly used cross-linking fixatives. For the rapid evaluation of certain tissues, rapid freeze for fixation and sectioning can be employed.
2. *Embedding.* Tissue structures must be made rigid and more resistant to damage from sectioning by impregnating them with paraffin or resin. First, the tissue is dehydrated, often in an alcohol agent, to replace the water in the tissue with an organic solvent, termed clearing. The cleared sample is then embedded with paraffin or plastic resin by allowing these substances to penetrate intracellular spaces and replace the organic solvents, thus imparting structural rigidity to the sample.
3. *Sectioning.* Light microscope evaluation requires very thin slices of the tissue specimen such that they may be transilluminated. These fine slices, with thickness equivalent to a single cell in the range of 10 μm, are cut using a precise cutting instrument called a microtome. The thin slices are mounted on a series of glass slides.
4. *Staining.* As most tissues are colorless, staining with various chemical dyes allows differentiation of the components within the specimen. The two basic classes of dyes are acidic and basic. Tissue components rich in acid, such as nucleoproteins (DNA/RNA), glycosaminoglycans, and acid glycoproteins, will stain richly with basic dyes and are thus termed basophilic structures. Conversely, strong acid staining or acidophilic structures include cell mitochondria, secretory granules, and collagen. Acid–base dye combinations allow contrast between various components. The most commonly used combination is hematoxylin (base) and eosin (acid), termed H&E staining.

Light Microscopy

Since Anton van Leeuwenhoek's first observation of single-cell organisms using primitive microscopes in 1676, microscopy has formed the foundation of general pathological evaluation. Improvements in the quality of the lenses have resulted in an improvement in resolution, or resolving power, which is the smallest distance between two actual separate particles that can be visualized and still allows the particles to appear separate. The use of the conventional light microscope remains the basis for routine histological evaluation, and is sufficient for most diagnosis, while providing resolution in the range of 0.2 μm. More advanced forms of light-based microscopes utilized in specialized scenarios include: phase contrast, polarizing, confocal, and fluorescence microscopy.

Frozen Sections

Intraoperative pathological tissue evaluation is often utilized by surgical oncologists to obtain further information, such as confirmation of tissue diagnosis or evaluation of margins that can guide real-time operative decisions. This is most commonly done with frozen sectioning, which has a turnaround time of minutes compared to the day it takes to prepare a permanent section. Tissue is frozen to render it hard enough to section with a special frozen space microtome called a cryotome, and then stained and evaluated. While good for quick coarse evaluation, the usefulness of a frozen section for evaluating finer details is inferior to that of a permanent section, and does not replace the latter.

4.5. CYTOLOGICAL EVALUATION

Cytological evaluation is another frequently utilized technique for quick cellular evaluation, and it is often used in intraoperative settings and in clinical settings, where rapid confirmation of the presence of malignancy is sought. Cytological specimens can be prepared either through imprint or scrape-smear methods. Imprint preparations are produced by directly applying the glass slide to the cut tissue surface being evaluated, while a scrape-smear involves grazing the tissue with the edge of the glass slide and subsequently smearing the accumulated scraped cells across the glass.

Cytological preparations and aspirates are also routinely applied to slides and smeared for clinical evaluation of malignancy. Cytological preparations are used as the basis of Pap smears to screen for cervical dysplasia. Fine-needle aspiration is commonly employed for undiagnosed masses, such as breast or pancreatic cysts, thyroid nodules, and enlarged lymph nodes. Fluids obtained through thoracocentesis (sampling of pleural fluid) and paracentesis (sampling of ascites fluid) can confirm the presence of malignant pleural effusion and intraperitoneal carcinomatosis, respectively.

Cytology preparations are advantageous in that they allow quick preparation and confirmation of the presence of malignancy, can allow evaluation of cellular details, and can be obtained when minimal tissue is present. However, cytologic preparations do not allow the evaluation of tissue architecture, which is vital for diagnosis in many malignancies, such as lymphoma, and the preparation method can crush or damage the cells. Often, the greatest utility of cytologic preparations is the confirmation of presence or absence of malignant cells, such that further diagnostic steps can be planned.

4.6. IMMUNOHISTOCHEMISTRY

Cellular tissues can be differentiated and malignant processes identified by the relative presence or absence of various macromolecules within the specimen. Cells are coated with a range of highly specific macromolecules, termed antigens, that permit the recognition and differentiation of one cell from another. These antigens include molecules such as hormones, receptors, cell adhesion molecules, proteins, and immunoglobulins that have altered expression in many types of tumors and cancers. Immunohistochemistry refers to the use of special antibodies to recognize and bind to various cellular antigens and subsequently visualize and demonstrate them in pathological specimens.

In the most common application of immunohistochemistry, labeling antibodies are utilized (Figure 4.1). The body will have produced a specific antibody to recognize and bind a specific antigen on a type of cell. The sectioned sample is then incubated with a secondary labeled antibody preparation that will bind and recognize the primary antibody of interest. These labeling antibodies are prepared with a coupling agent (such as a fluorescent compound, an enzyme, or a colored electron scattering component), that will subsequently allow visualization and localization of the areas of interest with microscopic techniques. A similar labeling technique can be used with special labeled sequences of nucleic acid, called

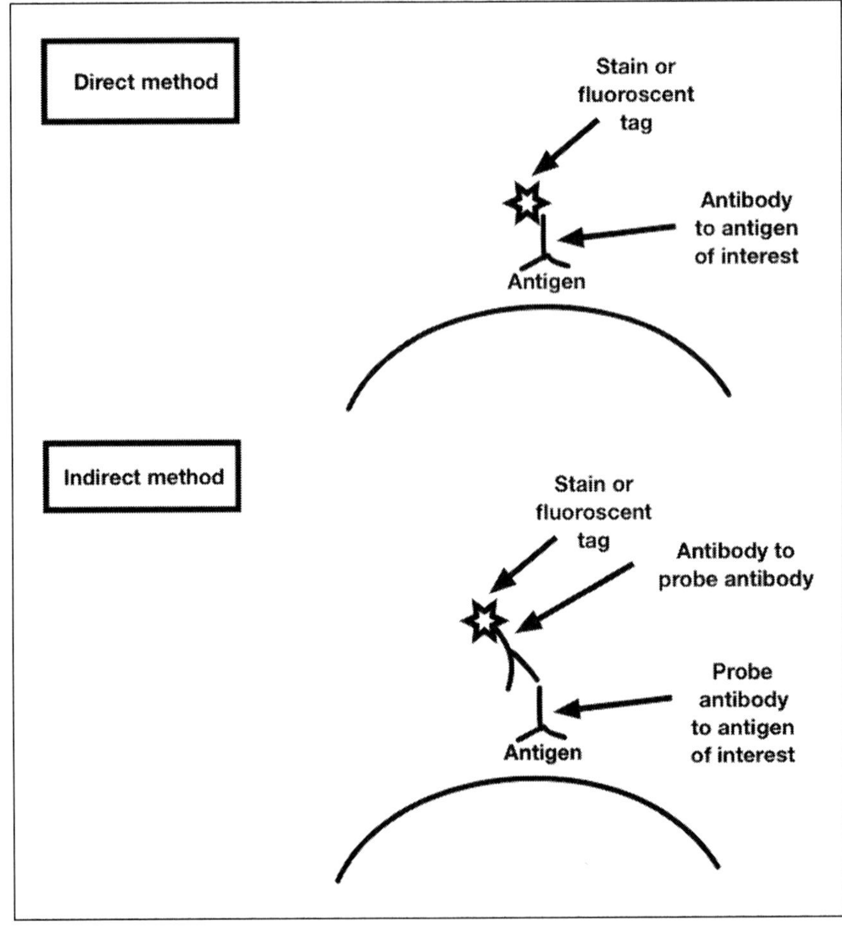

FIGURE 4.1 Immunohistochemistry

probes, used to recognize and bind specific sequences of DNA and RNA. This procedure is known as hybridization labeling.

Immunohistochemistry is vital to oncological pathology and characterization of unknown tumor masses. It is particularly helpful in settings where the initial biopsy contains a suspected metastatic deposit, and can be utilized to help determine the primary. Furthermore, in very poorly differentiated tissues or when the class of tissue origin is uncertain (i.e., epithelial vs. lymphoid origin), antibodies can allow for more specific diagnosis. The degree of expression of certain markers within cells can also have prognostic relevance, and is increasingly being used to help predict utility of certain targeted treatments in a variety of tumors.

4.7. ELECTRON MICROSCOPY

Electron microscopy is a highly specialized method of cellular evaluation that can achieve resolution significantly > a conventional light microscope. Images are obtained through the differential interactions of electrons with the tissue components, and can achieve a resolution of 0.001 μm. The tissue sample is embedded into extremely hard epoxy plastic and is sectioned to very thin slices, 10 to 15× thinner than a traditional slice. The three types of electron microscopes are:

1. *Transmission.* The thin tissue section is impregnated with a heavy metal, which acts as a stain, while a beam of electrons is passed through the sample, allowing visualization of the small structures and intracellular components.
2. *Scanning.* A thin metal coating is applied to the surface of the sample, and the electron beam is sequentially scanned over points within the specimen, creating an almost three-dimensional surface rendering.
3. *Analytical.* Allows the chemical composition of the components of the specimen to be determined.

Although electron microscopy can provide a significant amount of information regarding a tissue specimen, it is slow, very expensive, and labor intensive, and thus is primarily used as a research tool. It can be employed in selective clinical cases, where more information than can be provided with light microscopy is required to make a diagnosis. For tumor pathology, visualization of cellular ultrastructure can help in the classification of poorly differentiated neoplasms and other certain tumor types that exhibit specific subcellular hallmarks.

4.8. TERMINOLOGY

Abnormalities of Cellular Growth

Aberrant cell growth within tissue is classified according to the nature of the change, and can be broadly classified as alterations in the number of cells, the size of cells, and the maturity of cells. Terminologies used to describe these alterations are:

1. *Change in number*
   - Aplasia: decreased number of cells and absence of tissue.
   - Hypoplasia: decrease in tissue/organ mass due to decreased cell number (prior to cell maturity).
   - Hyperplasia: increase in tissue/organ mass due to increased cell number.
2. *Change in size*
   - Agenesis: congenital absence of a particular cell type.
   - Atrophy: acquired decreased tissue/organ mass after full maturity due to decrease in size of cellular components.
   - Hypertrophy: acquired increased tissue/organ mass after full maturity due to increased size of cellular components.
3. *Change in maturity*
   - Metaplasia: acquired change of one mature cell type to another mature cell type.
   - Dysplasia: changes in the maturation and development of a cell within a tissue/organ system.
   - Neoplasia: abnormal cellular proliferation resulting in new growths.
   - Anaplasia: neoplastic tissue with highly undifferentiated (immature) cells; a hallmark of malignant neoplasms.

Oncology primarily concerns itself with growths and masses secondary to neoplasia, termed neoplasms. Neoplasia can be differentiated from hyperplastic cellular proliferation in that neoplasia is typically spontaneous, occurs secondary to abnormal or unknown stimulus, is not proportional to the stimulus, and can proceed/develop in the absence of stimulus. Conversely, hyperplasia is cellular proliferation that is secondary, proportional to a normal stimulus (such as overstimulation as a response to repair tissue injury), and usually ceases on absence of the stimulus signal.

Neoplasms, or tumors, are classically differentiated into benign and malignant processes, although this dichotomous definition is understood to be simplistic given that carcinogenic changes tend to occur on a spectrum of premalignant to malignant masses. However, this distinction is still clinically relevant to both patient and oncologist, as cancer implies the presence of malignant growth. The basic differences associated with benign and malignant tumors are (Figure 4.2):

1. *Benign neoplasia.* Abnormal new growth of cells that is usually noninvasive, surrounded by a capsule, well differentiated (microscopic appearance resembling the cell of origin),

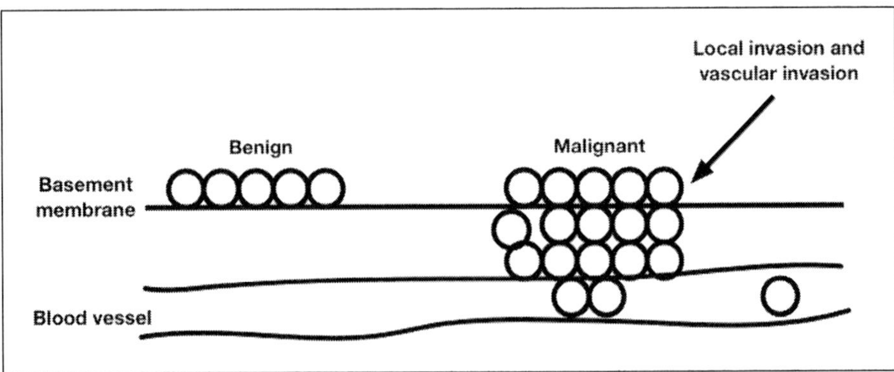

FIGURE 4.2 Benign versus malignant neoplasms

slower growing, has a lower rate of division (mitotic index), and does not typically spread (metastasize) to other sites.

2. *Malignant neoplasia.* Abnormal new growth of cells that is generally invasive into surrounding tissues, not encapsulated, varies in the degree of lack of differentiation, is more rapidly growing with a higher rate of division (mitotic index), and will often spread to secondary sites.

Tumor Nomenclature

Classification of tumor subtypes is typically on the basis of their cellular tissue type and organ system of origin, and a basic differentiation of benign and malignant neoplasia. Although general rules are applied to nomenclature, multiple exceptions and historical naming conventions still exist. Generally, benign tumors are denoted with the suffix -oma, and a prefix indicating the cellular type of origin (i.e., a benign tumor of fatty adipose tissue is a "lipoma"). There are multiple exceptions to this rule, such as lymphomas, melanomas, and seminomas, all of which are malignant growths. Malignant growths of epithelial (skin, glands, mucous membranes), mesenchymal (connective tissue, bone, muscle, vessels), and embryonic origin are generally noted with suffixes specific to their cellular type of origin:

1. Epithelial—"carcinoma"
   - Glandular or ductal—"adenocarcinoma"
   - Stratified squamous—"squamous cell carcinoma"
   - Mixed glandular-squamous—"adenosquamous carcinoma"
2. Mesenchymal—"sarcoma"
3. Embryonic—"blastoma"

Common tumor cell origins and their benign and malignant naming conventions are listed (note some malignant tumors have no benign counterpart) in Table 4.1.

TABLE 4.1 Tumor Nomenclature and Naming Conventions

Cell/Tissue Origin	Benign Tumor Name	Malignant Tumor Name
EPITHELIAL		
Squamous	Squamous cell papilloma	Squamous cell carcinoma
Transitional	Transitional cell papilloma	Transitional cell carcinoma
Basal	Basal cell papilloma	Basal cell carcinoma
Glandular	Adenoma	Adenocarcinoma
	Cystadenoma	Cystadenocarcinoma
Liver (mixed)	Hepatocellular adenoma	Hepatocellular carcinoma
Kidney (mixed)	Renal cell adenoma	Renal cell carcinoma
Bile duct	Bile duct adenoma	Cholangiocarcinoma
Melanocyte	Nevus	Malignant melanoma
MESENCHYMAL		
Fibrous tissue	Fibroma	Fibrosarcoma
	Dermatofibroma	Dermatofibrosarcoma
	Myxofibroma	Myxofibrosarcoma
Nerve sheath	Neurofibroma	Malignant nerve sheath tumor
Adipose (fat) tissue	Lipoma	Liposarcoma
Smooth muscle	Leiomyoma	Leiomyosarcoma
Skeletal muscle	Rhabdomyoma	Rhabdomyosarcoma
Cartilage	Chondroma	Chondrosarcoma
Bone	Osteoma	Osteogenic sarcoma
Vessels	Hemangioma	Hemangionsarcoma
Brain meninges	Meningioma	Malignant meningioma
EMBRYONIC		
Retinoblasts		Retinoblastoma
Kidney		Nephroblastoma
Liver		Hepatoblastoma
Notochord		Chordoma
Neuroblasts	Ganglioneuroma	Neuroblastoma
HEMATOPOEITIC		
Lymphatic tissue		Lymphoma
Lymphocytes, myeloid cells		Leukemia
Plasma cells	Plasmacytoma	Multiple myeloma

(*continued*)

TABLE 4.1 Tumor Nomenclature and Naming Conventions (*continued*)

Cell/Tissue Origin	Benign Tumor Name	Malignant Tumor Name
GERM CELL		
Testes		Seminoma, dysgerminoma, teratoma
Ovaries	Serous/mucinous cystadenoma	Serous, mucinous, papillary cystadenocarcinoma
	Benign cystic teratoma	Malignant teratoma
NERVOUS SYSTEM		
Astrocytes/glial cells		Glioblastoma multiforme
Schwann cells		Schwannoma

Chapter 5

Radiation Pathophysiology

KEY POINTS

- Radiation lesions are classified as: parenchymal, vascular, and connective/stromal and can be expressed in various timeframes (acute—within days to a few weeks, subacute—a few weeks to a few months, and late—3 or more months).
- Dose–volume histograms (DVHs) are used to graphically depict the dose–volume relationships of various cancer targets and normal tissues. DVH reduction parameter (dose [D] or volume [V]) points abstracted from the DVH curve can be used to judge radiation plan quality, target coverage, and normal tissue toxicity risk.
- Internationally generated standards in DVH parameters have been published by multiple investigators and have been recently summarized by the Quantitative Analyses of Normal Tissue Effects in the Clinic (QUANTEC) group. Specific QUANTEC DVH parameters for various normal tissues are summarized in this chapter.

5.1. TISSUE AND ORGAN RADIATION INJURY

The modern enterprise of radiotherapy balances adequate dosage to the cancer target(s), while respecting the tolerance of various nearby normal tissue structures. Radiation injury can be classified according to the timeframe of development (immediate: within 24 hours; acute: within days to a couple of weeks; subacute: several weeks to several months; and late: 3 or more months) as well as severity (acute and reversible, acute nonreversible—otherwise known as consequential injury, late non–life-threatening or severe, and late life-threatening or severe with loss of organ function). Appropriate radiotherapy decision making and planning strive to avoid situations where treatment failure both in terms of tumor control and extreme toxicity occurs.

Various types of lesions are commonly seen in relation to radiation injury at the tissue and/or organ level. They are defined below:

1. *Parenchymal*

- Cellular/Tissue Atrophy—Loss of cells due to necrosis and apoptosis leading to reduced number of cells and thinning of tissue structure.
- Cellular Atypia—Distortion of the cell cytoplasm and nucleus.
- Dysplasia—Abnormal cell development demonstrating preneoplastic findings such as a decrease in mature cell number and an increase in immature cells typical of the source tissue.
- Metaplasia—The replacement of one differentiated cell type by another differentiated cell type.
- Necrosis—Detrimental premature cell death (as opposed to apoptosis—programmed cell death).
- Secondary Cancer—Radiation exposure can be carcinogenic and can lead to the development of cancers within (or at the edge) of radiation volumes years after exposure.

2. *Vascular*

- Small Vessel Injury—Intimal macrophage infiltration, vessel fibrosis, fibrin deposition with cell necrosis.
- Medium Vessel Injury—Intimal fibrosis and macrophage infiltration, and vasculitis.
- Large Vessel Injury—Myointimal proliferation, vessel thrombi, and vessel dissection/rupture.

3. *Connective/Stromal*

- Fibrosis—Formation of excess connective tissue within an organ or tissue potentially leading to scar formation (confluent fibrosis impairing organ/tissue architecture and function).

5.2. DOSE–VOLUME HISTOGRAMS

A dose–volume histogram (DVH) is a commonly employed quality assurance tool to provide the clinician a graphical two-dimensional representation of the three-dimensional dose distribution related to a radiotherapy plan. This radiation plan is calculated on a computerized treatment planning system based on the CT simulation scan, target and normal tissue contours, and knowledge of radiation deposition. The DVH is generated by first determining dose bin ranges (e.g., Bin#1 0.00–0.50 Gy, Bin#2 0.51–1.00 Gy, and so on). The DVH is then generated by graphing a relative or absolute volume on the y-axis versus dose bin group on the x-axis. By making the bins infinitely small, more continuous curves can be generated. Clinicians can assess treatment quality by assessing the DVH curve versus predefined dose–volume points that are known to be related with a known risk of normal tissue toxicity and/or adequate target coverage. Two graphical DVH formats are available (Figure 5.1):

1. *Differential DVH.* A differential DVH appears like a traditional histogram graphing relative/absolute volume versus dose bin on the x-axis.
2. *Cumulative DVH.* Similar to a differential DVH; however, y-axis reflects relative/absolute volume associated with the x-axis bin dose or greater. By definition, the first and lowest dose bin will have maximum absolute volume or 100% relative volume. Similarly, zero volume (and 0% relative volume) will occur beyond the last dose bin of the target or organ at risk under consideration.

DVH and Radiation Toxicity

DVHs can be generated for all targets and organs at risk that are relevant for any particular treatment (Figure 5.2). Various organ-at-risk DVH parameters/metrics (parameters

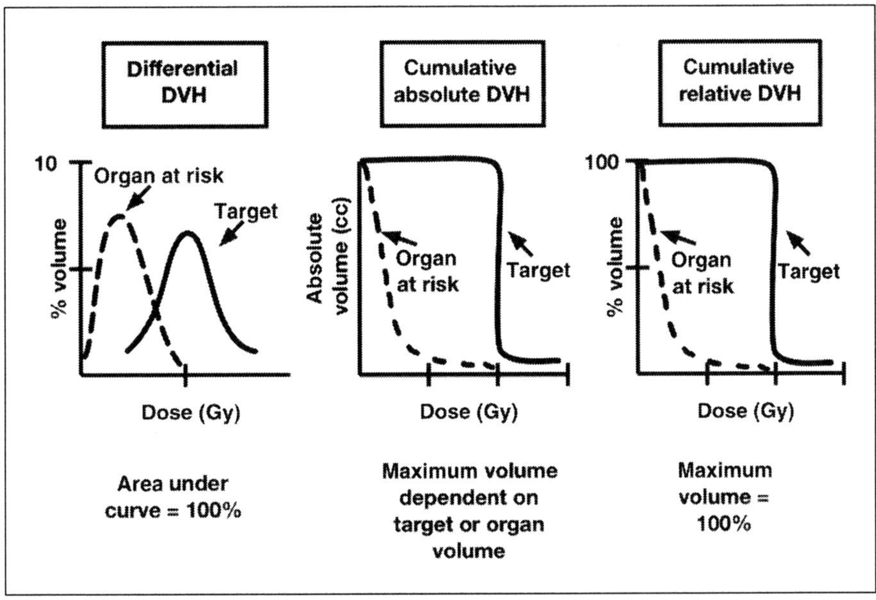

FIGURE 5.1 Dose–volume histograms

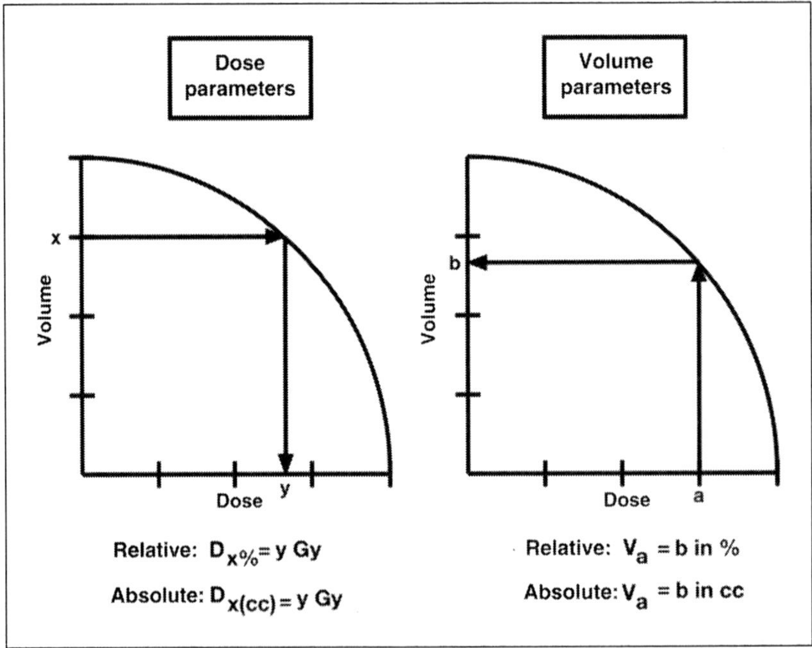

FIGURE 5.2 Dose–volume histogram reduction parameters

abstracted from DVH curves, e.g., rV_{20Gy} bilateral lung—relative percentage of bilateral lung volume receiving 20 Gy or higher) have been shown to be associated with or predictive of toxicity outcomes (e.g., radiation pneumonitis and rV_{20Gy} bilateral lung). The Quantitative QUANTEC group (QUANTEC Group, 2010) has published recommendations for dose–volume limits for a variety of normal tissues, which will be discussed in the remainder of this chapter.

5.3. BRAIN

Tissue Structure and Radiation Injury

Various cells within the central nervous system are vital to the normal functioning of the brain and are potentially sensitive to radiation injury:

1. *Neurons.* Approximately 10 billion nondividing neurons are in the adult human. Impairment of these cells by radiation can lead to disturbances, which can affect global and/or focal neurological functioning. Radiation injury can also lead to brain necrosis.
2. *Astrocytes.* Supporting network of cells with a variety of functions including neurological structure support, endothelial cell/blood–brain barrier support, and synaptic modulation. Radiation injury can lead to gliosis (cerebral scarring).
3. *Oligodendrocytes.* Myelin-producing supporting cells to aid with nerve conduction. Radiation injury can lead to focal demyelination plaques.
4. *Endothelial cells.* With the support of other important vascular cells including smooth muscle and fibroblasts, endothelial cells ensure vascularization of all neural tissues. Radiation injury can lead to cerebral edema (due to disruption of the blood–brain barrier), ischemia, and infarction.

Dose–Volume Histogram Parameters

The primary brain toxicity endpoint is symptomatic brain necrosis. To generate the brain DVH, the whole brain is contoured as one organ. QUANTEC maximum brain dose (in 1.8–2 Gy/day fractions) parameters for 5% and 10% risk of primary endpoint injury are 72 and 90 Gy, respectively. Partial brain radiotherapy at 60 Gy in 1.8 to 2 Gy/day should result in $< 3\%$ risk of symptomatic brain necrosis. Maximum dose to children should be 18 Gy or less (using a late neurocognitive function endpoint). In the context of stereotactic radiosurgery, V_{12Gy} should be kept to < 5 to 10 mL in order to ensure $< 20\%$ risk of symptomatic brain necrosis.

5.4. OPTIC NERVE AND CHIASM

Tissue Structure and Radiation Injury

The optic nerve is a structure that transmits visual information from the retina to the brain. All these nerve tracts converge in the X-shaped optic chiasm, where the medial tracts cross over (decussation) to the contralateral side in order to support stereoscopic vision. Both of these structures are considered to be similar to other peripheral nerves; yet, these two structures are embryologically related to the central nervous system, so the nerve fibers are covered with myelin from oligodendrocytes as opposed to Schwann cells (related to peripheral nerves). Other supporting structures for the nerve and chiasm include meningeal layers and vascular structures. Optic fibers begin at the retinae of the orbit and terminate in the lateral geniculate nucleus, pretectal nucleus, or suprachiasmatic nucleus.

Damage to the optic nerve can cause mono-ocular visual loss; whereas, optic chiasm injury can lead to bilateral partial or complete vision loss. Types of radiation injury (radiation-induced optic neuropathy) are similar to brain lesions and can include: necrosis, gliosis, and demyelination.

Dose-Volume Histogram Parameters

The primary endpoint for optic nerve and chiasm injury is blindness. Contouring of the optic nerve and particularly the chiasm can be challenging on CT with observed intra- and interphysician variations. Magnetic resonance imaging (MRI) can assist in the more accurate delineation of these structures. QUANTEC (1.8–2 Gy/day) maximum optic nerve/chiasm doses are listed as < 55 Gy (< 3% risk), 55–60 Gy (3%–7% risk), and more than 60 Gy (7%–20% risk). In the context of stereotactic radiosurgery, a maximum dose of < 12 Gy in a single dose will lead to < 10% risk of blindness. A maximum dose of 8 Gy or less will lead to rare risk of complications.

5.5. BRAINSTEM

Tissue Structure and Radiation Injury

The brainstem is located in the posterior part of the brain and is continuous with the spinal cord caudally. The function of the brainstem is critical in the regulation of cardiac, respiratory, and consciousness/sleep functions. This organ is responsible for the motor and sensory function of the face/neck through the related cranial nerves. Also, all major connections between the brain and the rest of the body pass through the brainstem. These include the corticospinal tract (motor function), posterior column-medial lemniscal pathway (proprioception, vibration, fine touch), and the spinothalamic tract (pain and touch). Anatomically, the brainstem is divided into the medulla oblongata, pons, and midbrain. Similar to other neurological tissues, the brainstem contains neurons, astrocytes, oligodendrocytes, and vascular networks that can express radiation injury in an analogous fashion as described in Section 6.4.

Dose-Volume Histogram Parameters

The QUANTEC primary endpoint for brainstem injury is brainstem necrosis and/or cranial neuropathy. Contouring the brainstem on CT imaging can be routine; yet, attention to the cranial and caudal extent of the volume is required. The cranial aspect of the brainstem can be indistinct from cerebellar and cerebral anatomy. The caudal aspect of the brainstem terminates at the level of the foramen magnum. The QUANTEC (1.8–2 Gy/day) brainstem tolerance is 54 Gy to the entire organ, 59 Gy to 1–10 mL of the brainstem, and 64 Gy to a point dose of < 1 cc in volume. These parameters will lead to < 5% risk of suffering the primary QUANTEC endpoint. In single-fraction stereotactic radiosurgery, a maximum brainstem dose of 12.5 Gy should lead to < 5% risk of necrosis and/or cranial neuropathy.

5.6. SPINAL CORD

Tissue Structure and Radiation Injury

The spinal cord consists of motor and sensory neurons with supporting cells such as astrocytes, oligodendrocytes, microglia, and vascular networks. All these cells are encased in fibrous dura and pia-arachnoid tissue and surrounded by the thecal sac and spinal canal. The spinal cord originates at the level of the foramen magnum and terminates at the upper lumbar spine with peripheral nerves in the lower lumbar and sacral spine (cauda equina).

Similar to other neural tissues, the spinal cord can be subject to various injuries including necrosis, gliosis, demyelination plaques, and vascular lesions. Collectively, these late radiation-related spinal cord injuries are denoted as spinal cord myelopathic lesions. Clinically, patients with spinal cord myelopathy can present with various symptoms including motor and sensory deficits, incontinence, and paralysis. Of note, L'Hermitte's syndrome is related to a transient demyelination of the spinal cord causing a shock-like sensation upon flexion of the neck. It is benign in its course and is seen in many patients receiving radiotherapy to the spine, such as lung cancer, head and neck cancer, and lymphomas.

Dose-Volume Histogram Parameters

The QUANTEC primary endpoint for spinal cord damage is spinal cord myelopathy. The spinal cord can be contoured either as the organ, the organ with 2 to 3 mm margin, the thecal sac and content, or the spinal canal. In the context of traditional 3DCRT planning at 1.8 to 2 Gy/day, the following maximum cord doses for full cord irradiation are related to associated estimates of spinal cord injury risk: 50 Gy (0.2%), 54 Gy (1%), 60 Gy (6%), 61 Gy (10%), and 69 Gy (50%). In the context of stereotactic radiosurgery, partial cord maximum doses of 13 Gy (one fraction) and 20 Gy (three fractions) are related to < 1% myelopathy risk.

5.7. INNER EAR/COCHLEA

Tissue Structure and Radiation Injury

The inner ear consists of a bony hollow structure within the temporal bone of the skull with two main sections: the cochlea and the vestibular system. The function of the cochlea is related to hearing, while the function of the vestibular system (containing the vestibule and three canals) is related to balance. The cochlea translates pressure waves from sound into neurological impulses by means of intermediary interactions between the fluid and membranes of the cochlea. Radiation injury to this organ is likely related to the damage of the cochlear neurons, sclerosis of vascular arterioles, and osteoradionecrosis of the temporal bone. Other structures that can express radiation damage include the skin of the ear, ossicles, tympanic membrane, and other soft tissues of the outer, middle, or inner ear.

Dose–Volume Histogram Parameters

The primary QUANTEC toxicity endpoint for inner ear/cochlear damage is the presence of sensorineural hearing loss. Given the small volume nature of the inner ear and cochlea, a DVH analysis relating dose–volume relationships with outcome is challenging. However, the cochlea can be contoured by utilizing both thin slice CT (1 mm) and appropriate window-level settings. The mean dose to the cochlea should be limited to < 45 Gy (preferably < 35 Gy) to reduce the risk of toxicity to below 30%.

5.8. PAROTID GLAND

Tissue Structure and Radiation Injury

The primary glands responsible for salivary function in the head and neck area include the parotid, submandibular, and sublingual glands. Other innumerable minor salivary glands also exist to support salivary function. These glands contain two types of secretory cells known as serous (clear enzyme-containing fluid) and mucinous (glycoprotein-containing fluid for lubrication) subtypes. Of note, the parotid gland is primarily a serous-cell–type gland, whereas the minor salivary glands are primarily mucinous. The submandibular and sublingual glands have both cell types. Structurally, these organs are organized with acini and ducts surrounded by myoepithelium and connective tissue (supported by vascular and neurological structures as well). From a radiotherapy point of view, the acinar serous cells are particularly radiosensitive, which can lead to cellular/tissue apoptosis and necrosis. The typical radiation response to salivary tissue includes an early inflammatory phase followed by a late glandular atrophy with fat replacement and possible tissue fibrosis.

Dose–Volume Histogram Parameters

The primary QUANTEC endpoint of interest is xerostomia (altered taste and/or mouth dryness). Contouring of the external surface of the parotid and submandibular glands can be routinely performed using CT simulation scans. Mean radiotherapy dose (at 1.8–2 Gy/day) for one or both parotid glands should be below 20 and 25 Gy, respectively, in order to keep the risk of clinically significant xerostomia < 20%. If possible, maintaining a mean submandibular dose of < 35 Gy can also assist in preserving salivary function.

5.9. LARYNX AND PHARYNX

Tissue Structure and Radiation Injury

The larynx, the organ responsible for phonation, is divided into the supraglottis/epiglottis, glottis, and subglottis. The pharynx, which surrounds the larynx, supports vocal, digestive, and respiratory functions. The epithelium of the larynx is squamous and columnar in nature, with other cell types including mucous and serous glandular cells, connective tissue, and smooth muscle. From a radiotherapy point of view, the targets for potential injury can include the vasculature, epithelium, and cartilage. In the acute phase, inflammation and edema are common. Late injury consists of tissue atrophy, tissue necrosis, sclerosis, vascular injury, as well as possible osteonecrosis and chondronecrosis. Pharyngeal injury is similar with early-phase edema and mucositis with late necrosis, fibrosis, and vascular injury.

Dose–Volume Histogram Parameters

There are various QUANTEC endpoints that are relevant to the treatment of the laryngeal and pharyngeal anatomy. They include laryngeal edema, dysphagia/aspiration, and vocal dysfunction. The contouring of the laryngeal anatomy is not completely defined, but should generally include the larynx from the top of the epiglottis to the bottom of the cricoid. Optional areas for contouring can include the base of the tongue, lateral pharyngeal walls, upper esophagus, pre-epiglottic space, and false vocal cords, as these areas are also critical for vocal dysfunction. DVH recommendations from the QUANTEC document include a maximum dose of < 66 Gy (1.8–2 Gy/day with chemo) to keep vocal dysfunction to < 20%. Other parameters include mean dose < 50 Gy (30% risk of aspiration), mean < 44 Gy (20% risk of edema, nonchemotherapy), and V_{50Gy} (20% risk of edema).

5.10. LUNG

Tissue Structure and Radiation Injury

The lung is a bilateral branching organ designed to support gas (oxygen and carbon dioxide) exchange at the level of alveoli. The alveolar ducts and pouches contain type I (squamous cells) and type II (cuboidal) pneumocytes, as well as capillaries, arteries, and veins. A large variety of other cells exist in the respiratory system including: neuroendocrine cells, goblet cells, mucous/serous glandular cells, fibroblasts, smooth muscle, and other supporting cell lines. Early radiation-induced lung injury consists of intra-alveolar edema with various inflammatory cells present. Injury is usually focused on the capillaries and type II pneumocytes, leading to various changes including cell swelling and cell detachment. Late radiation effects include progressive alveolar septal fibrosis and arterial intimal thickening. Clinically, three syndromes have been recognized in the literature: radiation pneumonitis (subacute), radiation fibrosis, and acute respiratory distress syndrome (abscopal effect of radiotherapy—severe acute radiation damage well outside radiation ports).

Dose-Volume Histogram Parameters

The primary QUANTEC endpoint that is relevant for pulmonary injury is symptomatic pneumonitis (usually requiring steroids). Bronchial stricture is also a relevant endpoint for high-dose radiotherapy. Lung contouring is usually performed as a joint organ on a 3DCT, using an external contour that excludes either gross target volume or planning target volume. In terms of central airways, maximum dose of 80 Gy is recommended to avoid bronchial stricture. In terms of radiation pneumonitis, the V_{20Gy} parameter should be kept under 30% to 35%, or the mean dose should be < 20 to 23 Gy to keep the primary symptomatic pneumonitis risk to < 20%. Mesothelioma or pneumonectomy situations require more stringent dose parameters such as V_{5Gy} < 60% and V_{20Gy} < 4%–10% to ensure minimal risk of severe or fatal radiation pneumonitis.

5.11. HEART

Tissue Structure and Radiation Injury

The heart is an organ specifically targeted toward the support of blood circulation as part of a larger cardiovascular system. The structure of the heart consists of various tissues including: the pericardium (fibrous sac), epicardium (fibrous tissue and mesothelial cells and containing vascular, neurological, and lymphatic tissues including the coronary arteries), myocardium (muscle supporting the cardiac pump), and endocardium (inner fibrous tissue and cardiac valves). Many of these structures can manifest radiation-induced injuries including: acute pericarditis and various late syndromes such as congestive heart failure, coronary artery disease/ischemia, valvular lesions, myocardial fibrosis, and myocardial infarction.

Dose-Volume Histogram Parameters

The primary QUANTEC endpoints for cardiac damage from radiation injury are pericarditis (acute) and cardiac mortality (late). Contouring the heart can be accomplished by the use of CT simulation; however, excluding various structures such as the diaphragm, liver, and large vessels can be challenging. For acute pericarditis, V_{30Gy} (in 1.8–2 Gy/day) should be $< 46\%$ and the mean heart dose should be < 26 Gy to keep toxicity rates under 15%. However, these dose limitations may need to be exceeded in order to treat highly aggressive cancers such as lung and esophageal tumors.

5.12. ESOPHAGUS

Tissue Structure and Radiation Injury

The esophagus is a tubular muscular organ with the function of taking food from the head and neck area into the digestive system. Various cell structures are contained within the esophagus including: a lining of squamous epithelium, lamina propria (connective tissue), muscle, vasculature, and nerves. In terms of radiotherapy injury, the targets of early changes are the epithelial cells, leading to a form of mucositis. Other early effects can lead to connective tissue edema, cell necrosis, and vessel thrombi. Late effects on the esophagus are mediated by either cell necrosis or tissue fibrosis, leading to macroscopic findings of esophageal ulcers or esophageal stricture. Late bleeding from radiotherapy can also be a result of telangiectasia formation within the esophagus.

Dose–Volume Histogram Parameters

The primary QUANTEC endpoint for radiation injury is considered to be either grade 2 or greater (requiring medical intervention) acute esophagitis. Some controversy exists in the contouring of the esophagus on CT with or without barium contrast. Typically, an external contour of the esophagus starting from the cricoid cartilage to the gastroesophageal junction (below the tumor if applicable) is used. In the context of 1.8 to 2 Gy/day chemoradiotherapy, a mean dose of 34 Gy or less should lead to a severe (grade 3 or greater) acute esophagitis risk of 5% to 20%. In terms of grade 2 (moderate) esophagitis, the following DVH parameters should lead to < 30% risk: $V_{35Gy} < 50\%$, $V_{60Gy} < 40\%$, and $V_{70Gy} < 20\%$.

5.13. LIVER

Tissue Structure and Radiation Injury

The liver is responsible for multiple functions including: metabolism, elimination of waste/detoxification, bile production, biochemical synthesis, and glycogen storage. The liver is a branching organ with various lobules containing hepatocytes, the functional and fundamental unit of the liver. The function of the liver is supported by vasculature (hepatic artery and portal vein and its branches), bile ducts, lymphatic tissue, and nerves. Acute radiation injury is manifested by vaso-occlusive disease (damage to the endothelial cells of the venous sinusoids and lobular veins). The hepatocytes are not the primary target, but can demonstrate radiation effects of atrophy and necrosis. This vaso-occlusive disease can lead to various clinical manifestations including liver enzyme abnormalities, hepatomegaly, and ascites. Late radiotherapy findings can include vascular fibrosis, as well as lobular collapse or distortion.

Dose–Volume Histogram Parameters

The primary QUANTEC endpoint for liver toxicity from radiotherapy is classic radiation-induced liver disease (RILD). Classic RILD is defined as hepatomegaly and ascites with elevated alkaline phosphatase in the absence of preexisting liver disease. This usually occurs 2 weeks to 3 months after radiation therapy. In the setting of 1.8 to 2 Gy/day therapy, DVH limits depend on the level of preexisting liver disease: no preexisting disease (mean dose < 30–32 Gy for < 5% risk and < 42 Gy for < 50% risk), and Child–Pugh A/hepatocellular carcinoma (mean dose < 28 Gy for < 5% risk and < 36 Gy for < 50% risk). Various stereotactic DVH parameter limits also exist for primary liver tumors (< 13 Gy in three fractions and < 18 Gy in six fractions) and liver metastases (< 15 Gy in three fractions and < 20 Gy in six fractions) to keep classic RILD risk under 5%.

5.14. STOMACH AND SMALL BOWEL

Tissue Structure and Radiation Injury

The stomach and small bowel are primarily concerned with the breakdown of food and the absorption of its constituent nutrients to support life. Radiation injury of the stomach is primarily manifested by the development of a radiation ulcer due to cell necrosis. Radiation injuries of the small bowel are classified into early (due to mucosal/villous damage leading to various biochemical malabsorption effects) and late injuries (due to vascular and connective tissue injuries leading to reduced blood flow and a potentially narrowed lumen). Severe complications can include a bleeding gastric ulcer and partial/complete bowel obstruction.

Dose-Volume Histogram Parameters

The primary QUANTEC endpoint for the stomach is late stomach ulceration. It can be contoured on CT simulation scans; yet, stomach shape and size can vary depending on the contents. Use of a limit of 45 Gy (1.8–2 Gy/day) to the entire stomach should limit the toxicity rate to < 7%. In terms of small bowel, the primary QUANTEC endpoint is grade 3 or greater (i.e., severe) acute toxicity requiring medical intervention. Similar to the stomach, small bowel contouring can be challenging due to variable filling and peristaltic motion. Recommended dose limits for small bowel at 2 Gy/day include: $V_{15Gy} < 120$ mL (small bowel contoured) or $V_{45Gy} < 195$ mL (peritoneal space contoured as a surrogate to account for small bowel motion).

Chapter 6

Imaging

KEY POINTS

- Medical imaging refers to a set of generally noninvasive techniques where images of the human body are generated for clinical or research purposes. Various two-dimensional (2D), three-dimensional (3D), and four-dimensional (4D) techniques are available to generate both anatomical and functional patient information to support cancer diagnosis, staging, treatment, and follow-up.
- A projectional radiograph is a medical image created by the assessment of x-rays after transmission through an object (patient). Fluoroscopic techniques utilize a cine display to show multiple images over time (e.g., respiratory motion in lung cancer). Classical radiation oncology planning heavily utilized fluoroscopic techniques to support radiotherapy targeting.
- Ultrasonography (US) is a nonionizing imaging technique that uses the detection of high-frequency sound waves to capture various anatomic structures. In radiation oncology, ultrasound has been used in the image guidance of prostate cancer and for the staging of potential liver metastases.
- Computed tomography (CT) is an ionizing medical imaging technique that can reconstruct 3D or 4D anatomical information from a series of 2D x-ray projections produced around an axis of interest. CT is extensively utilized in the staging and follow-up of cancer patients, as well as in the image-guided treatment of highly conformal radiotherapy. CT simulation is routinely utilized to define cancer targets and normal tissue structures and to perform radiotherapy dose calculations.
- Magnetic resonance imaging (MRI) is a nonionizing anatomical and functional imaging technique that exploits the property of atomic nuclei magnetic field alignment and relaxation to produce high-quality imaging. Similar to CT, MRI can be used for the staging and follow-up of cancer patients, as well as for target delineation of various tumors including the central nervous system, genitourinary, and head and neck systems.
- Single photon emission computed tomography (SPECT) technique is an ionizing 3D functional imaging technique that utilizes radiopharmaceuticals to assess various metabolic functions. Specifically, in radiation oncology, SPECT imaging has utility for staging (bone and thyroid scans), as well as specialized applications including pulmonary ventilation and perfusion assessment.
- Positron emission tomography (PET) is an ionizing functional imaging technique that detects positrons after decay of positron emitter–labeled radiopharmaceuticals. The type of functional imaging depends on the nature of the radiopharmaceutical (most commonly utilized is 18FDG for metabolic imaging of selected cancers including lung cancer). PET is commonly registered with CT in order to improve the anatomical interpretation of functional images.

6.1. MEDICAL IMAGING OVERVIEW

What is Medical Imaging?

Medical imaging refers to a set of techniques that generate images of the human body for either clinical or scientific purposes. With respect to clinical medical imaging, the use of imaging is performed to aid in the screening, diagnosis, or posttreatment follow-up of a variety of pathological conditions. Various medical disciplines are involved with the production of medical images including diagnostic radiology, nuclear medicine, pathology, and radiation oncology. Most medical imaging is considered to be of a noninvasive nature (i.e., does not penetrate the skin or other tissues); however, modern imaging with modalities such as CT and MRI can have important biological, chemical, and physical effects on biological systems such as those found in the human body.

Pixels, Voxels, and Signal Intensity

A pixel refers to the smallest finite surface area that can be placed on a single point in a two-dimensional (2D) coordinate system of an image (Figure 6.1). Each picture element (or pixel) has a unique address on the 2D coordinate system and also has an associated intensity value corresponding to an underlying parameter that is being measured within the surface area of the pixel. As an example, in photography, each pixel would be associated with various signal intensities of red, green, and blue colors (RBG color system), in order to display a final color of that specific picture element. In total, an entire set of pixels would comprise a planar digital image (a digital picture).

In medical imaging, relevant signal intensities will depend on the modality being utilized, which can include the Hounsfield unit (HU [CT]), proton density (proton MRI), or flow rate (Doppler ultrasound). Each imaging modality will have its own conventions regarding the display of high-intensity or low-intensity values for the signal; yet, both grayscale

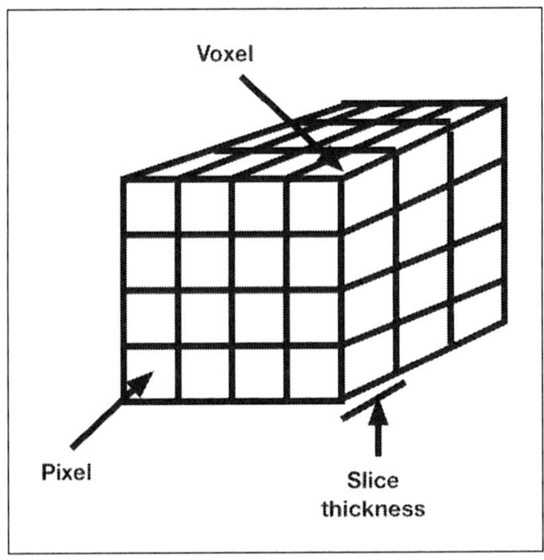

FIGURE 6.1 Pixels and voxels

(e.g., CT and MRI) and color (e.g., Doppler ultrasound) visual representations of intensity data are commonly utilized. These conventions will be discussed in the following imaging modality–specific sections of this chapter.

By definition, each pixel has an infinitely small thickness; its applicability to medical imaging is therefore limited to digital images of patient anatomy/pathology created by digital cameras, as well as the visual representation of full three-dimensional (3D) medical images on 2D computer monitors. Two-dimensional imaging such as projectional radiographs (i.e., x-rays) are also represented in a 2D pixel format; yet, the signal intensity associated with each pixel represents a cumulative signal of a volume consistent with the projection ray passing from the source, through the pixel, and to the detector (see Section 7.2). In medical imaging, a 3D concept analogous to the pixel is required for two reasons. First, many procedures require full-volume images of patient anatomy, so infinitely thin pixels cannot be utilized for this purpose. In addition, all volumetric imaging procedures, including ultrasound and radiographs, obtain signal intensities that represent some finite thickness (including microscopic or millimeter scales) of patient anatomy. A voxel (volume element) is used as an analogous construct to the pixel to represent a finite volume within a 3D grid in space (Figure 6.1). Associated with each voxel are a location (x, y, and z), volume (length, width, and height), as well as signal intensity associated with the modality being utilized.

Therefore, a basic medical image set will contain information regarding the 2D/3D grid with a definition of the origin, pixel/voxel size, as well as pixel/voxel locations and signal intensities for each unique pixel/voxel in the imaging dataset. Modern imaging digital file structure allows for additional information to be captured, including various patient- and modality-specific parameters under the Digital Imaging and Communication in Medicine (DICOM) standard. This will be discussed later in the chapter.

Structural Versus Functional Imaging

Another important consideration related to the modality of imaging to be utilized is the type of patient information that the modality is designed to acquire. Traditionally, medical imaging revolved around the imaging of normal anatomy and the detection of abnormal anatomy indicative of a pathological process. This form of medical imaging, otherwise known as structural (or anatomical) imaging, is still commonly used today and forms the backbone of medical imaging. Signals associated with structural imaging techniques are related to the underlying anatomical structure (e.g., very high CT HU signal intensities equating to the presence of bone, and very low values indicating air). Functional imaging can provide additional and complementary information regarding various physiological processes such as metabolic rate, lung ventilation, or blood flow. Often, images from functional imaging procedures such as positron emission tomography (PET) can be combined with structural imaging to provide improved diagnostic ability to users of medical imaging (e.g., PET-CT). The fusion of structural and functional imaging can allow for an augmented ability to localize functional changes back to patient anatomy, assisting in the diagnosis and treatment of patients. This is particularly important in some functional imaging techniques that have known low resolution such as PET and single photon emission computed tomography (SPECT).

6.2. PROJECTIONAL RADIOGRAPHS AND FLUOROSCOPY

Projectional Radiographs

A projectional radiograph is a medical image obtained by capturing x-rays that are transmitted through an object after x-ray exposure (Figure 6.2). These projectional radiograph x-rays can be converted into various media to be read including: photographic films, solid-state detectors, or phosphor screens. Projectional radiographs are particularly useful in clinical scenarios where bone or soft-tissue pathology may exist. Specific projectional radiographs that are used in medicine include: bone x-rays, chest radiographs, abdominal radiographs, mammograms, and dental radiographs.

Kilovoltage energy diagnostic x-rays are attenuated depending on the atomic number and density of the underlying material. Bone (with both high atomic number and density) is highly attenuated and will appear white on radiographs when backlit. Conversely, air (with relatively low atomic number and density) attenuates x-ray radiation to a far smaller degree and will appear black on radiographic images (more exposed on photographic film).

Fluoroscopy

The fluoroscopy imaging technique is related to a projectional radiograph, but utilizes a cine display (multiple images over time). A digital imaging device is required to update the displayed image depending on patient or physiological motion or the introduction of contrast agents that may change the x-ray attenuation of specific anatomical structures such as vasculature (Figure 6.2). These devices are either an image intensifier (e.g., cesium iodide–coated vacuum tube) or array detector (e.g., pixelated photon or electron detectors). Specific clinical applications of fluoroscopy include various angiographic techniques, double contrast (barium swallow/enema and air), as well as the simulation of classical radiotherapy fields.

Until the recent advent of CT simulation in the mid-1990s, conventional simulation, which utilized a medical fluoroscope mounted in a similar manner as the linear accelerators for treatment (i.e., the same degrees of freedom for the device as well as the patient couch), was the dominant method by which both radical and palliative radiotherapy planning was executed. The conventional fluoroscopic simulator has the advantage of real-time imaging including assessment of respiratory motion, low cost, and simplicity of operation; yet, major disadvantages are lack of axial imaging, dosimetric calculation limitations, and large uncertainty margins. These issues converge to limit radiation dosage due to large treatment volumes, particularly in the setting of radical radiotherapy (see Section 12.4).

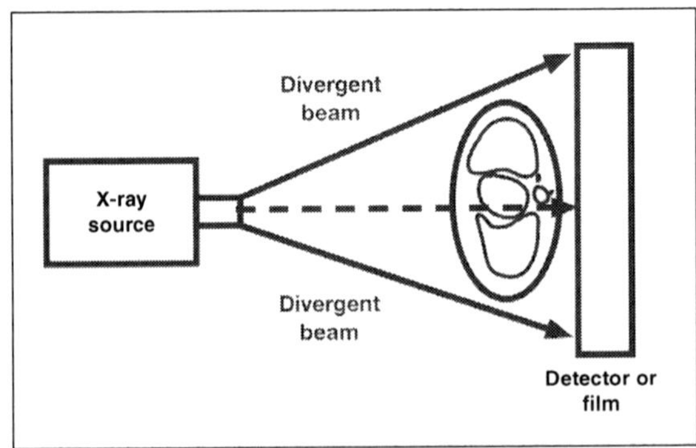

FIGURE 6.2 Projection radiographs and fluoroscopy

6.3. ULTRASOUND

Medical Ultrasound Technique

Medical ultrasonography (US) refers to an imaging technique that uses high-frequency ultrasound waves (between 2- and 18-MHz range) to image various anatomic structures such as vascular structures, abdominopelvic structures (e.g., liver, ovary, testis, and uterus), and musculoskeletal (MSK) tissue (e.g., muscle, tendons, and joint spaces). Pathological lesions can also be detected; thus, ultrasound can be utilized for cancer diagnosis and staging. Medical applications of ultrasonography include obstetrical (e.g., fetal development), cardiovascular (e.g., cardiac echocardiogram—cardiac valvular abnormalities, Doppler US—deep-vein thrombosis, carotid US—stenosis), and gastrointestinal (e.g., solid-organ assessment including gallbladder, liver, kidneys, and pancreas) among other applications.

The US technique uses a piezoelectric transducer that transforms electrical energy into high-frequency sound waves by the use of a transducer ring (Figure 6.3). Echoes from the internal anatomy of the patient are reflected back and acquired by the transducer. The relative amount of US echo versus transmission depends on tissue density. An image can then be formed by mathematically assessing changes in tissue density, the echo time lag, and the focal length of the US probe at the specific frequency being utilized. Various US functional modes are available that can generate 2D and 3D information, as well as specialized techniques such as Doppler mode to visualize blood flow. General advantages of the US technique include good imaging of MSK structures, excellent safety due to the nonionizing nature of the modality, the ability to acquire real-time images that demonstrate changes in tissue structure, and low cost. Disadvantages include lack of penetration, operator dependency, and bone/air artifacts.

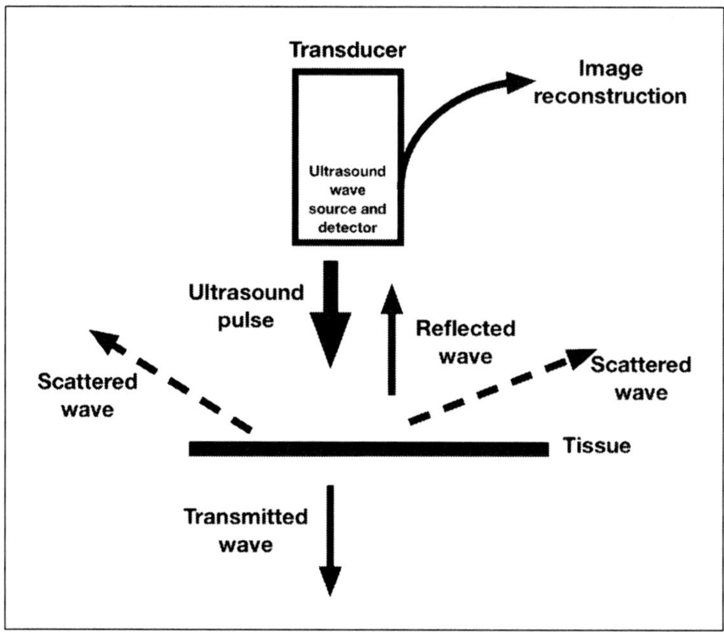

FIGURE 6.3 Medical ultrasound

Role of Ultrasound in Radiation Oncology

Ultrasound imaging can be used to assist in the diagnosis of multiple cancers including abdominal tumors (liver, gall bladder, pancreas, and kidney), genitourinary (GU) tumors (testicular and bladder), as well as MSK malignancies such as soft-tissue sarcomas. Similarly, for many solid tumors, ultrasound can be utilized in staging these same organs. In radiation oncology, the primary use of ultrasound has historically been related to the image guidance of prostate cancer radiotherapy (see Section 12.5), whereby daily on-treatment ultrasound is utilized to make small adjustments to patient positioning in order to adapt treatment to daily fluctuations in prostate location and rectal/bladder filling.

6.4. THREE- AND FOUR-DIMENSIONAL COMPUTED TOMOGRAPHY

Computed Tomography Imaging Technique

CT (also known as CAT, computed axial tomography, x-ray CT) is a medical imaging methodology, whereby a series of 2D x-ray projections produced around a specified axis is reconstructed into a 3D or four-dimensional (4D, cine series of CT over time, e.g., over a respiratory cycle) image by the use of a mathematical algorithm (Figure 6.4). The diagnostic use of CT in medicine can include the anatomic imaging (of any body site) of many disease processes including tumors, infections, hemorrhage, and trauma (among others).

The advantage of CT techniques (over simpler 2D methods) include: elimination of image superposition (i.e., the overlay of more than one structure in the image, see Section 6.2), 3D and 4D imaging that can be displayed, small contrast differences in tissue that can be resolved, and imaging reformatting, which can occur with axial, coronal, sagittal, as well as nontraditional slice orientations. Additionally, oral and intravenous contrast agents can also be utilized to improve the operating characteristics of diagnosis. CT can also be fused with other imaging modalities to assist in diagnosis (e.g., PET-CT, see Section 6.7). The disadvantages of CT imaging include radiation dose exposure, contrast reactions, as well as various imaging artifacts (streak—metal implants, ring—detector malfunction/miscalibration, noise—thin slice or low x-ray power, blurring—insufficient slice thickness, and motion—due to patient or physiological motion).

CT scans are obtained by having an x-ray source rotating around the patient with an array of detectors (various generations of detectors have been used including: cesium iodide scintillation, xenon ion chambers, and photodiode detectors). The scan information from all the x-ray projections is subjected to a mathematical algorithm (e.g., filtered back projection) in order to generate a 3D image. A CT pixel is related to relative x-ray radio density on the HU scale (ranging from low attenuation −1024 to high attenuation +3071). By definition, water has an HU value of 0 and air is −1000. Other structures can have variable values but the following are known representative values: bone (+400), titanium (+1000), and cranial bone (+2000).

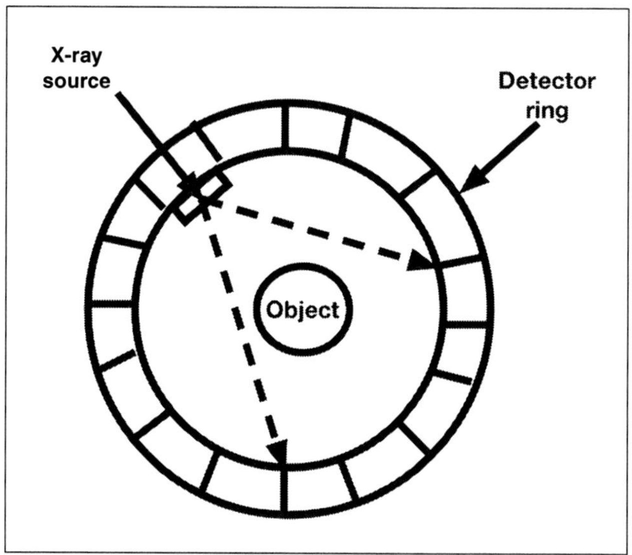

FIGURE 6.4 Three-dimensional computed tomography

Utility of Computed Tomography in Radiation Oncology

Within the context of radiation oncology, use of CT serves three major purposes. Firstly, CT imaging can be diagnostic and can assist in the determination of the intent and extent of required radiation treatment by completing patient staging. Secondly, a CT simulation scan can be performed in order to define radiotherapy targets and normal structures (either alone or with fusion imaging such as MRI or PET/CT). Thirdly, the HU information from the CT simulation is vital for the calculation of planned dose to the anatomy, since megavoltage radiation dose is deposited in a manner directly proportional to electron density (see Section 1.4). Furthermore, electron density can be calculated from a linear transformation of the HU. Therefore, CT information is currently vital for modern radiation planning (i.e., other imaging technologies including MRI can inform targets but cannot be used for dose calculation). In addition, 4D CT (a respiratory-based cine loop obtained from CT imaging with a respiratory surrogate device to collect respiratory phase information) is commonly used to plan radical radiotherapy of thoracic tumors (see Section 12.4 and Figure 6.5).

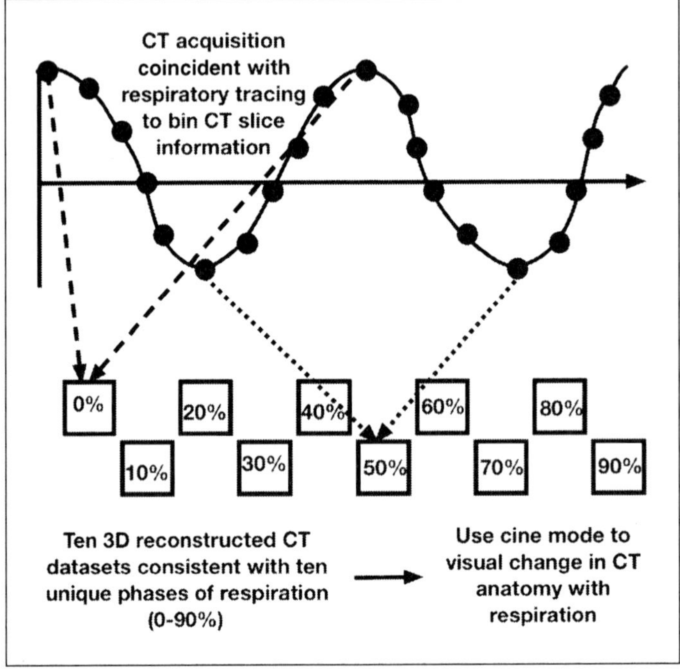

FIGURE 6.5 Four-dimensional computed tomography

6.5. MAGNETIC RESONANCE IMAGING AND SPECTROSCOPY

MRI Technique

The MRI technique exploits the property of nuclear magnetic resonance to obtain medical images. Essentially, an MRI uses a very strong magnetic field to change the nuclear polar alignment, which leads to a rotating magnetic field (Figure 6.6). The MRI scanning coil can detect these rotating magnetic fields as they relax back to a normal equilibrium (nonaligned) state. A mathematical algorithm is used to construct a 3D imaging dataset that can be visualized for anatomic and pathological diagnostic purposes. The primary paramagnetic atomic target for MRI scanning is the proton (^{1}H MRI). In biological tissue, water is a dominant constituent in cells. In addition, fat has high concentrations of protons within the hydrocarbon structures and provides an important signal in many MRI sequences (see Table 6.1). Paramagnetic contrast agents, such as Gadolinium, can be used to augment the imaging of vasculature, cancers, and various inflammatory processes.

The advantages of MRI scans include excellent soft-tissue contrast, nonionizing imaging, multiplane imaging reconstruction, as well as multiple available MRI sequences. Disadvantages include increased cost, risk with implanted paramagnetic materials/medical devices within the patient (e.g., metal in the eye, pacemakers), issues with possible claustrophobia, and motion artifacts when compared to CT techniques. CT is usually utilized in areas with possible motion artifacts (e.g., lung and upper abdomen), as well as tissues with high atomic numbers near other tissues with low atomic numbers (e.g., bone and surrounding soft tissue).

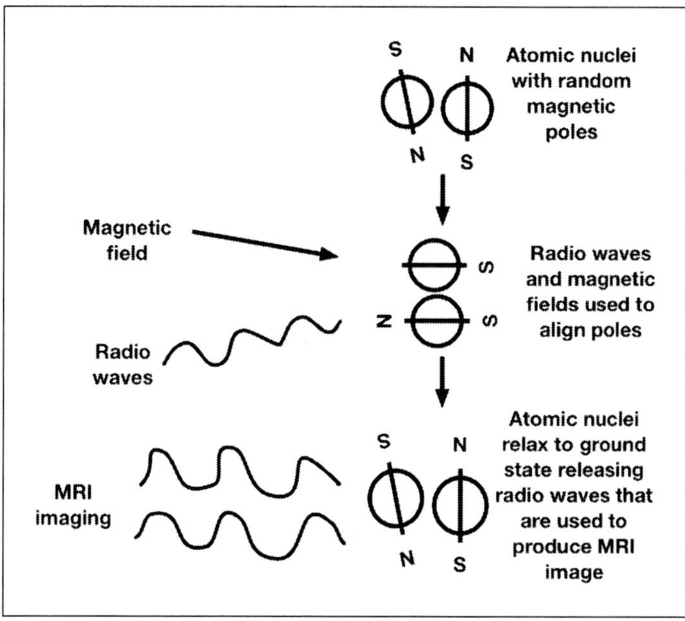

FIGURE 6.6 Magnetic resonance imaging technique

Utility of MRI Techniques in Radiation Oncology

Diagnostic MRI scanning is useful in the diagnosis and staging of various malignancies and metastatic sites including the brain, head and neck, liver, adrenals, sarcomas, GU (prostate and bladder), and gynecological (cervix) cancers. In addition, diagnostic MRI information is routinely fused with CT simulation scans in order to improve the anatomical localization of tumor and normal tissue targets. Attention to the MRI sequence, fusion methodology, and MRI artifacts are important to optimize MRI fusion utility in radiation oncology treatment.

TABLE 6.1 Clinical Utility of Various MRI Sequences and Techniques

MRI Sequence	Utility of MRI Sequence
T1-weighted	A standard scan with fat content of anatomy in a lighter color (good for CNS)
T2-weighted	A standard scan with fat content of anatomy in a darker color and water as a lighter color (good for edema)
T2*-weighted	A standard scan with increased contrast for venous blood but inferior air-tissue boundary delineation
Spin density–weighted	A standard scan probing mobile hydrogen atom variations, with fat/tumors showing up brightly and water darkly
Diffusion-weighted	Measures diffusion of water in tissue; therefore, edema and stroke lesions appear lighter on these scans
Fluid-attenuated inversion recovery (FLAIR)	Suppresses fluid signals, clinical utility in multiple sclerosis
MRI angiography	Use of a paramagnetic contrast agent such as gadolinium to highlight vascular stenosis or aneurysm lesions
MR spectroscopy	Use of a pulse sequence to highlight and image various biochemical agents in order to investigate normal and abnormal cellular metabolism including those related to tumors
Functional MRI	MRI technique to image neural activity by the assessment of the blood oxygen level–dependent (BOLD) effect
Cine MRI	Multiple dataset MRI over time to adapt for respiratory and cardiac movement
MRI simulation	Use of coregistered MRI with CT simulation scan to delineate tumors and normal tissues for the purpose of radiotherapy planning

CNS, central nervous system; CT, computed tomography.

6.6. SINGLE PHOTON EMISSION COMPUTED TOMOGRAPHY

Single Photon Emission Computed Tomography Technique

This nuclear medicine imaging technique is designed to obtain 3D functional information. The functional information that can be obtained from a SPECT scan will depend on the radiopharmaceutical utilized. A radiopharmaceutical is defined as a radioisotope attached to a ligand with specific binding properties to a tissue(s) of interest. Gamma emissions that occur from the radiolabeled drug of interest can be imaged using a planar gamma camera (Figure 6.7). A 3D image is reconstructed with a mathematical tomographic reconstruction algorithm that fuses multiple 2D image projections (obtained from multiple angles around the patient approximately every 3° to 6°) to create a full imaging dataset. Typical image resolution that can be obtained by SPECT scanning is in the order of around 1 cm. Advantages of this imaging technique include the relative availability of the technique, and the multifunctional nature of SPECT scanning (cardiac, neuropsychiatric, and oncology applications). Disadvantages include radiation exposure, artifacts, signal-to-noise concerns, scanning time, and low imaging resolution.

Utility of Single Photon Emission Computed Tomography in Radiation Oncology

SPECT scanning is routinely utilized in bone scanning (technetium-99m phosphonate or bisphosphonate) for the staging of many solid tumors including prostate, breast, lung, and colorectal cancers. Thyroid scans with iodine-123–labeled metaiodobenzylguanidine can be used to investigate and stage several tumor subtypes such as pheochromocytomas and neuroblastomas. Normal tissue functional perfusion and ventilation imaging (e.g., quantitative

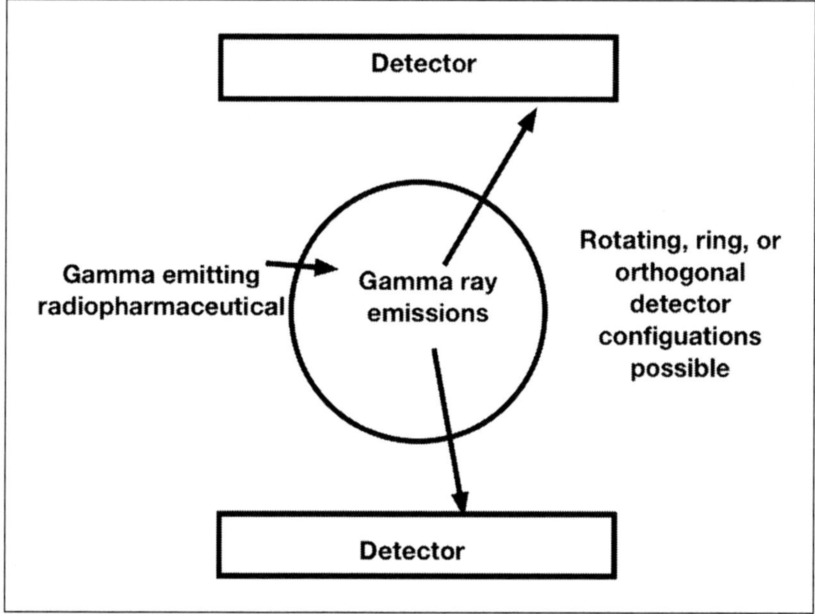

FIGURE 6.7 SPECT technique

ventilation/perfusion scan) can also assist the thoracic radiation oncologists and surgeons in the management of lung cancer patients with borderline pulmonary function that may be managed by radical radiation or surgery. This information can identify areas of highly (or poorly) functioning lung that can be used to estimate posttreatment respiratory function. Various ventilation (xenon- or technetium-labeled diethylene triamine penta-acetic acid) and perfusion (technetium-macroaggregated albumin) agents are available to obtain this qualitative and quantitative lung functional information.

6.7. POSITRON EMISSION TOMOGRAPHY

Positron Emission Tomography Technique

PET is a functional medical imaging technique that can detect radiopharmaceuticals designed to assess a specific metabolic function. These radiopharmaceuticals are tagged with radionuclides that produce positrons after positron radioactive decay (see Section 1.3). These positrons are not stable and suffer a matter–antimatter annihilation event, whereby all mass from the positron and an electron from the surrounding medium are transformed into an identical pair of photons travelling in nearly opposite directions. These coincident photons can be detected by a ring of photomultiplier/photodiode scintillation detectors and are registered by the computer system for processing (Figure 6.8). Photons not detected in pairs are ultimately ignored by the system. Image reconstruction occurs by the use of a "line of coincidence" analysis, whereby thousands of decay events are summed up to generate an image.

PET images routinely have poor signal-to-noise ratios; yet, this can be improved by the acquisition of a CT during the same imaging session. Fusion of the PET with CT allows for improved image quality due to the combination of functional imaging overlaid with anatomically accurate CT information, as well as allowing for attenuation correction of the PET imaging. The main disadvantages of PET imaging can include short radionuclide half-life, infrastructure costs (such as a cyclotron to generate radionuclides), signal-to-noise concerns, and low sensitivity and specificity of PET for diagnosis. The operating characteristics of PET can highly depend on the quantitative thresholds utilized (standardized uptake value [SUV]). The SUV, which equals maximum/mean intensity divided by weight-adjusted radiopharmaceutical dose, is commonly used for this purpose.

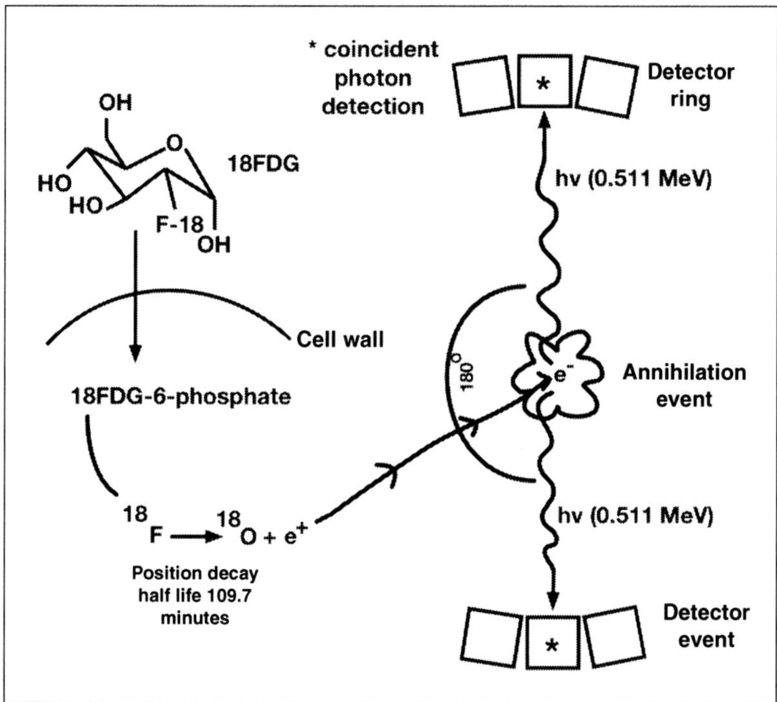

FIGURE 6.8 PET technique

Radionuclides and Radiopharmaceuticals

Various positron-emitting radionuclides can be used for PET imaging. These include: ^{11}C ($t_{1/2}$: 20.3 minutes), ^{13}N ($t_{1/2}$: 9.9 minutes), ^{15}O ($t_{1/2}$: 122.2 minutes), and ^{18}F ($t_{1/2}$: 109.7 minutes). These radionuclides can be included in various biochemicals such as fluorodeoxyglucose (FDG, metabolism tracer) and choline (marker of malignancy), as well as simple molecules such as water and ammonia. Ultimately, almost any metabolic process/pathway can be imaged with PET as long as a biochemical can be labeled with a positron emitter such as those listed above.

Utility of Positron Emission Tomography in Radiation Oncology

Fluorine-18 FDG PET scanning has multiple uses in oncology, including the staging of lung cancers and lymphomas. In the context of radiation oncology, lung PET/CT also has the additional utility of guiding radiation therapy in the setting of lung tumors with atelectasis and/or mediastinal lymph nodes. Often, accurate delineation of a target can be challenging in the context of lung tumors, causing collapse of the entire or partial lung. Similarly, inclusion of borderline-sized lymph nodes (< 1.5 cm) can be a challenge in radiotherapy planning. PET/CT scans can be fused with planning CT simulation scans in order to better define treatment targets.

6.8. MEDICAL IMAGING INFORMATICS

Picture Archiving and Communication System

A picture archiving and communication system (PACS) allows for the efficient storage and access to digital images and their associated reports. This approach circumvents the need to store, retrieve, and transport physical media such as film, paper, and disks. The PACS system consists of four major components in order to achieve all of its mandated functions including: imaging information, a secure network for transfer of information, an archive for queries to submit and receive information, and workstations for requesting and displaying imaging (Figure 6.9). The four main uses for a PACS system are:

1. *Radiology workflow management.* Allows for the efficient capture and storage of patient imaging for future reporting and physician usage.
2. *Image integration platform.* Allows for cross-integration with other hospital systems including the electronic medical record, practice management software (e.g., billing software), and a hospital information system (medical, legal, and administrative management system).
3. *Remote access.* Allows for the viewing of radiological images off-site in order to better coordinate care by supporting alternative models of care, such as telemedicine and teleradiology.
4. *Physical media replacement.* Allows for the replacement of physical media with its disadvantages of cost, physical storage requirements, and lack of instant access.

Modern PACS systems can handle a variety of images for various types of radiology equipment including oncology-intense technologies such as CT, MRI, and PET. A PACS

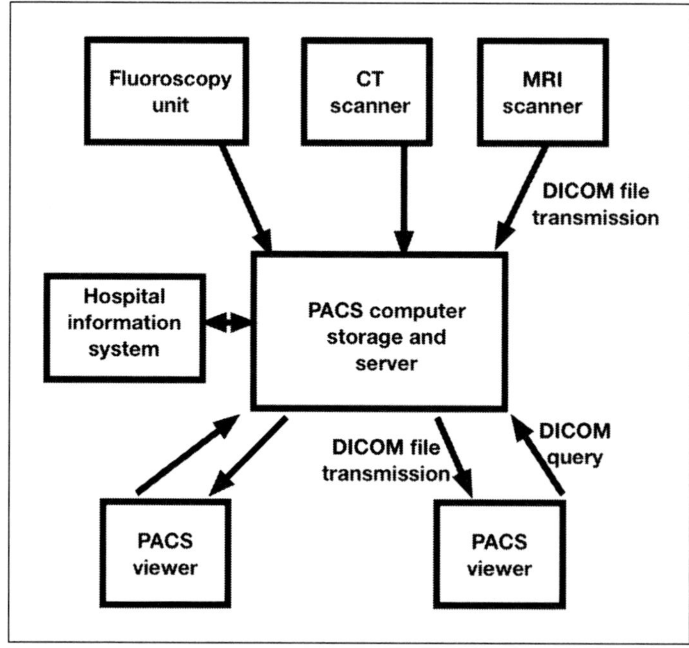

FIGURE 6.9 Medical imaging informatics

network consists of a variety of radiology equipment producing medical imaging. When produced, these medical images are sent to a PACS archive (data storage and transmission computer) via a quality assurance workstation (to allow for maintenance of the PACS database). Physicians can query the PACS archive by using other workstations in order to review medical images and reports.

Digital Imaging and Communications in Medicine

DICOM is an imaging standard (from the National Electrical Manufacturers Association—NEMA) for the storage, data exchange, and handling of a variety of forms of medical imaging information. This standard contains specifications regarding the file format to store both text and images contained within an imaging encounter, as well as a transmission control protocol and internet protocol to facilitate communication between PACS systems. Important characteristics of the DICOM format are that each individual DICOM file is generally associated with one image (e.g., one orthogonal film or one CT/MRI slice although cine loops can also be encoded into one DICOM file), and that a naming convention exists, so that the filename for each slice references the patient identification number (Figure 6.9). Within each DICOM file, a header exists that codes textual or numerical information related to the image including such attributes as patient name, ordering physician, study date, and so forth. In addition, one attribute of the file relates directly to the imaging (pixel or voxel) information for the slice/cine loop of interest. DICOM is a standard that is broadly supported, yet, DICOM compatibility issues can still arise that can limit the intercommunication between PACS and other imaging systems. In terms of radiotherapy, another related standard is the DICOM-RT standard. This standard encodes radiotherapy point-of-interest (i.e., isocenter), volume-of-interest (i.e., contours), and dose (i.e., isodose) information coregistered on the same coordinate system as DICOM information from the associated CT and/or MRI simulation imaging. Other radiation contouring standards exist to support contour and dose information exchange including Radiation Therapy Oncology Group and region of interest file formats.

PART II: CLINICAL SCIENCE CONCEPTS

Chapter 7

Clinical Epidemiology and Biostatistics

KEY POINTS

- Evidence-based medicine (EBM) is a set of procedures to systematically interpret and assess various forms of medical evidence to assist in decision making. One important aspect of EBM is the calculation of the therapeutic ratio related to an intervention: the number of patients needed to treat (NNT) to benefit one patient versus the number needed to harm (NNH) one patient.
- Randomized controlled trials (RCTs) are the current gold standard for the assessment of new diagnostic and therapeutic approaches for disease (including cancer). The reduction of bias is paramount in well-conducted RCTs and can include such maneuvers as random assignment, blinding, and placebo control.
- RCT sample size is related to several factors including: statistical power, type 1 error rate, type 2 error rate, effect size, baseline endpoint variance, and expected loss to follow-up.
- The successful administration of clinical trials involves the production of a complete clinical trial protocol and appropriate trial oversight by trial investigators/staff, sponsors, regulatory agencies, institutional review boards (IRBs), and data safety monitoring committees. Best practices regarding clinical trial registration and reporting exist in order to ensure proper dissemination of ongoing and completed clinical trials.
- Critical appraisal of the medical literature is concerned with the systematic evaluation of the clinical trial findings as it relates to patient care decision making in the domains of study methodology, results assessment, and external validity. The assessment of potential bias(es) that may impact clinical trial results is an important aspect of critical appraisal.
- Various endpoints are important in cancer clinical trials (and patients) including: survival, mortality, tumor response, disease-free survival, time to treatment failure, health-related quality of life, symptom improvement, and change in tumor markers.
- Estimates of patient survival can be created using life tables and Kaplan–Meier curves, which use discrete and infinitely small time intervals to calculate survival characteristics, respectively. Both systems take into account patients lost to follow-up prior to reaching the endpoint of interest (censoring).
- Various knowledge translation documents summarizing clinical trials exist and include: review articles, systematic reviews, meta-analyses, practice guidelines, and consensus statements.
- A predictive factor is a variable that is related to treatment response. A prognostic factor is a variable that is related to patient outcome irrespective of treatment regimen utilized (reflective of natural history of the disease).

7.1. EVIDENCE-BASED MEDICINE

Overview

Evidence-based medicine (EBM) is an approach to systematically interpret and assess available medical evidence to assist in clinical decision making. This approach can be used for the assessment of prognostic, diagnostic, and treatment interventions in a variety of clinical scenarios. Various forms of evidence can be used to inform the EBM process, which include summary knowledge translation documents (meta-analyses and systematic reviews of randomized controlled trials [RCTs]), single RCTs, prospective cohort studies, retrospective studies, expert opinion, and conventional wisdom.

References to EBM have been found in early texts in ancient Greece, yet, the modern introduction of these methodologies was in the 1970s by Dr. Archie Cochrane (Scotland). This led to an international movement to summarize medical evidence in the Cochrane Collaboration. Specific methodologies for the critical appraisal of medical evidence were published by Drs. Gordon Guyatt and David Sackett of McMaster University (among others). Critical appraisal methodologies assess various issues such as trial design and execution, patient generalizability, statistical power, patient follow-up, and endpoint selection/ascertainment.

The advantage of the EBM approach is that rational clinical decision making is more likely to be based on evidence as opposed to other factors. Various limitations to the EBM approach exist including: significant cost of clinical trials, publication bias of positive trials, significant time-lag between trial initiation and reporting, and external generalizability of trial results to more general patient populations.

Levels of Medical Evidence

Various systems exist in the medical literature to grade the level of evidence behind any specific medical recommendation. Two well-known systems include the US Preventive Services Task Force (Level I: one or more RCTs; Level II: (a) non-RCT, (b) cohort/case-control, (c) time series; and Level III: expert opinion) and the UK National Health Service (Level A: RCT or cohort study; Level B: retrospective study, case-control, outcomes research; Level C: case series; and Level D: expert opinion).

Statistical Methods

Various statistical concepts exist that are important in the context of EBM (Figure 7.1):

1. *Number needed to treat/harm.* Defined as the number of individuals that have to be exposed to an intervention (compared to standard of care intervention or placebo) to either obtain a desired benefit (NNT—number needed to treat) or an undesired clinically important negative event (e.g., death, number needed to harm [NNH]).
2. *Receiver–operator curves.* In the context of diagnostic tests where various cutoff points are possible (each with a unique sensitivity and specificity for each cutoff value), a receiver–operator curve graphing sensitivity (i.e., the true-positive rate) versus specificity (i.e., the false-positive rate) can be performed. The area under the receiver–operator curve is

proportional to the general usefulness of the test (with area under curve of 1 being a perfect test and 0.5 being no better that random chance).

3. *Likelihood ratio.* As a result of Bayes' theorem, a pretest probability of a diagnosis can be modified by the likelihood ratio of either a positive or negative test in order to calculate a post-test probability. This post-test probability, therefore, takes into account both the test result, as well as the prevalence of the disease in the patient population being assessed. The likelihood ratio is mathematically related to other concepts such as sensitivity, specificity, positive/negative predictive value, and accuracy.

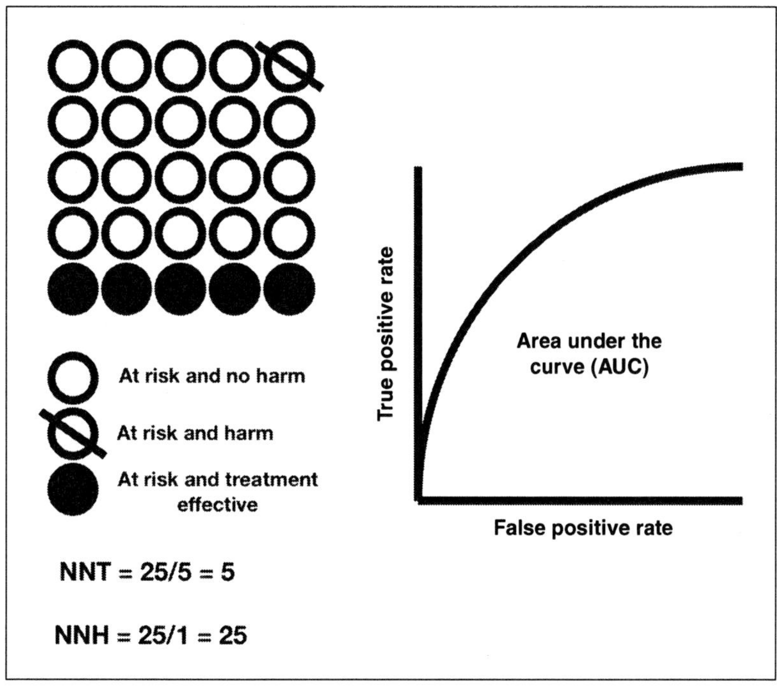

FIGURE 7.1 Statistical methods in EBM

7.2. CLINICAL TRIAL DESIGN

Introduction to Clinical Trials

A clinical trial is a form of medical research that investigates the impact of various technologies (e.g., drugs, diagnostic/prognostic tests, and medical devices) on human health. The general goals of such clinical trials are to obtain efficacy and safety information of new technologies. The scope of clinical trials can range from small pilot safety studies (often derived from preclinical animal or laboratory studies) to large multi-institutional RCTs comparing new technologies versus a standard of care approach (e.g., current standard or placebo if no standard exists).

The reported use of clinical trials has been documented as far back as biblical times, in which a clinical trial of a vegetarian versus meat diet was recounted in the Book of Daniel. Other historical milestones regarding the experimental method for clinical trials included: Avicenna's *The Canon of Medicine* in the 9th century in which experimental methods for drug testing where described, James Lind's 16th century experimentation of the effect of citrus fruit on Vitamin C deficiency (scurvy), Louis's 19th century trial on blood-letting in pneumonia, and Hill's RCT on streptomycin therapy for tuberculosis.

Types of Clinical Trials

There are multiple classifications for clinical trials. Trials can be classified by: level of intervention (observational vs. interventional), technology to be assessed (prevention vs. screening vs. diagnostic vs. therapy), phase (I—safety and dose finding study, II—preliminary efficacy study, III—definitive RCT, and IV—postmarketing safety monitoring for rare side effects), design (parallel group assignment vs. factorial trials vs. crossover study vs. cluster trials), hypothesis (superiority vs. equivalence vs. noninferiority), and trial aim (explanatory vs. pragmatic trials).

Clinical Trial Design Features

Clinical studies in EBM can include observational studies including: cohort studies (nonrandomized assessment of one or more defined patient groups of an endpoint or endpoints of interest) and case-control studies (identification of endpoint of interest with matching of negative controls to assess prognostic variables of interest). The most robust evidence for confirming or changing medical practice usually comes from well-designed and reported RCTs. These trials can have the following design features to reduce bias (Figure 7.2):

1. *Randomization.* Patients are randomly assigned to the active intervention arm or the control (standard of care/placebo) arm of the study. Statistical and logistical procedures exist to ensure that the randomization occurs in an unbiased manner. Various modifications of this approach include block randomization (repeated randomization of small groups of study subjects to minimize imbalance) and stratification (partitioning of patients depending on known significant prognostic groups to ensure equal representation between experimental and control arms). Ultimately, randomization procedures will create very similar groups for comparison in terms of both known and unknown risk factors. If any

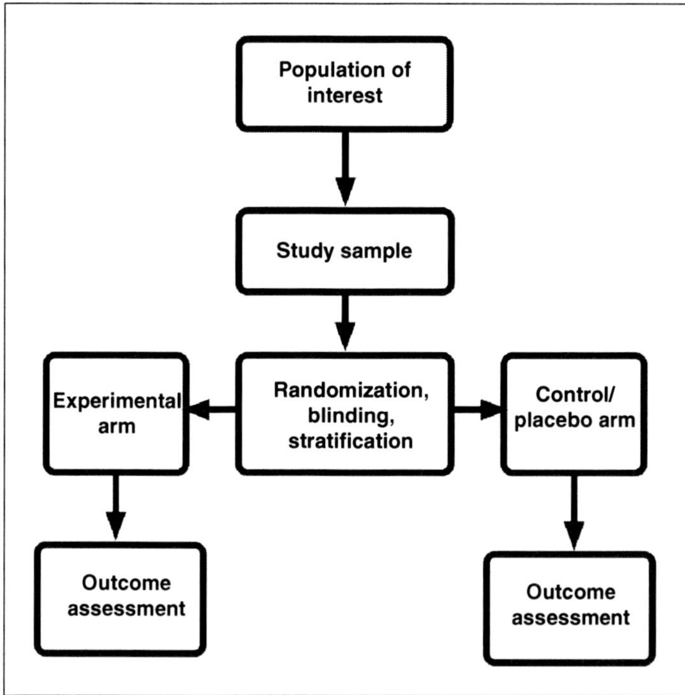

FIGURE 7.2 RCT design

bias between groups occurs after randomization, that bias would have been generated in a random fashion and can be adjusted by various statistical techniques.

2. *Blinding.* Blinding procedures attempt to reduce or eliminate any bias that can occur because of the knowledge of treatment assignment. This can apply to patients, investigators, clinical trial endpoint assessors, and statistical personnel. Depending on the clinical trial question being asked as well as the nature of the proposed treatments or tests, blinding of all or some of these individuals should be considered. Various terms are used in the literature and include: single-blind (patient blinded to intervention), double-blind (patients and researchers blinded to intervention assignment), triple-blind (patients, researchers, and endpoint assessors), and quadruple-blind (triple-blind but with statistical personnel included in the blinding procedures).
3. *Placebo control.* In studies where a new intervention is proposed where a standard-of-care therapy or test is not in place, the use of a placebo-controlled trial may be considered. The main advantage of the use of placebos is the fact that often the mere act of an intervention occurring can provoke a positive (or negative) response that can be related to the endpoint(s) of interest. The appropriate use of placebos can disentangle the act of intervention from the inherent benefits (and risks) of the intervention itself.

7.3. CLINICAL TRIAL SAMPLE SIZE

Sample Size Components

In the context of an RCT, a set of hypotheses are generated regarding the influence of an intervention on the primary outcome of interest. In a typical two-arm comparative study, the null hypothesis is stated as the default or status-quo position as it exists prior to conduct of the clinical trial (e.g., that no difference exists between the intervention and control groups in terms of the primary outcome of interest). The alternative hypothesis depends on the type of study, but can be one of the following: superiority study—that the intervention arm is superior, or noninferiority study—that the intervention arm is not inferior to the control arm. Equivalence trials are designed to prove that the intervention and control arms are identical. They generally have larger sample size requirements due to the narrow confidence intervals required for such studies.

Sample size determination (for an RCT) can be calculated by mathematical formulae, tables, and computer calculators depending on the following parameters:

1. *Statistical power.* This is defined as the probability that a study will reject the null hypothesis in favor of the alternative hypothesis. Generally, most well-designed studies will have power of at least 80% (sometimes ranging as high as 95%).
2. *Type I (α) error.* This error is the false-positive rate of the trial, in which the study does find a difference between the intervention and control groups where no true difference exists. Typical type I error rates are in the range of 5% or less as clinical trialists attempt to reduce the possibility of finding a false benefit of an intervention. It is important to note that based on this statistical construct, around 5% of well-designed positive clinical trials may have reported false-positive results.
3. *Type II (β) error.* The type II error rate is the probability that a study will not find a difference when a true difference between the control and intervention arms exists. This is otherwise known as the false-negative rate, which is mathematically related to the power probability by the following equation: power = $1 - \beta$.
4. *Effect size.* This is the magnitude of the expected difference between the intervention and control groups. If the expected difference of the intervention is expected to be large, then sample sizes tend to be smaller.
5. *Baseline endpoint variance.* This is related to the precision of endpoint assessment. In situations where the endpoint of interest is not precisely measured, larger sample sizes are required to resolve differences between groups, in order to ensure accurate determination of the mean endpoint estimates of both intervention and control groups.

Other Sample Size Considerations

Another important consideration with regards to sample size determination includes an adjustment for the proportion of individuals that will be lost to follow-up on their own accord or will not be followed up entirely due to other parallel events (e.g., 6-month cancer survival trial, but a proportion of patients may die prior to this timeframe due to other illnesses). In this case, a loss to follow-up adjustment is required, whereby the initial calculated sample size should be adjusted by the expected proportion lost to follow-up in order to calculate the final sample size for the clinical trial.

7.4. CLINICAL TRIAL ADMINISTRATION

Clinical Trial Protocol

A clinical trial protocol is a document created to provide background information, objectives, hypotheses, inclusion/exclusion criteria, intervention and control treatment details, as well as statistical considerations (including primary and secondary endpoints and sample size determination) of a clinical trial. In addition, clinical trials will also have information related to the reporting of adverse events, as well as an informed consent document for patients to review and sign. The purpose of the protocol is to ensure that all individuals follow a common set of procedures to ensure that the final results of the trial can be properly interpreted.

Clinical Trial Oversight

Various parties are responsible for the appropriate oversight of clinical trials. They generally include:

1. *Study sponsor.* The sponsor of a clinical trial can consist of a private enterprise, university, or another entity responsible for the conduct of the study. Some studies are directly sponsored by physicians and/or scientists funded by peer-reviewed grants or other granting opportunities internal or external to the location where the research takes place. Study sponsors have the responsibility to ensure that patients and investigators are aware of relevant information regarding the interventions and control treatments being utilized in the clinical trial. This is done by the creation of a clinical protocol, informed consent document, as well as communication of important adverse events. Many studies also use the services of a data safety monitoring committee to assess either blinded or unblinded data to ensure the ongoing safety and nonfutility of the clinical trial.
2. *Investigators.* Physicians and other scientists are responsible for the day-to-day conduct of the clinical trial to ensure protocol compliance, appropriate patient informed consent, staff supervision, patient safety, and the review and reporting of adverse events. Serious events need to be reported to the study sponsor and the IRB by predefined time periods and procedures.
3. *IRB (ethics).* IRBs review clinical protocols and informed consent documentation to ensure that patient safety, clinical trial ethics, and privacy are assessed and protected. Clinical trials routinely undergo periodic review to ensure that patient safety and privacy continue to be protected. Also, significant adverse events need to be reported to the IRB in order for an ongoing assessment of the relative benefits and risks of clinical trial continuation.
4. *Regulatory agencies.* Depending on the jurisdiction of the clinical trial and the nature of the intervention, various regulatory agencies can be involved with the approval of clinical protocols and the review of evidence from such protocol prior to either protocol activation or intervention approval for clinical use. In the United States, the Food and Drug Administration (FDA) serves this role for the evaluation of new drugs and medical devices.

Clinical Trial Registration

Increasingly, clinical trials are required to be registered on a publicly available registry (such as a Web site), in order to qualify for publication in a variety of high-impact journals. This is done in order to facilitate information transfer between investigators and institutions, to avoid duplication of effort, and to assist in the creation of knowledge transfer documents such as meta-analyses. Historically, clinical trials were performed and many trials were not published if the intervention was not found to be of benefit. This has led to a publication bias in the literature where negative results are underrepresented. Ultimately, the registry movement has been created to improve the validity and transparency of the published (and unpublished) medical literature.

Clinical Trial Reporting Standards

Another issue of importance with regard to clinical trials is the unbiased and accurate reporting of completed clinical trials in the medical literature. Reporting standards allow for a standardized approach to prepare clinical trial reports in order to improve readability, reduce bias, and facilitate critical appraisal. Different reporting standards do exist; the dominant approach utilized by major medical journals is the Consolidated Standards of Reporting Trials (CONSORT). The 2010 version of the CONSORT statement consists of a 25-item checklist listing the technical requirements for the reporting of trial design, patient flow, results, and interpretation (www.consort-statement.org).

7.5. CRITICAL APPRAISAL

Fundamental Concepts in Critical Appraisal

The critical appraisal of medical literature is concerned with the methodological and systematic assessment of the strength, reproducibility, and applicability of evidence to a clinical scenario or patient population. In general, the main domains that need to be assessed for clinical trials include study methodology, results assessment, and an external assessment of the results as they apply to a patient population or disorder of interest. During a critical appraisal encounter, a focus on potential issues that may have led to biased or incorrect results needs to be performed, in order to assess the strength of the conclusions that can be drawn from the evidence. Also, an understanding of other similar literature (e.g., clinical trials, knowledge translation documents) needs to occur in order to put the individual study in appropriate context. Various educational resources are available to teach critical appraisal techniques, including the Centre for Evidence-Based Medicine (www.cebm.net).

Critical Appraisal of Clinical Trials

Different approaches exist for the evaluation of various forms of evidence including RCTs, prognosis studies, diagnostic studies, and meta-analyses. In the context of RCTs, the following approach as detailed by Guyatt is routinely used.

1. *Assessment of internal validity.* This section of the critical appraisal requires an assessment of the fundamental methodology utilized in the clinical trial. A focus on the following questions is helpful in determining the internal methodological validity:

   - Was a well-defined population of patients recruited for the study?
   - Were the patients randomized to the intervention and control groups?
   - How was the randomization performed? Was there any possible bias with the randomization procedures?
   - Were all patients in the trial accounted for and analyzed in the assigned group (e.g., intent-to-treat analysis)?
   - Were blinding procedures for the patients, investigators, outcome assessors, and statistician(s) utilized in the trial?

2. *Assessment of results.* The second section of critical appraisal assesses the statistical and clinical significance of the study results by calculation of the size and precision of the treatment effects.

   - Treatment effect size can be calculated by one of four parameters including: relative risk (ratio of outcome in intervention vs. control group, with RR = 1 meaning no difference between groups), absolute relative risk (ARR, risk of outcome in control minus intervention group, with ARR = 0 meaning no difference between groups), relative risk reduction (RRR, the ARR divided by the control risk rate which allows for an assessment of the relative change in risk due to the intervention), and the NNT (which is the inverse of the ARR and reflects the number of patients that need to be exposed to the intervention to prevent one primary outcome event). A related concept to NNT is

the NNH, which calculates the number of patients that are exposed to an intervention that will lead to one negative outcome of interest. The comparison of NNT and NNH can be a useful exercise to assess the clinical utility of an intervention.
- Treatment effect precision can be assessed by looking both at the point estimate and the variation of intervention and control outcomes. This is usually reported as a 95% confidence interval. If the point estimate of an intervention falls within the 95% confidence interval of the control group outcome, then the trial will be reported as a negative trial, as the null hypothesis was not rejected on statistical grounds.

3. *Assessment of external validity.* In this final phase of critical appraisal, the individual must assess whether or not the clinical trial results apply to the management of the patient at hand, other related clinical trial evidence, the feasibility of such treatment in terms of treatment availability, logistics, funding, and toxicity, as well as the therapeutic ratios (i.e., the benefits versus the harms of the intervention).

Forms of Bias in Clinical Trials

There are several forms of bias in clinical trials. Randomization, stratification, and blinding can address many of them if successfully employed. Some common forms of bias are listed herein:

1. *Assessment bias.* Improper assessment of primary or secondary study outcomes.
2. *Ascertainment bias.* Patient assignment is known within a blinded study (e.g., due to specific side effects of the intervention), which can lead to biased outcome reporting.
3. *Performance bias.* Systematic differences in nonprotocol treatment (i.e., co-interventions) between control and intervention groups.
4. *Attrition bias.* A difference in length of follow-up between intervention and control groups.
5. *Allocation bias.* Systematic differences in baseline prognostic factors between control and intervention groups.

7.6. CANCER CLINICAL TRIAL ENDPOINTS

A variety of traditional (e.g., survival), nontraditional (e.g., health-related quality of life), and surrogate (e.g., response rate) endpoints exist to support the construction and interpretation of cancer clinical trials. Approvals of interventions do not necessarily need to be based on the traditional survival endpoint, as other clinically important endpoints have been used to justify the approval and use of various interventions in oncology. A list of common endpoints used in oncology clinical trials are presented herein:

1. *Survival.* This is usually calculated from the date of death (or last follow-up) to the date of diagnosis, start of treatment, or end of treatment.
2. *Mortality.* Similar to survival time, mortality rate is a percentage of individuals surviving to a fixed period of time.
3. *Tumor response.* This endpoint can be expressed as a proportion of patients achieving a level of either cross-sectional or volumetric response to treatment. Related endpoints include the response duration (total time in which a response was observed) or time to tumor progression (time between tumor progression and treatment initiation/completion). A commonly used system for the assessment of solid tumors is the Response Evaluation Criteria in Solid Tumors (RECIST) criteria (Therasse et al., 2000) that have specific rules for measurable and nonmeasurable lesions/disease to classify patients into complete response (CR—complete resolution), partial response (PR—at least 30% cross-sectional sum reduction), stable disease (SD—neither PR or PD), and progressive disease (PD—at least 20% cross-sectional sum increase).
4. *Disease-free survival.* This is defined as the time a patient survives with no sign of any disease. A related but different concept is the progression-free survival. Progression-free survival is the time that a patient may have a disease that is clinically and/or radiologically apparent but progression has not occurred (see RECIST defined previously).
5. *Time to treatment failure.* Defined as the time of treatment initiation to treatment discontinuation.
6. *Health-related quality of life.* Various general, treatment-specific, disease-specific, and symptom-specific health-related quality-of-life (HRQOL) instruments have been validated for clinical use in the medical literature. HRQOL is a relevant primary or secondary endpoint, particularly in trials assessing symptom palliation and metastatic patient populations.
7. *Symptom improvement.* Various symptom scores (e.g., 10-point pain scale) relevant to the manifestations of malignancy and the effects of treatment are available in the literature. Selection of these endpoints must be done carefully in order to ensure that the symptom assessment is unbiased and clinically relevant to the disease process and mechanism of action of the intervention.
8. *Tumor markers.* Several cancer processes are related to the detection of tumor markers. These marker levels can be proportional to the underlying burden of disease and can indicate tumor response and progression. Examples of tumor markers in clinical use include CA-125 (ovarian), PSA (prostate), as well as alpha-feto protein and beta-HCG (germ cell tumors).

7.7. SURVIVAL ANALYSIS

Overview

Survival analysis allows for the graphical or tabular depiction of the estimated survival curve function of percentage survival (or other cancer outcome) versus survival time. Another more general term for survival analysis is a time-to-event analysis, in which any event can be assessed versus event time. As the sample size of a patient population increases, the estimated function approaches the true function of the population of interest. A tabular representation of survival analysis is otherwise known as a life table and the graphical representation is known as a Kaplan–Meier curve.

Life Tables

A life table depicts the proportion of patients surviving, experiencing events, and patients censored during predefined time periods (intervals). Using this approach, the probability density (probability of failure per time period) and the hazard rate (probability that a patient alive at the beginning of a time interval will die during that interval) are calculated. A cumulative proportion surviving curve (the life table survival function) can be generated by the product of the proportion of the original population (at time zero) that are alive at the beginning of the time interval and the interval survival rate (Figure 7.3).

Kaplan–Meier Curves

In the context of a Kaplan–Meier curve, as events occur, the survival curve "ticks" off events by reducing the percentage survival (y-axis) by the proportion of events versus total patients at risk during that period of time (Figure 7.4). Conceptually, a Kaplan–Meier curve can be

Interval (years)	Number at risk	Number dying	Number removed alive	Probability dying	Probability of interval survival	Probability of overall survival
0	100	–	–	–	–	1
0.001 –1.0	100	10	10	0.1	0.9	0.9 (1x0.9)
1.001 –2.0	80	8	7	0.1	0.9	0.81 (0.9x0.9)

→ Multiplicative factors

FIGURE 7.3 Life tables

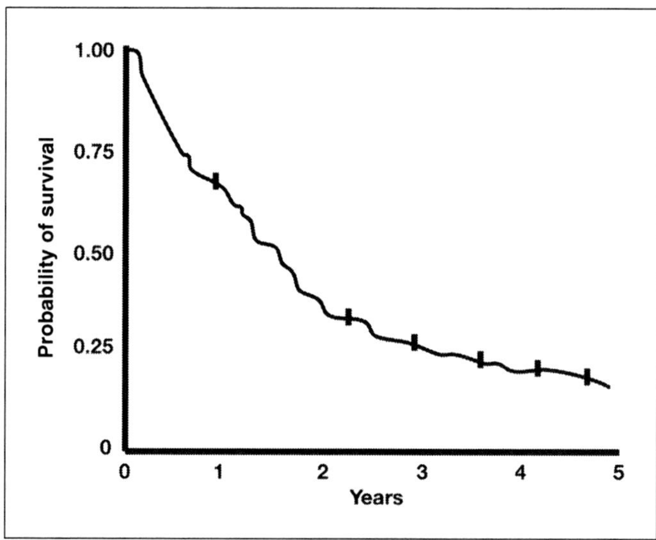

FIGURE 7.4 Kaplan–Meier curve

considered to be a life table with infinitely small time intervals. Patients who have not experienced the event (i.e., death in a standard survival curve) are considered to be right-censored (noncomplete information) and are graphically depicted as a hash mark and no longer contribute to the number of patients at risk of future events. The comparison of two survival curves can be performed with the parametric Cox proportional hazards test or a nonparametric-based log-rank test.

7.8. KNOWLEDGE TRANSLATION

Review Articles

Review articles are written in order to summarize the knowledge on a topic of interest. Generally, review articles synthesize, interpret, and summarize research findings as previously reported by other research teams, as opposed to presenting new research results. Review articles are usually classified as either narrative (literature) reviews or systematic reviews. A literature review logically presents referenced medical evidence in an unbiased manner to provide a summary of present knowledge and concepts for future research.

A systematic review is a more rigorous form of literature review, in which a set of study inclusion and exclusion criteria are created to guide the review process. Often, the level and quality of evidence can be assessed by existing instruments or checklists. In addition, a search strategy is utilized in order to ensure a complete list of abstracts and papers for review. A well-known group that conducts systematic reviews is the Cochrane Collaboration. The Cochrane methodology for the creation of systematic reviews utilizes an eight-step process: (a) review question(s) and study criteria development, (b) study search, (c) study selection and data abstraction, (d) bias assessment, (e) data analysis with possible meta-analysis, (f) reporting bias assessment, (g) summary results/findings, and (h) interpretation and conclusions.

Meta-analysis

A meta-analysis is a statistical methodology in which multiple studies assessing a similar hypothesis are combined together to estimate an effect size related to an intervention. The main advantages of this approach include: increased statistical power, assessment of study variation, assessment of possible publication bias, and improved decision making due to multiple versus single study assessment. Known disadvantages of the meta-analysis methodology includes: incomplete assessment of bias and possible lack of study quality assessment. Information obtained from meta-analysis can be presented in different ways; however, the forest plot is a common method to graphically display the odds ratio of the intervention versus control of all studies included in the meta-analysis (Figure 7.5).

Practice Guidelines and Consensus Statements

A practice guideline differs from literature reviews, systematic reviews, and meta-analyses, in that medical evidence is gathered in order to provide guidance to medical practitioners based on expert consensus after review of the best available evidence to guide practice. Consensus statements are documents similar to practice guidelines, where a group of experts review medical evidence on a topic of interest and draft a list of evidence-based or expert opinion statements that are designed to guide medical practitioners. Practice guidelines and consensus statements are usually coordinated by various organizations that are interested in the topic to be studied. In oncology, the American Society of Clinical Oncology, the National Comprehensive Cancer Network, and the American Society of Radiation Oncology (among other organizations) have created practice guidelines and consensus statements for a variety of tumor sites and treatment scenarios.

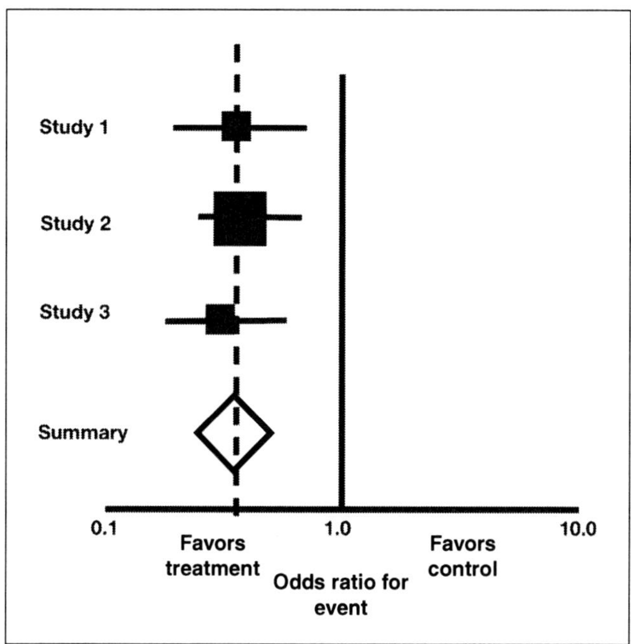

FIGURE 7.5 Meta-analysis forest plots

7.9. PREDICTIVE AND PROGNOSTIC FACTORS

Overview

Although frequently used interchangeably, the terms *predictive factors* and *prognostic factors* refer to separate but related concepts important to medicine (and oncology).

1. *Predictive Factor.* A predictive factor is a patient or disease-related variable that has been shown to be related to the response (or lack of response) to a defined treatment course. Such predictive factors may demonstrate that a differential response to treatment exists (e.g., one group will benefit while the other does not or has inferior response).
2. *Prognostic Factor.* A prognostic factor is a patient or disease-related variable that has been shown to be directly related to patient outcome irrespective of treatment regimen delivered (e.g., absence of therapy or standard therapy given). These factors are more related to the natural history of the disease.

Predictive and prognostic factors can be statistically calculated by the use of logistic (for binary outcomes) or Cox regression (for continuous time-to-event outcomes) techniques. In addition, various statistical constructs exist with the relationship between predictive factor and outcome/disease status in the context of diagnostic testing (Figure 7.6).

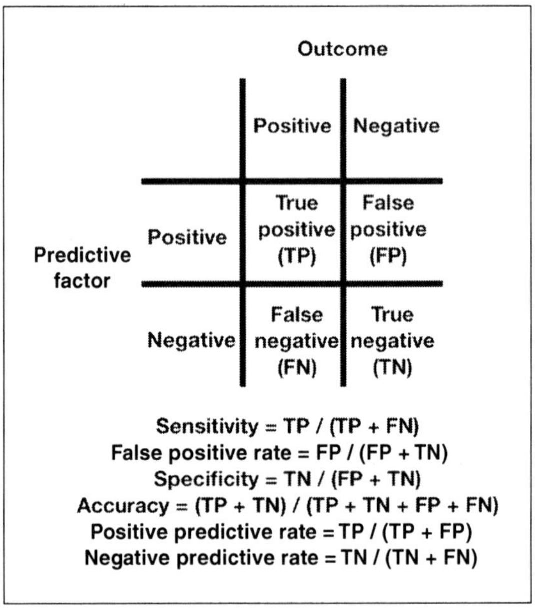

		Outcome	
		Positive	Negative
Predictive factor	Positive	True positive (TP)	False positive (FP)
	Negative	False negative (FN)	True negative (TN)

Sensitivity = TP / (TP + FN)
False positive rate = FP / (FP + TN)
Specificity = TN / (FP + TN)
Accuracy = (TP + TN) / (TP + TN + FP + FN)
Positive predictive rate = TP / (TP + FP)
Negative predictive rate = TN / (TN + FN)

FIGURE 7.6 Predictive factor statistical considerations

Chapter 8

Cancer Epidemiology

KEY POINTS

- Factors that are found to be related with an outcome of interest are known to be "associated" with each other. Causality is highly difficult to prove; yet, the following features are considered to increase the evidence of causation: strength of association, consistency, specificity, temporality, biological gradient, plausibility, coherence, analogy, and experimental evidence.
- Cancer incidence is the number of new cases of a specific cancer over a specified period of time per unit of population. Cancer prevalence is the number of patients (new and preexisting, but alive) with a specific cancer at a period of time per unit of population. Cancer mortality can be expressed as a survival rate at a specified time frame or as a mortality risk for a fixed time period per population unit.
- Known cancer risk factors include age, sex, geography, genetic susceptibility/family history, ethnicity, and socioeconomic status.

8.1. EPIDEMIOLOGICAL PRINCIPLES

Epidemiology is a branch of medicine concerned with the incidence, distribution, and control of disease. The word is derived from the Greek language roots *epi* and *demos*, literally translating into "the study of what is upon people." It can be more accurately defined as the study of the distribution and determinants of health-related states or events in specified populations, and the use of this knowledge to address health and disease concerns. In the previous chapter, we introduced the multidisciplinary science of clinical epidemiology and the associated types of clinical studies. In this chapter, we focus our attention on the application of this science to cancer research to define cancer risk factors, prognostic factors, and trends that continuously refine the clinical practice of oncology.

Causation and Causality

Determining the cause of disease allows identification of the factors that can ultimately lead to disease prevention, and the goal of linking risk factors to cancer remains central to cancer epidemiology. Causation within the scope of cancer epidemiology generally implies that there exists sufficient evidence to say with a degree of certainty that reducing exposure to a particular risk factor would be followed by an eventual observable reduction in the frequency of a particular cancer. Causal inferences typically rely on two components: an observed association between the proposed causal factor and the probability of the outcome, and a plausible proposed mechanism to explain the observed association.

The concept of causation remains difficult to define as it is impossible to say with certainty that one event causes another because often we cannot physically observe the actual production of the effect, but can only say that one event is followed by the other. For example, we know excessive alcohol consumption is a risk factor for laryngeal cancer because we can observe the association that many of those who get laryngeal cancer have a history of excessive drinking. Conversely, we know this cancer occurs less frequently in those who do not drink. However, we cannot say definitively that alcohol always causes laryngeal cancer because there are many individuals who drink excessively who do not get laryngeal cancer, and there are some nonconsumers of alcohol who develop this cancer. Potentially, there are one or more outside factors, either known or unknown, that also affect the probability of the outcome, known as confounders. In the case above, a known confounder would be smoking, whereas unknown confounders could include genetic and environmental factors not yet known for laryngeal cancer. Furthermore, we cannot manipulate this potential cause and accurately predict a change in the outcome/disease probability (i.e., cannot accurately predict the effect of reducing alcohol consumption from 10 to 4 beers/day and predict the reduced likelihood of cancer). Determination of causes of cancer is made particularly difficult as it is now recognized that most cancers are multifactorial in their nature, meaning they have multiple causes that work together to increase the probability of cancer developing. Therefore, a working definition of causation in epidemiology means that a causal factor is associated with a difference in the probability of the outcome.

Multiple criteria and models for causality have been proposed over the years. One of the earliest and most famous examples stemmed from Robert Koch's research into bacteria as the causation of disease. Published in 1890 and recognized with a Nobel Prize in 1905, Koch postulated a set of criteria for determining whether a particular bacteria (organism) caused a disease:

1. The bacteria must be present in every case of the disease.
2. The bacteria must be isolated from the host with the disease and grown in pure culture.

3. The specific disease must be reproduced when a pure culture of the bacteria is inoculated into a healthy susceptible host.
4. The bacteria must be recoverable from the experimentally infected host.

Numerous further modifications and refinements of these rules followed, but the postulates above do reveal the goal of empirically identifying a causal association and the reproducibility and consistency of the association, and the ability to prove that association within experimental conditions. The aspects of association to be considered to determine causation were further refined by Sir Bradford Hill in 1965 and form the criteria commonly used to judge causality today (Figure 8.1):

1. *Strength.* Statistical strength and magnitude of the association. A larger measured effect makes it less likely that the effect results from chance, confounding, or moderate bias.
2. *Consistency.* The association between exposure and outcome is a persistent finding in multiple observations and studies conducted by different investigators, in different settings.
3. *Specificity.* A cause having very few observed effects, and conversely, an effect having a low number of causes increases the specificity claim. This remains difficult given the multifactorial nature of cancer causes.
4. *Temporality.* The cause must occur before the outcome or effect of question.
5. *Biologic gradient.* An increase of strength/exposure of the purported cause results in a finding of a graded increase in the observed effect. Observed biologic or dose–response gradient strengthens the case for causality as most confounders should not exhibit a closely linked gradient.
6. *Plausibility.* An observed association should be explained by substantive biological arguments.
7. *Coherence.* A causal association should not violate laws of science and should remain consistent with fundamentally accepted knowledge.
8. *Analogy.* If a proposed exposure and outcome relationship is very similar to an already observed and accepted causal association, then it is suggested that the standards of evidence required to make the similar association is reduced.
9. *Experiment.* Randomized evidence that test the cause and effect association will strongly impact the ability to judge the truth of the causation claim. However, randomized experiments on humans are often not possible or ethical.

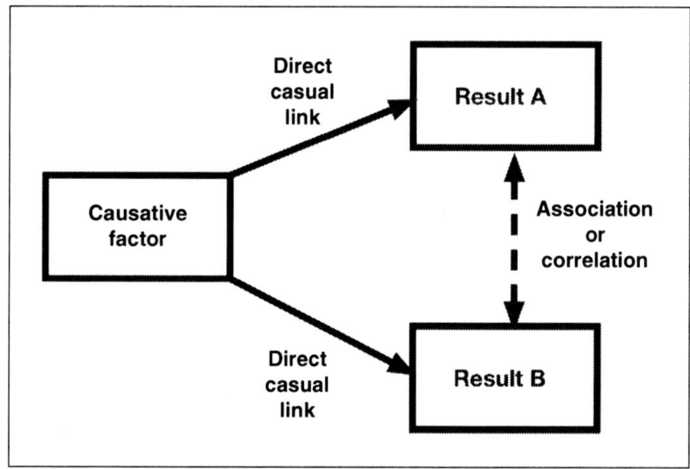

FIGURE 8.1 Association versus causation

8.2. INCIDENCE AND SURVIVAL

Cancer Incidence

The incidence of cancer is the number of new cancer cases occurring in a population at risk for the disease over a specified period of time, usually 1 year, per 100,000 individuals in that population (Figure 8.2). The cancer incidence rate is a measure of the absolute risk of getting the disease and a method of expressing the cancer burden within a particular population at risk.

Cancer incidence rates can be expressed as crude or age-adjusted rates. Crude incidence rate represents an average risk for an entire population and is essentially the number of new cancer cases per 100,000 individuals. An age-adjusted incidence rate can be a more useful comparator to different populations as it accounts for variations of incidence in different age brackets by expressing incidence as a weighted average. This allows for a comparison between populations that differ significantly in composition (i.e., one town where 40% of the population is over the age of 60, compared to another where only 10% is over the age of 60).

Cancer incidence is on the rise, and the World Health Organization reports that the expected new global cancer diagnoses will grow to 15 million by the year 2020. The leading causes of cancer incidence worldwide are lung, breast, and stomach cancer. However, there is huge geographic variation as a result of various genetic, environmental, and cultural/behavioral risk factors.

Cancer Prevalence

Also known as point prevalence, cancer prevalence is defined as the number of cases of cancer present in a population at a specific point in time, divided by the number of individuals

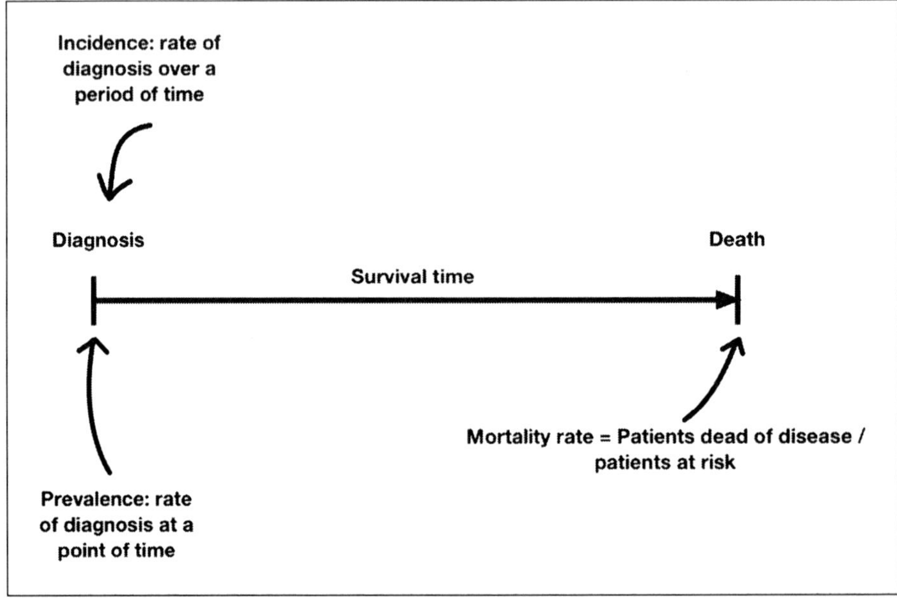

FIGURE 8.2 Cancer incidence, prevalence, survival, and mortality

in the population (or per unit population, Figure 8.2). These represent individuals who have been previously diagnosed with a cancer and are still alive at a given point of measurement, whether their cancer is active or in remission. If one counts only those diagnosed in the last 5 years, this is termed a partial prevalence. The most prevalent cancers worldwide are breast, colorectal, and prostate, likely attributable to their significant incidence coupled with better prognosis.

Cancer Survival

Survival rates are usually referred to as the relative proportion of individuals from a particular cancer cohort still alive at a given time point past their diagnosis. It is a very important measure used in clinical trials to report clinical outcomes of cancer therapies (see Section 7.7). Although cancer survival is generally reported at a 5-year interval, shorter or longer intervals can be more appropriate for a given cancer type (Figure 8.2). For example, for most head and neck squamous cell carcinomas, a 2- or 3-year survival measure is considered significant given that these cancers tend to be very aggressive, with the majority of relapses occurring within the first 2 to 3 years post treatment. Similarly, a 10-year survival interval would be more appropriate for most low-risk prostate cancers, given the slow and prolonged nature of the disease.

Common measures of expressing survival are overall survival and disease-free/cancer-specific survival. Overall survival in oncology is the number of individuals, with a given cancer, free of death from any cause at a time point after their diagnosis. Generally, overall survival is measured from the time of diagnosis until the event of death from any cause, including cancer. Disease-free survival is the number of individuals considered cured or in remission from a cancer, and is usually from a given time point (most often diagnosis, to the time that a cancer recurrence is confirmed). A related measure is progression-free survival, where the event of cancer progression is variably defined by various researchers (i.e., development of a new area of metastases, growth of a tumor by 20% on CT scan).

8.3. MORTALITY

Cancer Mortality

The annual cancer mortality rate is the number of deaths from cancer in a 1-year period divided by the population at risk during that period, expressed as per 100,000 individuals (Figure 8.2). A similar and more commonly reported measure is the death rate, which is an expression of the cancer mortality as the number of deaths from a given cancer annually per 1,000 people with that specific cancer.

The leading causes of cancer mortality worldwide are lung, stomach, and liver cancers. In the United States, combined cancer death rates have continued to decline since the 1990s, driven largely by improved outcomes in screening and treatment of common cancers such as breast, colorectal, and prostate cancers, and a decline in lung cancer incidence (Annual Report to the Nation on the Status of Cancer, Eheman et al., 2012). A similar downward trend in cancer mortality has been reported in Canada, but these pooled statistics can mistakenly be taken to imply that there have been improvements in mortality for all cancers, which is incorrect given that mortality from cancers such as pancreatic and liver cancers have been shown to increase in that time period, likely related to increasing incidence. However, studying cancer mortality rates allows one to understand the longer term impact(s) of screening, diagnostic, and treatment interventions, and the effects of shifting patterns of cancer risk factors.

8.4. PREDISPOSITION AND GENERAL CANCER RISK FACTORS

According to the American Cancer Society, the lifetime risk of developing an invasive cancer is 45% for males and 38% for women, while the risk of dying of these cancers is 23% and 20%, respectively. As discussed earlier in this chapter, epidemiologists have long understood the strong association between certain behaviors and risk factors, such as tobacco consumption and the development of various cancers. However, given that not all individuals who smoke will ultimately develop a malignancy, it is realized that carcinogenesis is a multifactorial process. Individuals can be thought of as having a given baseline set of general risk factors, with some having greater predisposition to the risk of developing or dying of cancer. Those baseline predisposing factors that have been studied for many years are most commonly related to age, sex, geography, ethnicity, genetic susceptibility, and socioeconomic status. The latter factor of socioeconomic status ties in to more recent research into the lifestyle choices that increase cancer risk. In this section, these general baseline risk factors are briefly explored, while modifiable lifestyle factors (such as obesity) and infectious causes are discussed in Section 9.1.

Age

The risk of developing cancer is most strongly correlated to increasing age, and increases sharply after age 50, likely related to an accumulation of risk factors and genetic damage that increases the likelihood of carcinogenesis. In developed countries, over 60% of all cancers are diagnosed in individuals over the age of 65, and a third in those over the age of 75. This is influenced by the predominance of the most common cancers (with prostate, breast, colorectal region, and lung being most prevalent) in older age groups.

Sex

Overall rates of cancer incidence and mortality have a slightly male predominance of M:F ratio of 1.2:1 and 1.5:1, respectively. Cancers that most differentially occur in males are head and neck (especially larynx and pharynx) and bladder, while breast, gallbladder, and thyroid malignancies occur more commonly in women.

Geography

Significant geographic variations exist in cancer incidence and mortality and are likely a reflection of large variations in underlying risk factors (i.e., genetics, ethnicity), changes in infectious patterns of disease, cultural and behavioral practices, availability and access to health care (including cancer screening, diagnostic services, and treatment), and reporting of cancer outcomes.

Genetic Susceptibility and Family History

Genetic syndromes that predispose individuals to cancer development are thought to contribute toward 5% to 7% of human cancers. The syndromes and the underlying genetic abnormalities were discussed in Section 2.10. The most common known hereditary cancer syndromes are hereditary non-polyposis colorectal cancer (HNPCC, aka Lynch syndrome), familial adenomatous polyposis (FAP), neurofibromatosis Type 1 (NF-1), and hereditary breast ovarian cancer (most commonly *BRCA1* and *BRCA2*). The number of known cancer syndromes likely pales in comparison to the vast number of still unknown genetic variants and mutations that predispose certain individuals and families to malignancy. It is generally accepted that individuals with a family history of cancer have a risk of developing a malignancy equal to that of a person 5 to 20 years older (Goossens and DeGreve, 2010). For example, an individual with a family history of colorectal cancer would on average have the same risk at age 40 as an individual without family history does at age 50. Genetic testing, when available, should be discussed with patients with significant family histories of cancer, from identifiable high-risk groups, multiple primary malignancies, or with unusually young age of presentation.

Ethnicity

Observed differences in incidence and mortality of various cancers amongst individuals of different ethnic backgrounds are currently thought to only be a partial reflection in differences of genetic susceptibility. For example, women of Ashkenazi Jewish background have high prevalence of *BRCA* alleles, predisposing them to breast and ovarian cancers. However, the majority of observed differences related to ethnicity are likely confounded by socioeconomic differences, cultural practices, diet, and environmental risk factors. For example, south Asians have a high incidence of oral cancers, likely related to the common cultural practice of chewing betel nuts, a known carcinogen linked to oral cancers.

Socioeconomic Status

Socioeconomic status is considered one of the major predictors of all health outcomes. Within a developed population, lower socioeconomic status and educational level is generally associated with a higher rate of cancer incidence and death. This is likely related to a higher prevalence of health-related risk factors (i.e., smoking, obesity, poor nutrition), and decreased access to health-care services and treatments. More affluent populations tend to have better access to screening and diagnostic tests that can result in earlier detection and treatment. Multiple studies confirm that lower socioeconomic status is associated with significant differences in overall survival and cancer-specific survival. A Canadian study of community median income in the province of Ontario revealed substantial differences in 5 years overall survival for most cancers between the poorest and richest communities, with the most pronounced absolute survival difference being 16% for cervical cancer (Booth et al., 2010).

8.5. MOLECULAR EPIDEMIOLOGY AND CANCER

Molecular epidemiology is a relatively new and rapidly expanding field that is shaping the understanding of human cancer by studying the underlying genetic patterns of both individuals with cancer, as well as malignant cells themselves. Studies made possible by the complete sequencing of the human genome (first completed in 2003 as the Human Genome Project) and advances in laboratory techniques have spawned this new area of research, which was broadly applied to all diseases, and subsequently to cancer genomics (Hartman et al., 2010). Similar to the epidemiological study of a disease attempting to associate habits and risk factors with disease causation, molecular epidemiologists have scoured the human genome in large-scale studies to identify patterns of genetic variation linked with the development of cancer.

The initial basis of molecular genetics studies was the identification of gene alleles that varied by a single nucleotide, but still have a prevalence of more that 1% within the population. These variations are termed single nucleotide polymorphisms (SNPs), and their presence within a gene can alter its function, predisposing one to the presence of disease. The ability to type multiple SNPs at a single time gave way to large studies aiming to identify SNPs within the genome that imparted a greater susceptibility to cancer development. However, over 7 million SNPs have been identified in the human genome, while only a handful have thus far been associated with various cancers. Beyond SNPs, other areas of variation in the human genome, such as epigenetics (variation in DNA methylation patterns), are undergoing intensive oncological study.

Aside from the testing of individuals, testing of malignant tumors using DNA microarrays has allowed the identification of given molecular markers within malignant cells that are involved in cell division and metabolic pathways. Identifying and understanding the various patterns of expression of molecular markers will allow subclassification of tumor types on the basis of genomics, and not just histology. Ultimately, this may be used for prognostication and clinical decision making to determine the likelihood of response to a given treatment and also to determine new targets for therapeutic medications. For example, in the treatment of lung adenocarcinoma, a patient's tumor can be routinely tested for two known mutations in the gene for the epidermal growth factor receptor (EGFR), with deletions at exon 19 and substitutions at exon 21. These are highly predictive of response to targeted treatment with tyrosine kinase inhibitors. More recently, expression assays testing gene signatures of between 16 and 97 known variants have been developed for the subclassification and prognostic stratification of breast cancers and are used in clinical practice to aid treatment decisions.

As whole genome testing becomes more cost-effective and commonplace, understanding of cancer from cellular to molecular processes will drive the development of new screening tests. These will allow prognostic risk stratification of newly diagnosed individuals and will ultimately shape future oncological practice.

Chapter 9

Prevention and Screening

KEY POINTS

- Modifiable risk factors to reduce the risk of a cancer diagnosis include: smoking status, alcohol intake, obesity/diet/physical activity, sexual practices, contaminated injections, and environmental exposures.
- Various active cancer prevention strategies for high-risk patient populations exist and include: drug chemoprevention, breast cancer surgical prophylaxis, gynecological surgical prophylaxis, and colorectal surgical prophylaxis. Cancer screening attempts to identify patients at an earlier stage of disease to improve outcomes at both the individual and population level (e.g., breast, prostate, colorectal, and gynecological).
- Various viruses have been shown to be related to cancer risk, which include hepatitis B virus (HBV) and human papillomavirus (HPV). Vaccination strategies are available for these viruses in order to reduce potential infection and potential cancer development.

9.1. RISK FACTOR AVOIDANCE

Although advances in cancer therapeutics dominated the oncology focus in the late 20th century, in recent years, the focus has shifted sharply to reducing the overall burden of cancer through preventative and screening measures. It is claimed that one-third of all cancers could be prevented by behavioral changes, and early detection of many cancers could lead to superior outcomes (Danaei et al., 2005). Other estimates of this collective environmental risk, based on twin studies that control for genetic factors, have suggested a 50% contribution to cancer development. For example, the decline in lung cancer mortality in men in the Western hemisphere is largely attributable to a decrease in lung cancer incidence, secondary to successful efforts to decrease smoking rates rather than significant therapeutic advances in cancer treatment. While certainly not all cancers can be prevented through behavior modification, it has been estimated that one-third of cancer deaths worldwide can be directly attributed to modifiable risk factors.

Smoking

Use of tobacco is currently considered the number one avoidable risk factor for cancer development, and is linked to the development of approximately 21% of the world's cancers, and nearly 1.5 million cancer-related deaths annually (Danaei et al., 2005). Given that nearly one in five North American adults are smokers, continued efforts and education for smoking cessation are crucial to reducing cancer incidence.

Alcohol Intake

Excess consumption of alcohol is linked as a primary risk factor in 5% of all human cancer cases, and is most commonly linked to head and neck and liver malignancies. Recently, focus has shifted to a link between alcohol consumption and increased breast cancer risk. An observational study of over 105,000 women found even those with cumulative low lifetime consumption of alcohol (three to six drinks per week) had a 15% relative risk increase of developing breast cancer, although the effect that confounding factors, such as mammography screening and exercise, had on the results is unclear (Chen et al., 2011). A safe level of alcohol consumption has yet to be established, as this link continues to be studied.

Obesity

Given the rising incidence of obesity as an epidemic in the developed world, it is a particularly concerning cancer risk factor. Studies of obesity in the United States have linked increased risk of becoming obese with lower socioeconomic and educational status; groups unfortunately are also considered to be at slightly higher risk for adverse global health outcomes. Being overweight (body mass index [BMI] > 25) or obese (BMI > 30) is associated as a prime risk factor in approximately 2% of all cancer cases, most commonly linked to the development of colorectal, postmenopausal breast, endometrial, esophageal, kidney, and pancreatic malignancies (Eheman et al., 2012; Danaei et al., 2005). The mechanism is likely complex and multifactorial related to changes in sex hormones, growth factors, insulin, and immune responses, which can all contribute to the cascade of carcinogenesis. Evidence from meta-analyses suggest that each increase in BMI of 5 can be associated with a 30% to 60% increased risk of endometrial, kidney, and esophageal cancers and a 13% to 18% increased risk of colorectal, pancreatic, or breast malignancies (Eheman et al., 2012). Furthermore, excessive weight may be associated with adverse survival impact amongst patients with breast and colorectal cancers. A focus on developing healthy eating habits and preventing onset of obesity in childhood and adolescence has been advocated to prevent the long-term incidence of oncological and other diseases.

Diet

Low fruit and vegetable intake has been associated with approximately 5% of human cancer cases, most commonly those affecting the aerodigestive tract. A suggested mechanism for this benefit relates to increased fiber intake as the primary factor resulting in increased stool bulk and decreased colonic transit time (thus reducing the exposure of the digestive mucosa to possible ingested carcinogens). Furthermore, increases in intake of folate and antioxidants could decrease the likelihood of cancer development. Lastly, individuals with increased fruit and vegetable intake are less likely to be overweight and physically inactive. Recent studies have suggested a modest benefit of decreased cancer risk, favoring those with higher dietary vegetable intake (Boffetta et al., 2010). A recent meta-analysis suggested that a vegetable and fruit intake threshold of between 100 and 200 g/day could be associated with an estimated 10% decreased risk of colorectal cancer (Aune et al., 2011). In addition to increased fruit and vegetable intake, reduced consumption of red or charred meats, avoidance of foods exposed to pesticides, hormones, and antibiotics, and reduced consumption of heavily processed products have all been proposed as part of a healthy diet that could minimize consumption of potential carcinogens and conceivably reduce overall cancer risk.

Physical Activity

Similar as a risk factor, and linked with the development of obesity, lack of physical activity is still considered an independent cancer risk factor, and ongoing research is examining the link between exercise and cell cycle changes. For adults, guidelines for physical activity have recommended 75 minutes of vigorous or 150 minutes of moderate aerobic activity per week. For U.S. children, 60 minutes of cardiovascular activity a day, 7 days a week has been proposed as a goal. Lack of physical activity has been associated with an approximate 30% to 40% increase in the risk of colorectal, postmenopausal breast, and endometrial malignancies (Eheman et al., 2012).

Sexual Practices

Unsafe sexual practices, primarily unprotected intercourse, are a major risk factor for the transmission of human cancer viruses, most specifically human papillomavirus (HPV), hepatitis B and hepatitis C, and HIV. Unsafe sexual practices contribute to 3% of worldwide cancer cases, but most concerning is the major risk factor for the development of cervical cancer, one of the most preventable female malignancies. For full discussion on infectious etiologies of cancer and prevention, see Section 9.3.

Contaminated Injections

Similar to unsafe sexual practices, the use of virus-contaminated injection apparatus in a healthcare setting is a particularly significant cancer risk factor in the developing world. Rates of infection when exposed to percutaneous injury with infected blood are estimated to be 6% to 30%, 1.8%, and 0.3 % for hepatitis B, hepatitis C, and HIV, respectively. Safe needle handling precautions and disposal guidelines should be strictly followed for reduction of risk to healthcare workers. Healthcare workers should be vaccinated against hepatitis B. In countries where resources exist, healthcare workers exposed to blood products through needle-stick injuries should follow postexposure prophylaxis procedures, if indicated, to reduce the risk of infection. In addition to cleansing of the site, the virus status of the source of the blood should be identified and or tested, if possible. Local occupational health guidelines should subsequently be followed to determine whether individuals exposed to possible HIV or hepatitis B infected blood should be offered postexposure prophylaxis in the form of highly active antiretroviral therapy or hepatitis B immunoglobulin, respectively. There is no currently available effective postexposure prophylaxis for hepatitis C virus.

Environmental Air Pollution and Household Smoke Exposure

Exposure to carcinogens in the air from industrial sources and second-hand smoke is a significant risk factor for the development of lung carcinoma. An estimated 10% to 25% of lung carcinomas worldwide occur in never smokers, with cumulative exposure before age 25 posing the highest risk. Living in close proximity to factories, oil refineries, high traffic areas, and other sources of airborne carcinogens, such as formaldehyde, benzene, carbon tetrachloride, polycyclic aromatic hydrocarbons, naphthalene, and 1,3-butadiene, have been associated with a 1.3 to 1.7 relative lung cancer risk increase as found by case-control and cohort studies (Stewart, 2012). While community air pollution is a difficult risk factor to modify for many individuals, second-hand smoking exposure is a potentially modifiable risk factor through increased antismoking regulations and decreased exposure of children to second-hand smoke in the home and in vehicles.

9.2. THERAPEUTIC PREVENTION STRATEGIES

Surgical Prophylaxis

The use of surgery for prophylaxis of cancer development is most established in the management of individuals with very high genetic risk of inherited cancer syndromes. While the use of prophylactic surgery in many instances is still controversial, it has been well established in the management of patients at high risk for colorectal, breast, and gynecological malignancies.

Colorectal Cancer Surgical Prophylaxis

The most common hereditary syndromes associated with the development of colorectal cancers are familial adenomatous polyposis (FAP), MYH-associated polyposis (MAP), and Lynch syndrome (aka hereditary nonpolyposis colorectal cancer). FAP is characterized by numerous adenomas within the colon, and a near 100% risk of developing colorectal cancer by age 40. Given this high penetrance, total colectomy ± proctectomy is generally recommended as early as is feasible to reduce the risk of cancer development. While this surgery is potentially curative, there is still up to a 45% lifetime risk of developing cancerous adenomas at the site of anastomosis; these patients must therefore still undergo lifetime colonoscopy surveillance. Patients with genetically confirmed MAP are generally recommended to undergo annual colonoscopy surveillance for polyp removal, and are recommended for colonic resection if polyp size, burden, or histology becomes increasingly concerning. Patients with Lynch syndrome have an 80% lifetime risk of colorectal cancer development. For patients with confirmed Lynch syndrome, the use of prophylactic colectomy is more controversial, because frequent colonoscopies at an interval of between 1 and 2 years should identify most cancers and premalignant polyps. This approach is thought to confer a better quality of life in patients who are amenable to surveillance.

Gynecological Cancer Surgical Prophylaxis

The lifetime risk of ovarian cancer development in patients with *BRCA1* and *BRCA2* gene mutations is 25% to 40% and 15% to 25%, respectively, much higher than the baseline risk of 1.5%. Therefore, patients with known *BRCA* mutations should have a discussion regarding prophylactic risk–reducing bilateral salpingo-oophorectomy, which has been shown in studies to reduce ovarian cancer risk up to 96%. Further studies have suggested a decreased breast cancer risk of 50% in patients of this population undergoing the procedure. While the procedure is relatively safe and cost-effective, the side effects include induction of early menopause and loss of fertility. While the optimal timing of the procedure is not fully established, it is generally recommended that women have the procedure once childbearing is complete, and typically before age 35 for *BRCA1* and age 40 for *BRCA2*. Lynch syndrome also increases the risk of ovarian cancer, as well as endometrial cancers. Although prophylactic bilateral salpingo-oophorectomy should be discussed with patients with Lynch syndrome, its role has not been fully explored. Lynch syndrome does confer a lifetime risk of endometrial cancer between 20% and 60%. Although hysterectomy has been shown to prevent the development of endometrial cancer, given that it is a cancer that is often diagnosed early and managed, a survival benefit to prophylactic hysterectomy has not yet been established. In patients with Lynch syndrome undergoing surgical colectomy, discussion should occur with the patient about the possibility of concomitant hysterectomy and salpingo-oophorectomy.

Breast Cancer Surgical Prophylaxis

Patients at high risk of breast cancer are typically identified by the presence of a known genetic syndrome (most significantly, but not limited to *BRCA1* and *BRCA2*) or by a significant family history of breast cancer that suggests a possible hereditary component and strong individual risk. Although recent studies are suggesting an increased role for MRI surveillance for early detection of breast cancer development, the long-term results of such approaches are still unknown. Patients at high risk of breast cancer or with known *BRCA* mutations should have a discussion regarding the use of prophylactic mastectomy, as this surgical approach has been demonstrated to prevent up to 90% of breast cancers, and up to 95% when combined with bilateral salpingo-oophorectomy. However, given the obvious physical and potential psychological ramifications of prophylactic mastectomy, the decision to undergo this procedure versus enhanced surveillance should undoubtedly be based on individual risk factors and the result of informed shared decision making between patient and physician.

Chemoprevention

The use of pharmaceuticals, vaccines, or nutrient supplements to prevent the development of precancerous lesions or halt the progression of these lesions to malignancy is termed *chemoprevention*. The success of vaccinations in the prevention of cancers related to infectious agents is discussed in Section 9.3. Pharmaceutical agents studied for these properties often include anti-inflammatory agents (i.e., acetylsalicylic acid for colorectal cancer risk), hormonal targets (i.e., selective estrogen receptor modulators for breast cancer), or modulators of cell growth cycles and growth factors (i.e., metformin, which may affect breast cancer risk through modulation of insulin-like growth factors). Unfortunately, only a minority of agents have been proven as effective chemotherapeutic agents in phase 3 trials and received approval from the Food and Drug Administration for this purpose (listed in Table 9.1, as recently described by Davis and Wu, 2012).

TABLE 9.1 Selected Chemopreventative Therapies

Disease Site	Lesion Type	Therapy
Premalignant		
Genitourinary	Bladder Dysplasia	Intravesical BCG or anthracycline (Valrubicin)
Gynecological (cervical, vulvar cancers)	Dysplasia/Intraepithelial neoplasia	Vaccination against HPV
Gastrointestinal (esophageal, anal cancers)	Esophageal Dysplasia	PDT (porfirmer sodium based)
	Anorectal Dysplasia	Vaccination against HPV
Skin	Actinic Keratosis	Masoprocol, 5-FU, Diclofenac Sodium, 5-ALA + PDT
Malignant		
Breast	DCIS, Atypical ductal/lobular hyperplasia	Selective Endocrine Receptor Modulators (Tamoxifen, Raloxifene)

9.3. VACCINATION PREVENTION STRATEGIES

Infectious Agents Associated With Cancer

In 2002, it was estimated that almost 18% of cancers worldwide (approximately 1.9 million cases) were associated with an infectious etiology, whether it be a virus, bacteria, or parasite. The idea of an infectious agent as a carcinogen is based on the understanding that the infection contributes to the development of malignancy through carcinogenesis by a combination of genetic alteration of the cell and/or impairment of immune function. Typically, cancer-associated infectious agents are characterized by the establishment of chronic rather than acute infections, and a prolonged period of time between the onset of infection and development of malignancy. However, the majority of those infected do not ultimately develop malignancy.

A period of prolonged infection can establish an environment for carcinogenesis through three broad mechanisms: virus-induced transformation (by either causing alterations in the regulation of the cell cycle including activation of oncogenes or inhibition of tumor suppressors), local effects of chronic inflammation (leading to higher proliferation of tissue, direct DNA and cell membrane damage, and increased potential for DNA mutagenesis through release of cytokines and reactive oxygen species), or immunosuppression (altered cytotoxic lymphocyte responses and inability to manage malignant precursor cells). Infectious agents associated with human cancers are listed in Table 9.2.

Cancer Vaccination

Recent efforts at cancer prevention have focused on vaccination as a strategy to reduce the risk of contracting oncogenic infections. With regard to prevention, the two most widespread

TABLE 9.2 Common Infectious Agents and Associated Sites of Human Malignancies

Virus	Cancers
Human papillomavirus (HPV)	Cervical, anal, oropharyngeal cancers, and small proportion of mouth, penile, vulvar, and vaginal cancers.
Hepatitis B virus (HBV)	Hepatocellular carcinoma
Hepatitis C virus (HCV)	Hepatocellular carcinoma
Epstein-Barr virus (EBV)	Nasopharyngeal cancer, Burkitt lymphoma, Hodgkin lymphoma, posttransplant lymphoproliferative disorder
Human herpesvirus 8 (HHV8, also known as Kaposi's sarcoma-associated herpesvirus (KSHV))	Kaposi's sarcoma, typically found in conjunction with HIV-infected individuals
Human T-lymphotropic virus 1 (HTLV-1)	Adult T-cell lymphoma
Southeast Asian liver fluke (*Opisthorchis viverrini*)	Cholangiocarcinoma (bile duct)
Schistosoma (blood flukes)	Bladder cancer
Helicobacter pylori	Gastric cancer
HIV	HIV-related immunosupression linked with the development of HHV8-related Kaposi's sarcoma, and increased risk of non-Hodgkin lymphoma

strategies have focused on reducing the transmission of hepatitis B virus (HBV) and the HPV through vaccination programs. It is estimated that global vaccination programs aimed at these two viruses alone will prevent over 1 million cancer deaths per year.

Hepatitis B Virus

HBV is associated with a significantly increased risk for the development of hepatocellular carcinoma (HCC), which is within the top two causes of male cancer death worldwide. Chronic infection in the carrier state for HBV is thought to lead to a state of chronic inflammation, which causes an environment predisposed to the development of malignancy. There are over 350 million carriers of HBV worldwide, with the virus being particularly endemic in sub-Saharan Africa and Eastern and Southeast Asia, where carrier rates approach 20%. Those who are carriers of HBV have an approximately 100 times greater risk of developing HCC than noncarriers. In highly endemic areas, vertical transmission perinatally or in early childhood predominates, whereas in countries of low carrier frequency, transmission is mainly horizontal in adult populations by sexual transmission or engagement in high-risk activities such as needle sharing. Although a therapeutic vaccine for HBV has not yet been developed, a prophylactic vaccine against infection was first brought to market in 1982 that was shown to prevent transmission of infection in 90% of neonates and prevent contraction of HBV in 95% of children. Targeted worldwide vaccination strategies in endemic areas have already shown reduced carrier state rates from 8%–15% to 1%–2%, with a resultant decline in the rates of HCC development. Currently, over 90% of the world's countries, including Canada and the United States, have routine HBV vaccination programs.

Human Papillomavirus

There are nearly 100 strains (types) of HPVs, a sexually transmitted infection that can affect the epithelia of the anogenital area and upper aerodigestive tract, causing issues ranging from anogenital warts, dysplasia, and ultimately malignancy. Chronic HPV infection is believed to be the sole cause of cervical cancer, one of the leading causes of cancer death in woman worldwide, and more recently has been implicated in anal and oropharyngeal cancers in both males and females. Cervical HPV infection is common, and it is estimated that three-quarters of women in the United States will have at least one infection in their lifetime, though the majority are able to clear the infection on their own, and only a small fraction of those infected will go on to develop a cancer. The most prevalent high-risk HPV oncogenic virus types are HPV-16 and HPV-18, which code for oncoproteins, through viral genes E6 and E7 that inactivate tumor suppressor genes and provide favorable conditions for the development of dysplasia that may lead to carcinogenesis. Although the majority of cervical cancers are prevented in the developed world through screening, it is estimated that the majority of the 275,000 cervical cancer deaths a year occur in the developing world, where funding and lack of access to primary screening remain significant challenges. In 2006, vaccines that prevent infection of HPV-16 and HPV-18 have been used clinically after large phase 3 trials revealed between 98% and 100% efficacy in preventing the development of cervical intraepithelial neoplasia. The long-term efficacy in terms of protection beyond 6 years after administration, and the role of vaccination in females with already 5 to 10 years of sexual activity (increased likelihood of previous HPV exposure and/or infection) is debated. Another controversy of the vaccination program in developed nations is the type specificity of the vaccines, which does not prevent infection with other potentially serious HPV strains, and thus does not yet obviate the need for continued screening with Pap smears. Vaccination programs targeting adolescent females and more recently, males, have been enacted in industrialized countries, and global strategies to develop and deliver the vaccine to developing nations where the impact could be most profound are being advocated.

9.4. EFFECTIVE CANCER SCREENING

Secondary prevention of malignancy through the use of an intervention across a broad asymptomatic population to aid in the early diagnosis of the disease is called cancer screening. A screening intervention aims to establish whether an individual from an at-risk population is likely to have a given disease, by which further investigations could be indicated in hopes of diagnosing disease earlier in its natural history. The premise is that a cancer detected at an earlier or premalignant state could potentially be easier to cure or even prevent. Common cancer screening tests can take many forms including a physical exam maneuver (i.e., digital rectal exam), blood test (i.e., prostate-specific antigen testing [PSA]), diagnostic scan (i.e., mammogram), or even cytology (i.e., Pap smear). In this section, the use of screening in an oncological context is discussed in detail.

Principles of Cancer Screening

Cancer screening is itself an intervention that is applied to a largely asymptomatic population that is likely to be healthy and free of disease. Given that a screening intervention may have potential side effects, carries a risk of false diagnosis, and holds a risk of perpetuating further unnecessary interventions, one must justify the appropriateness and effectiveness of a screening program for a given malignancy. Principles to guide cancer screening were developed by the World Health Organization:

- A suitable screening test should exist that is accurate, safe, cost-effective, easy, and acceptable to apply to a population at large.
- Natural history of the cancer should allow for a detectable preclinical phase, which allows an opportunity for early detection.
- The disease should be an important public health problem in terms of frequency and severity.
- A treatment intervention for early detected cancer, which favorably improves the outcome and mortality from disease, should exist.
- A screening strategy indicating a target population and the timing and implementation of the screening test should exist and be based on scientific evidence.

Genetic Counseling

Cancer genetic counseling is a process by which an individual's cancer risk is assessed through an examination of family and personal cancer history, and discussion of possible genetic mutations and human cancer syndromes that could be implicated. Genetic counseling can often, but does not always, lead to genetic testing for known human cancer mutations, though the number of unknown mutations outweighs the relatively small number of identifiable mutations. Guidelines exist to identify individuals that may warrant referral for genetic counseling (Weitzel et al., 2011):

- Early onset of cancer (i.e., colon cancer before age 50)
- Individual with more than one primary cancer
- Cancers in multiple generations on same side of a family
- Constellations of cancers associated with cancer syndromes (i.e., breast + ovarian [*BRCA*], colon + endometrial [Lynch])

- Rare cancers (retinoblastoma, adrenocortical carcinoma)
- Unusual presentation of cancer (i.e., male breast cancer, ocular melanoma)
- Uncommon cancer histology (i.e., medullary thyroid carcinoma)
- Geographic populations known to be of high risk for hereditary cancer (i.e., Ashkenazi Jewish)
- Strong family history of a particular cancer
- Unusual or dysmorphic physical features

Based on these criteria, an individual will be referred. Typically, a genetic counseling session will fundamentally include a careful history with particular attention to family history of cancer, pedigree construction, and a careful physical exam with attention paid to the presence of possible dysmorphic or syndrome-associated findings. Synthesizing this information to conduct a risk assessment for an individual, one first seeks to estimate an individual or family member's risk of cancer, whether it could be caused by a single genetic mutation, and whether testing could conceivably identify the mutation. If the latter parameter is met, then DNA testing can be offered. DNA testing can potentially be beneficial in identifying key genetic mutations for individuals at risk, and can be subsequently used to make recommendations on screening and surveillance. However, there are numerous pitfalls to DNA testing, including the psychological impact of potentially carrying a mutation, the risk of false positives, confidentiality of results, and insurance ramifications. Therefore, appropriate genetic counseling should always guide decisions about pursuing genetic testing. Genetic counseling will continue to have a growing role in cancer care as increasingly sophisticated DNA testing techniques mature and become adept at identifying individual cancer mutations and molecular cancer risk profiles.

9.5. CANCER SCREENING EXAMPLES

Breast Cancer Screening

Mammography as a screening tool has been commonly implemented since the 1960s, and is based on the premise that the detection of nonclinically palpable breast tumors can lead to the diagnosis of tumors when they are smaller. The size of a breast tumor at diagnosis can affect the surgical management (breast conservation vs. mastectomy), decision regarding systemic treatment, and prognosis as smaller tumors are less likely to have spread to regional lymph nodes, or metastasized.

Multiple large-scale randomized clinical trials have demonstrated a survival benefit in favor of using mammography screening. A recent U.S. Preventative Services Task Force meta-analysis reveals that the relative risk of breast cancer mortality with mammography for women aged 40 to 49 and 50 to 59 are 0.85 and 0.86, respectively, while in the 60 to 69 year age groups, it is 0.68. Although the ~15% reduction in risk in the former age group seems significant, in the context of screening, this translates into having 1,904 women aged 40 to 49 undergo a routine mammogram to prevent one extra cancer death, whereas screening 377 women in the 60 to 69 age group would achieve the same effect. Screening for women aged 70 and older is controversial, and the aforementioned report found no evidence of benefit in this population, while the 2011 Canadian Task Force on Preventative Health Care report suggests screening women in the 70 to 74 age bracket every 2 to 3 years. The current U.S. and Canadian guidelines on screening are summarized in Table 9.3. The breast screening guidelines do not apply to high-risk populations, such as those with personal or first-degree family history of breast cancer, known *BRCA* mutations, or previous chest wall irradiation (i.e., childhood Hodgkin's disease).

Colorectal Cancer Screening

Screening for colorectal cancers has been associated with an approximately 16% decrease in mortality. This benefit is derived from identification of premalignant polyps (adenomas), which can be removed endoscopically before they progress to invasive carcinomas, thus significantly reducing colorectal cancer incidence. The average time from onset of a polyp to development of invasive malignancy is long, estimated at approximately 10 years.

The most commonly utilized screening tools are the fecal occult blood test and colonoscopy. Fecal occult blood tests measure for the presence of hemoglobin, which can indicate a gastrointestinal source of bleeding warranting endoscopy to find a possible polyp or cancer. A solitary fecal occult blood test is subject to a risk of false negative, and so screening is done with multiple (usually two or three) samples to increase the sensitivity of this test. Positive

TABLE 9.3 Breast Cancer Mammography Screening Guidelines

Age (yr)	40–49	50–59	60–69	70–74	>75
U.S. Preventative Task Force (2009)	Shared decision making	Every 2 years	Every 2 years	Every 2 years	Insufficient
Canadian Task Force on Preventative Health Care (2011)	Not recommended	Every 2–3 years	Every 2–3 years	Every 2–3 years	Not recommended

fecal occult blood testing necessitates the use of colonoscopy, a form of flexible endoscopy that allows visualization and assessment of the rectum and entire colon, and removal of any lesions encountered. Although colonoscopy has not been directly studied, use of one-time flexible sigmoidoscopy (which only allows assessment of the rectum and left colon) has demonstrated a 31% reduction in colorectal cancer mortality. Therefore, current guidelines are based on the premise that colonoscopy is likely superior to flexible sigmoidoscopy, as it allows assessment of the complete colon. Traditional colonoscopy is the preferred technique of surveillance for individuals at high risk of colorectal cancer, but its cost-effectiveness as a primary screening tool for the average-risk population is debated. While guidelines differ, a summary of the American College of Gastroenterology recommendations are presented in Table 9.4.

Newer techniques of colorectal assessment, including virtual computed tomographic colonoscopy and camera capsule endoscopy may not confer the procedural risk of traditional colonoscopy. However, they do not allow removal of polyps at the time of identification and may not be as sensitive in detecting small lesions. Therefore, their role as a screening tool is still being defined.

Prostate Cancer Screening

Given the very heterogeneous nature of the disease, which runs the spectrum of slow growing and indolent disease to very aggressive forms, screening for prostate cancer is a controversial topic with conflicting guidelines on the use of the two currently available screening tests. The two screening tests are the digital rectal examination (DRE) and PSA testing. PSA is a glycoprotein that is produced almost exclusively by the prostate and allows liquefaction of semen, and is usually elevated in prostate cancer. A test to measure its presence was developed in 1986, and has since been widely adopted as a screening tool for men at increased risk of prostate cancer. Adoption of the PSA test has been thought to be the main contributor to the significantly increased incidence of prostate cancer, given the increased detection of asymptomatic cases. Given that many men with prostate cancer are destined to have indolent disease and not die of their cancer even in the absence of treatment, concerns regarding overidentification of cases and hence overtreatment are becoming more

TABLE 9.4 Colorectal Cancer Screening Recommendations (American College of Gastroenterology, Rex et al., 2008)

Group	Comments	
Average risk	Preferred: colonoscopy for 10 years beginning at age 50 (45 in African-Americans) Alternative: flexible sigmoidoscopy for 5 to 10 years, CT colonography for 5 years, or annual fecal occult blood testing	
Positive family history in single first-degree relative	Age of relative ≥ 60 years	Same as average risk
	Age of relative < 60 years	Colonoscopy for 5 years beginning at age 40 years or 10 years younger than the age of onset of the youngest affected relative
FAP	Annual flexible sigmoidoscopy or colonoscopy until time of colectomy; thereafter flexible sigmoidoscopy for 6 to 12 months if retained rectum	
Lynch	Colonoscopy every 2 years beginning at age 20 to 25 years, then annually after age 40 years	

CT, computed tomography; FAP, familial adenomatous polyposis.

prominent. Two very large randomized control trials, the U.S. Prostate, Lung, Colorectal, and Ovarian (PLCO) Cancer Screening Trial and European Randomized Study of Screening for Prostate Cancer have found either a nonexistent or very small and minimal mortality benefit of screening, respectively. The European study found that one cancer death is prevented for every thousand men screened between the ages of 55 and 69 years.

Given that PSA screening will lead to a significant proportion of patients undergoing biopsy, and ultimately being exposed to the morbidity of surgery, radiation, or hormones, the utility of PSA as a screening tool has been questioned because the harms to the majority of men may outweigh the benefits to a select few. Based on this, in 2012, the United States Preventative Task Force made a highly publicized and controversial recommendation against all PSA screening. This recommendation has been recently criticized by the American Urological Association, which maintains its recommendation that all men with a life expectancy of > 10 years should be offered PSA testing and DRE, with a baseline at age 40, and rescreening intervals should be determined by the physician thereafter. This controversy is likely to exist until more substantial evidence is produced, or a better screening test becomes available.

Cervical Cancer Screening

The development of cancers of the uterine cervix can be identified through morphologic changes in the cervical tissue that indicate a premalignant lesion, termed *cervical intraepithelial neoplasia.* A prime example of an effective cancer screening program is the implementation of the Papanicolaou test, commonly called a Pap smear, which has resulted in a significant decline in cervical cancer incidence and mortality by approximately 80% since its adoption as a screening tool in the last 60 years. This cytological test, which has evolved over the years, involves using a brush to scrape cells from the endocervix, which can be studied for abnormal cytology. Based on the presence of atypical or dysplastic cells, patients can be referred for a more definitive method of evaluation termed *colposcopy*, where the lesions can be directly visualized and biopsied under magnification. In this way, early premalignant lesions are identified and removed before having the ability to develop into invasive malignancies.

Given that most cervical malignancies are HPV related (see Section 10.3), recent screening programs have attempted to incorporate the use of testing cytological specimens for HPV DNA of the high-risk HPV types. This has been suggested as a method for interpreting the results of indeterminate cytological specimens termed atypical squamous cells of undetermined significance. Despite increasing vaccination against HPV in the at-risk population, present guidelines still recommend that the vaccinated population undergo cervical screening. Current cervical cancer screening guidelines recommend cervical cancer screening with Pap smears starting at age 21 (or 3 years after age of first intercourse), and continuing to age 65. The latest recommendations from the American Cancer Society recommend Pap smear screening every 3 years for women between age 21 and 29 years, and every 5 years with an HPV DNA test from age 30 to 65 years. It has been recommended not to screen women over age 65 with a history of normal smears, or women who do not have a cervix due to previous hysterectomy for nonmalignant causes.

Ovarian Cancer Screening

Carcinomas of the ovaries are most commonly diagnosed at an advanced stage and are associated with a poor survival. The use of population-based screening for ovarian cancer has focused on the use of the CA-125 tumor marker and transvaginal ultrasound.

CA-125 is a glycoprotein that is secreted by serous papillary and other types of ovarian tumors. Elevation of CA-125 increases the chances of a patient having ovarian carcinoma. Transvaginal ultrasound allows visualization of the ovaries and fallopian tubes for morphological changes suggestive of disease. Given that definitive diagnosis generally requires an invasive surgical procedure (e.g., laparotomy), it is important for these tests to have a low false-positive rate to avoid exposing too many women to an unnecessarily risky procedure. The large randomized PLCO Cancer Screening Trial found that offering annual CA-125 testing for 6 years and annual transvaginal ultrasound for 4 years to women aged 55 to 74 years did not reduce ovarian cancer mortality (Buys et al., 2011). Currently, there is no accepted screening regimen for asymptomatic women. A large randomized trial of over 200,000 postmenopausal women conducted by the UK Collaborative Trial of Ovarian Cancer Screening Group (UKCTOCS) is ongoing and is hoping to answer this question.

Chapter 10

Cancer Staging

KEY POINTS

- Cancer staging is instrumental in obtaining information regarding the anatomical spread of cancer and to support appropriate decision-making. Stage information also helps in inter-physician/institutional communication and clinical trials. Various staging systems exist including those created by the American Joint Committee on Cancer and the International Union Against Cancer (UICC).
- Cancer diagnosis and workup attempt to answer several questions including: whether cancer is present, what type of cancer is present, and what is the extent of disease.
- The dominant system of stage classification for most solid tumors is the tumor nodes and metastases (TNM) system, in which each aspect of cancer staging is then combined to provide an overall stage grouping from stage I (highly localized) to stage IV (disseminated). Other factors, including pathological and tumor markers, are increasingly being used in cancer staging.
- A variety of staging rules exist to deal with clinical versus pathological staging, neoadjuvant/re-treatment, multifocal disease, and unknown staging among others.
- A variety of non-TNM staging systems exist and are commonly used for lymphomas, myeloma, gynecological cancers, colon cancers, melanomas, and testicular tumors.

10.1. INTRODUCTION

Cancer Stage

The extent of a cancer within an individual patient is defined as its stage. Thus, a cancer that has progressed and spread is defined as having an advanced stage. Advancing stage generally implies a poorer prognosis. Staging of cancers has traditionally and still remains largely based on anatomic extent of spread; yet, recent efforts have sought to incorporate other non-anatomical factors (e.g., tumor markers) affecting prognosis as modifiers of stage.

Staging cancer at the time of diagnosis and treatment decision has become a crucial descriptor by which physicians can clearly communicate a patient's disease status and on which appropriate decisions regarding treatment can be made. Furthermore, a consistent system of staging cancers facilitates the conduction of clinical research and the applicability of its results from one center to another.

Staging Systems

A desire to develop a systematic approach and language for assigning cancer stage led to the development of staging classification systems. These earlier efforts in 1929 have evolved into the most commonplace staging systems used today, with the primary system being updated and maintained by the American Joint Committee on Cancer (AJCC). The AJCC staging system is largely based on the tumor nodes and metastases (TNM) system developed by the International Union Against Cancer (UICC), and unifies other various site-specific systems that had been previously developed. The AJCC releases periodic updates to the staging system, making relevant changes on the basis of new evidence regarding factors affecting treatment and prognosis, with the most recent release of the seventh edition in 2010. The TNM system is described in depth in Section 10.3.

10.2. CANCER DIAGNOSIS AND WORKUP

Diagnosis of cancer can occur in a multitude of ways, but one way to dichotomize these various patient presentations is asymptomatic and symptomatic classifications. Diagnosis of asymptomatic malignancy in patients can occur through screening or incidentally through routine clinical examination or imaging for another purpose. Cancer screening, the use of a targeted intervention over a large population to diagnose malignancy in asymptomatic individuals, is discussed in depth in Chapter 9. Incidental primary tumors, known colloquially as "incidentalomas," have increasing presentation secondary to more widespread use and availability of cross-sectional imaging.

The path to a diagnosis of symptomatic malignancy is highly variable among patients. A clinician must retain a high index of suspicion for malignancy when clinical symptoms and patient risk factors warrant placing cancer high on the differential diagnosis. A clinical history, including risk factors for cancer and family history, and focused physical examination can be used to direct the clinical workup that may include blood tests, imaging (see Chapter 6), and referral for diagnostic interventions aimed at locating and defining a site of primary tumor. Once a possible primary tumor has been located, two essential questions must be answered: (a) what kind of tumor is present? and (b) if cancer is present, what is the extent of disease? Ideally, the presence of tumor must be confirmed pathologically through the use of biopsy or cytological techniques. Typically, a primary tumor is preferred to be sampled when it can be obtained safely and easily accessible nodes (i.e., neck, axilla) can often be sampled as well to obtain pathological information.

Once the presence of malignancy has been confirmed, then the focus of clinical workup is aimed at defining the extent, or "stage" of disease. Investigations that may be warranted include specific blood work, such as tumor markers, and imaging aimed at defining the extent of primary involvement, and also the presence of lymph node or distant metastases. Recommended clinical workup varies significantly according to the site of primary tumor, the clinical suspicion of early or advanced disease, patient symptoms, and local practices based on availability and timeliness of technologies and tests. For example, a computed tomography (CT) scan of the brain is often done routinely in the absence of neurological symptoms for workup of advanced small cell cancers of the lung given the high likelihood of brain metastases in these patients. However, a CT scan of the brain would not be done routinely for women with a small, very early primary tumor in the breast in the absence of neurological symptoms, given the low likelihood of finding metastatic disease. A fine balance must be struck between the increasing access to technologically advanced imaging modalities, such as positron emission tomography–CT scanning, and their cost effectiveness and evidence-based utility in staging and making clinical treatment decisions. Large oncological organizations, such as the National Comprehensive Cancer Network and Cancer Care Ontario, have developed practice guidelines based on reviews of the literature, which include recommendations on initial workup of newly diagnosed cancers.

10.3. TUMOR NODES AND METASTASES STAGING AND GROUPING

Tumor Nodes and Metastases Classification

The TNM staging system is an anatomic-based system first developed by the surgeon Pierre Denoix in the late 1940s, and subsequently evolved to form the foundation of the current AJCC cancer staging system. TNM stands for tumor (local tumor size/spread), nodes (regional nodal involvement), and metastases (distant spread of tumor beyond regional lymphatics). An individual cancer is assigned a numeric sub-classification (typically ranging from 0 to 4, or the unknown "X" denotation) for each of three categories (Figure 10.1). The general framework for this numeric sub-classification is:

1. *Tumor*
   - T0: no evidence of primary tumor.
   - Tis: in situ carcinoma.
   - T(1–4): increasing primary size or extent.
   - Tx: primary cannot be assessed (often used in cancers of unknown primary origin [PUK]).
2. *Nodes*
   - N0: no lymph node spread.
   - N(1–3): increasing number of nodes involved or extent/location.
   - NX: nodal status cannot be assessed.
3. *Metastases*
   - M0: no distant metastases.
   - M1: distant metastases present.
   - Mx: (unable to assess metastatic spread) has been removed from the AJCC 7th edition and M0 should be used in its place.

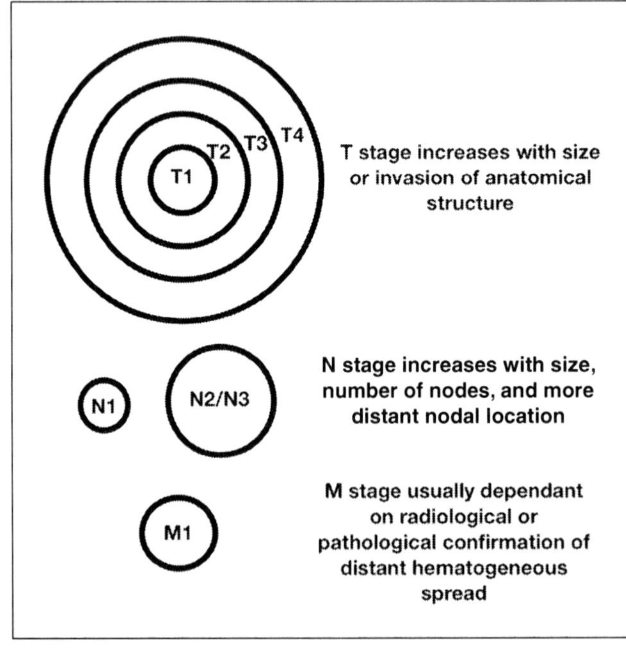

FIGURE 10.1 The TNM staging paradigm

Tumor Nodes and Metastases Stage Groupings

Based on this site-specific classification, a cancer typically will be grouped into one of four stage categories (I, II, III, and IV). The stage groupings seek to place TNM classifications with similar prognoses into the same bracket, varying according to tumor site. For example, a T2N1 breast cancer with N1 lymph node spread is a stage II grouping, whereas a T2N1 bladder cancer with N1 lymph node spread is considered stage IV, reflecting the differentially poorer prognostic implications of nodal spread in bladder cancer. Recent efforts have been made to incorporate non-anatomic factors into the stage groupings for various cancers (i.e., PSA, Gleason score as prognostic predictors for prostate cancer).

10.4. STAGING CONSIDERATIONS

Classification Prefixes/Designators

TNM classification is based on clinical (physical examination, imaging, and tests) or pathologic (at time of surgery, autopsy) evaluation (Figure 10.2). Given that the timing and information used to assign a stage is crucial for decision making, TNM classifications are often preceded by a prefix, typically "c" or "p" indicating clinical or pathologic staging (i.e., cT1N1M0). Special situations, including post-neoadjuvant treatment, re-treatment, and autopsy are noted below, though the latter two are used less frequently in clinical scenarios.

1. *Clinical (c).* Defined as stage before definitive treatment and within 4 months of diagnosis (pre-treatment), based on symptoms, physical examination, imaging, and investigations including diagnostic scopes and biopsies.
2. *Pathologic (p).* Staging based on surgical resection of the primary and/or lymph nodes and examination of the specimen by pathologist, and is generally given preference over clinical stage when it can be assessed, as it is more predictive of prognosis.
3. *Post-(neoadjuvant) treatment (y).* The y modifier is used to re-stage a patient to communicate response to a given therapy, and can be done either clinically (denoted as yc) or pathologically (denoted as yp).
4. *Re-treatment (r).* Used for re-staging of a recurrent or progressive tumor following initial therapy.
5. *Autopsy (a).* Assigned based on pathologic findings at time of autopsy, and most commonly used to document previously undiagnosed tumors.

As noted above, pathologic staging will trump clinical staging and can result in change to both the numeric sub-classifications, and thus overall stage groupings. This phenomenon

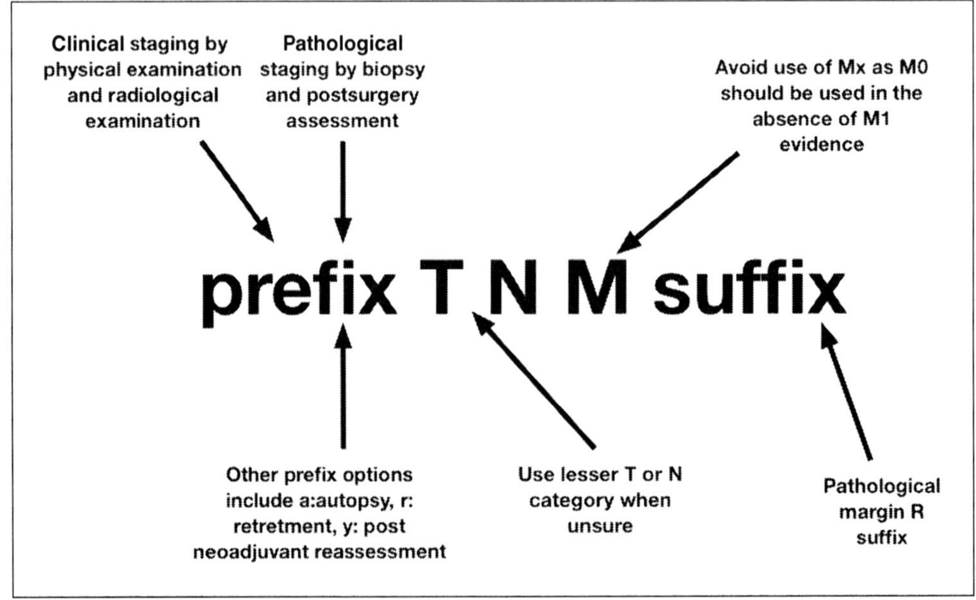

FIGURE 10.2 TNM staging rules

is known as "upstaging" or "downstaging," where the new information results in a worsened or improved prognosis, respectively. In common usage, clinical and pathologic staging information are often reported in a mixed fashion, especially given that metastatic status is often not documented pathologically, even following definitive surgery of the primary and lymph nodes. For example, a tonsil cancer staged clinically (e.g., stage II, cT2 cN0 cM0) on the basis of examination and CT scan undergoes definitive removal of the tumor and dissection of the lymph nodes. A larger tumor than initially thought and lymph node involvement are found pathologically, so the patient's stage is updated to accurately denote this (e.g., stage IVA (aka stage "four A"), pT3 pN2 cM0).

General Staging Rules

The AJCC has defined a set of standard rules used to guide TNM staging. As per the *AJCC Cancer Staging Handbook*, seventh edition, general rules to follow when staging are:

1. Confirm cancer presence through microscopic evaluation (i.e., biopsy, cytology) and classify according to the most recent International Classification of Diseases Oncology standard (currently ICD-O-3), with the exception of rare cases when such an evaluation cannot be undertaken.
2. Clinical staging utilizes all information prior to definitive treatment and within 4 months of diagnosis, whichever period is shorter, providing no progression has occurred.
3. Pathologic staging will include information gleaned from definitive surgery, either at the end of the first course of treatment or 4 months post-diagnosis, whichever period is longer.
4. In cases where neoadjuvant treatment has taken place (see above), report both the initial pretreatment clinical "c" stage, as well as the post-neoadjuvant treatment "yc" or "yp" stage for comparison of treatment effect.
5. If progression occurs between time of initial staging and start of definitive therapy, stage with information obtained prior to the documented progression.
6. When there is doubt as to a TNM sub-classification (i.e., T3 vs. T4 clinically) based on all the available information, or there is absence of measurement of a non-anatomic prognostic factor, default to the lesser category to favor the lesser stage.
7. Stage synchronous primary tumors in paired organs (i.e., bilateral breast cancers diagnosed at same time) independently. Stage metachronus tumors not thought to be recurrence in a single organ independently (i.e., histologically different left-sided breast cancers diagnosed 20 years apart).
8. Report T stage of multiple synchronous primary tumors in a single organ by the T stage of the most advanced tumor's characteristics, and use an (m) suffix denotation (i.e., T2(m)).
9. Use the "X" denotation for T and N as sparingly as possible. If a cancer is classified as TX or NX, a stage grouping can only be assigned if the grouping rules state "Any T" or "Any N." MX, a designation which existed in previous versions of the AJCC system, is no longer to be used clinically, because M0 is used as default in the absence of evidence supporting distant metastases.

Reporting of Surgical Margins

Following primary treatment, an R denotation is commonly used to report the clinical or surgical presence of residual primary tumor. Most commonly, this R denotation is applied following definitive surgery to comment on the status of surgical margins, and can incorporate both the surgeon's operative observations and the pathological findings. The R sub-classifications are:

- R0: no residual primary tumor
- R1: microscopic residual tumor
- R2: macroscopic residual tumor
- Rx: presence of residual primary tumor not assessed

10.5. COMMON NON-TNM SITE-SPECIFIC STAGING SYSTEMS

Numerous variances and historical staging systems exist for a variety of cancers. In this section, common non-TNM staging classification systems are presented for discussion.

Lymphoma (Hodgkin/Non-Hodgkin)

Given the unique nature of spread of primary hematogenous malignancies, classification of lymphomas does not use the TNM system, but rather a composite anatomical and clinical scheme known as the Ann Arbor Staging System. The staging system is based primarily on anatomical location of lymph node regions of involvement:

1. *Stage I.* Single nodal region.
2. *Stage II.* Two or more lymph node regions on same side of diaphragm, or one nodal region associated with spread to one extra-lymphatic site on the same side of diaphragm.
3. *Stage III.* Involvement of lymph node regions above and below diaphragm, which may include involvement of the spleen.
4. *Stage IV.* Diffuse involvement of one or more extra-lymphatic organs or spread to distant organ, including bone marrow.

Use of the suffix E denotes the presence of extra-nodal disease in other organs and viscera (i.e., skin, liver, and lungs), and includes bone marrow. Waldeyer's ring, thymus, and spleen are considered as part of the nodal regions, but splenic involvement is denoted with the suffix S. Each roman numeric stage is further sub-classified clinically as A or B, with the latter denoting the clinical presence of B-symptoms at the time of diagnosis (fever, drenching night sweats, and weight loss).

Multiple Myeloma

Given the nature of development of multiple myeloma, a TNM system is not utilized for this disease. Rather, a system incorporating serum blood work at the time of diagnosis called the Durie–Salmon system is used. The Durie–Salmon system is:

1. Stage I requires all of the following: Hb > 10.0 g/dL, serum calcium ≤ 12 mg/dL, normal bone x-rays or solitary bone lesions, immunoglobulin (Ig)G < 5 g/dL, IgA < 3 g/dL, urine M-protein < 4 g/24 hours.
2. Stage II does not fit stage I or III criteria.
3. Stage III requires one of the following: Hb < 8.5 g/dL, serum calcium > 12 mg/dL, three or more bone lesions, IgG > 7 g/dL, IgA > 5 g/dL, urine M-protein > 12 g/24 hours.
4. Subtypes: A or B for serum creatinine < or > 2.0 mg/dL, respectively.

A secondary staging system termed the international staging system for multiple myeloma has been developed more recently.

- Stage I: serum B2-microglobulin < 3.5 mg/L, serum albumin ≥ 3.5 g/dL.
- Stage II: Does not fit stage I or III.
- Stage III: serum B2-microglobulin ≥ 5.5 mg/L.

Gynecologic Malignancies

Staging systems for malignancies of the cervix, uterus, ovaries, fallopian tubes, vagina, vulva, and gestational trophoblastic malignancies have been traditionally maintained by the Féderation Internationale de Gynécologie et d'Obstétrique (FIGO). FIGO staging is similar to TNM staging in that it is anatomically derived based on the extent of spread of the primary tumor, nodal involvement, and metastases. However, rather than separately scoring each of these criteria, an overall roman numeric staging (from I to IV with substages denoted by letters A to C) is assigned. The most recent update to FIGO staging was released in 2009. The AJCC TNM staging for each site is set to match and coincide with the FIGO staging system.

Colon Cancer

While the TNM system is currently used for colorectal carcinomas, two historic classifications of note were used extensively prior to full adoption of the TNM system, and appear in previously published literature regarding the disease. The Dukes classification system was developed and named after a British pathologist in 1932. The Dukes Classification system is:

- Dukes A: invasion into, but not through the bowel wall.
- Dukes B: invasion through bowel wall, but no lymph node invasion.
- Dukes C: lymph node involvement.
- Dukes D: distant metastases.

A further refinement of the system is the Modified Astler–Coller classification:

- Stage A: mucosa only.
- Stage B1: extending into muscularis propria, but not penetrating through.
- Stage B2: penetrating through muscularis propria.
- Stage C1: extending into muscularis propria but not penetrating through, and nodal involvement.
- Stage C2: penetrating through muscularis propria, nodal involvement.
- Stage D: distant metastatic spread.

Melanoma

Melanoma currently utilizes the TNM staging system developed by the AJCC. The T staging of melanoma is based on the previous observations by Dr. Alexander Breslow in 1970 that the depth of invasion of melanoma was a significant prognostic indicator. The original Breslow stages, on the basis of depth of pathologic invasion were I = ≤ 0.75 mm, II = 0.75 to 1.5 mm, III = 1.51 to 2.25 mm, IV = 2.25 to 3.0 mm, *V* ≤ 3.0 mm. Similar in concept to the Breslow system, up until the latest TNM staging update, the system of Clark level was used to describe the anatomical level of invasion into the skin. The Clark levels are:

- I: in-situ disease confined to epidermis.
- II: invasion into papillary dermis.
- III: invasion into junction of papillary and reticular dermis.
- IV: invasion into reticular dermis.
- V: invasion into subcutaneous fat.

Recent studies have demonstrated that Clark level is the least correlative with prognosis, and both the Breslow staging and Clark level have been replaced by the current T staging system endorsed by the AJCC.

Testicular Cancer

In addition to the TNM anatomic staging for cancer of the testes, the AJCC has a fourth "S" criterion used for staging. The "S" criterion represents the serum tumor markers. Alpha-fetoprotein (AFP), human chorionic gonadotropin (hCG), and lactate dehydrogenase (LDH) are serum tumor markers commonly found elevated in testicular cancers. They are also potential markers of metastatic disease and can be followed post-primary treatment to determine if there has been response to treatment and to gauge the presence of residual disease.

The S sub-classifications are:

- SX: marker studies not available or performed.
- S0: marker study levels within normal limits.
- S1: LDH < 1.5 × upper limit normal, hCG < 5,000 mg/mL, and AFP < 1,000 ng/ mL.
- S2: LDH 1.5 to 10 × upper limit normal or hCG 5,000 to 50,000 mg/mL, or AFP 1,000 to 10,000 ng/mL.
- S3: LDH > 10 × upper limit normal or hCG > 50,000 mg/mL, or AFP > 10,000 ng/mL.

The serum markers should be measured at baseline pre-treatment, and also measured post-orchiectomy. If measured to be high post-orchiectomy, then serial measurements should be taken to ensure appropriate decrease of the values secondary to decay of the factors, otherwise residual disease should be suspected.

Chapter 11

General Cancer Treatment Considerations

KEY POINTS

- A variety of goals of cancer therapy exists and can include: survival-based endpoints, tumor control endpoints, health-related quality-of-life, and various palliative/symptom control endpoints.
- There are multiple roles for surgery in the management of cancer, which include: diagnosis, staging, primary treatment, palliation, and toxicity management.
- Chemotherapy is utilized as primary, adjuvant, and palliative treatment for a host of cancers. The mechanism of action of chemotherapy drugs depend on the nature of the drug utilized; yet, they commonly interrupt processes that support cell division and growth. Commonly utilized classes of chemotherapy include: alkylating agents, antimetabolites, cytotoxic antibodies, alkaloids, and topoisomerase inhibitors. Common side-effect classes include: myelosuppression/immunosuppression, organ damage, and various other acute/late effects.
- Hormonal therapy is a form of anticancer treatment that inhibits normal steroid production in the human body to interfere with gene expression and cell growth in various hormonally driven cancers such as breast cancer and prostate cancer. Various hormonal therapy classes exist: aromatase inhibitors, gonadotropin-releasing hormone (GnRH) analogs/antagonists, antiandrogens, and estrogen receptor modulators. Targeted therapy is a form of drug therapy that interferes with cancer cell growth by direct inhibition of cellular processes (instead of DNA replication) by the use of one of two classes: monoclonal antibodies and small molecules.
- Radiotherapy can be used as primary therapy in a variety of tumors including early stage larynx cancer, prostate cancer, liver cancer, early stage lymphomas, and non-melanoma skin cancer as well as an alternative to surgery and/or chemotherapy (central nervous system [CNS] tumors, head and neck cancers, lung cancer, gynecological cancer, gastrointestinal (GI) cancers, and bladder cancer). Radiotherapy modalities include: external-beam, brachytherapy, and radionuclide therapy. Radiotherapy can also be given for adjuvant (prior to or after definitive primary therapy) or salvage (after recurrent disease is identified) to improve clinically relevant cancer endpoints such as survival and recurrence-free survival.

- Radiotherapy and chemotherapy are commonly combined to improve results because of the potential additive anticancer effects (but can also cause possible additional toxicities). Chemoradiation has been shown to be of benefit in multiple cancer scenarios including: CNS gliomas, head and neck cancers, lung cancers, various gastrointestinal cancers, bladder cancer, and cervical cancer.
- Radiotherapy can also be used to palliate a range of symptoms related to various anatomical areas including the CNS, head and neck area, thorax, abdomen, pelvis, and the musculoskeletal system.

11.1. GOALS OF THERAPY

Overview

Definition of the goal of cancer treatment is important for three reasons. At the front end it greatly assists decision making among various treatment approaches and with a treatment modality (e.g., radical vs. palliative radiotherapy). After treatment, the definition of the goal of therapy will allow for an objective assessment of the success of treatment given and the requirement for further therapy. Additionally, the definition of the various possible goals of therapy and their respective endpoints are useful for clinical trial design and reporting as well as publication/dissemination of population-based cancer reports.

Survival-Based Endpoints

1. *Cure.* Defined as complete eradication of the cancer. Usually defined at a specific time period relevant to the natural history of the cancer.
2. *Survival prolongation.* Extended survival because of anticancer treatment over and above expected survival if patient not treated.

Tumor Control

1. *Tumor response and duration.* Assessment of the effect of anticancer treatment on disease burden. Response evaluation criteria in solid tumors criteria (www.recist.com, complete response, partial response, stable disease and progressive disease) are commonly used in clinical trials and inter-physician communication.
2. *Progression-free survival.* Time elapsed since treatment initiation where cancer has not clinically progressed. Some newer targeted agents are designed to extend progression-free survival time because of the cancer growth stasis properties of these agents.
3. *Local/regional control.* Similar to tumor response and duration but reflecting local and regional impacts of surgery and radiotherapy on the burden of cancer.

Palliative

1. *Symptom improvement.* Objective patient-reported improvement of a documented symptom prior to treatment initiation.
2. *Symptom prevention.* Prevention of possible symptoms can be an important goal of therapy. Examples include the use of radiotherapy to prevent either bronchial obstruction in a narrowing airway or neurological compromise from a tumor abutting against the spinal cord.

11.2. SURGERY

Overview

The role of surgery in the management of cancer patients stretches out from initial diagnosis and staging, primary treatment, as well as the palliation of cancer-related symptoms and treatment-related toxicities. These surgical cancer interventions are summarized below.

Diagnosis

Various surgical/radiological procedures can be performed to obtain cellular/tissue material for pathological assessment prior to cancer decision-making. These include: fine needle aspiration cytology, core needle biopsy, incisional biopsy (where part of the tumor is removed), and excisional biopsy (where all the tumors are removed).

Staging

Surgical interventions are commonly utilized to determine or confirm the extent of disease prior to definitive cancer decision-making. Examples can include: mediastinoscopy (lung cancer), sentinel node biopsy (breast cancer, melanoma), lymph node dissection (head and neck, breast, gastrointestinal [GI]), and laparotomy (gynecological cancers).

Definitive Treatment

Primary surgical treatment for cancer can be performed alone or in conjunction with presurgery or post-surgery chemotherapy and/or radiation therapy. Surgical considerations must include surgical resectability, medical operability, and anatomical patterns of spread/extent of surgical resection. Types of cancer surgeries that are commonly performed include: craniotomy, lobectomy/pneumonectomy, esophagectomy, gastrectomy, colectomy, prostatectomy, cystectomy, and hysterectomy. Various forms of each of these procedures exist and will depend on the instrumentation used (e.g., open vs. laparoscopic vs. robotic) and the extent of surgery (e.g., simple vs. radical vs. modified radical).

Palliative Treatment

Surgical maneuvers for the palliation of cancer patients can provide important clinical benefits. Various clinical scenarios that may benefit from palliative surgery can include: bypass stenting, bypass tubing (e.g., G-tube), draining of fluid, metastatectomy, recurrent disease resection, superior vena cava obstruction, spinal cord compression, pericardial tamponade, and bypass of lumen obstruction (e.g., bowel).

11.3. CHEMOTHERAPY

Overview

Chemotherapy refers to the use of standard drug treatment for the primary purpose of eliciting an anticancer response by reducing cancer cell number. Other non-cancerous diseases can be treated with chemotherapy drugs including various connective tissue disorders (rheumatoid arthritis, scleroderma, Crohn's disease). The early use of chemotherapy stemmed from the use of mustard gas from World War I, in which it was observed that this chemical class has significant myelosuppressive properties. The first clinical use of such therapy was in lymphoma patients in 1942.

Mechanism of Action

Chemotherapy drugs inherently interfere with many of the processes that cancer cells (and normal cells) rely upon for cell division and replication (Figure 11.1). In general, cells with high turnover (i.e., high growth rate) may be more susceptible to chemotherapy drugs as

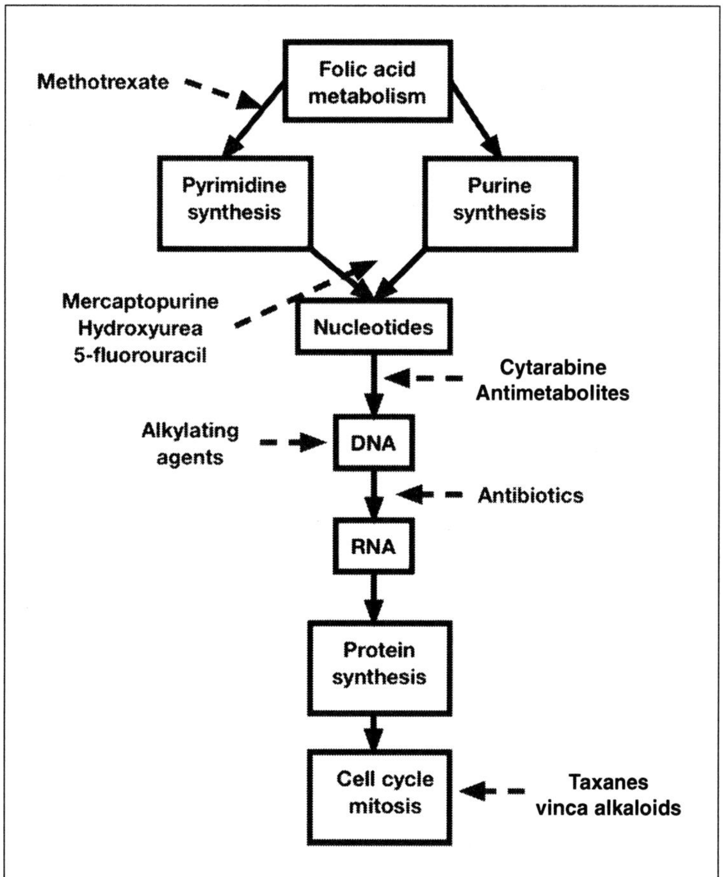

FIGURE 11.1 Chemotherapeutic mechanisms of action

a large proportion of cells may be in various mitotic phases that are directly or indirectly targeted by various chemotherapy drug classes. Cancers can become resistant to chemotherapy using a variety of mechanisms, including the presence of a *p*-glycoprotein that has been shown to pump intracellular chemotherapy out of the cell.

Chemotherapy can be delivered as single agents or in combination. When used in combination, complementary drugs are often combined to attack the cancer using different non-overlapping mechanisms of action. Additionally, the side-effect profile of the individual drug components may also be non-overlapping, improving patient tolerability to these chemotherapy treatments. Chemotherapy can be given alone or in combination with other treatments (usually surgery, radiotherapy, or both) to achieve the goal of treatment whether it is cure, adjuvant/salvage treatment, or palliation.

Chemotherapy Classes

1. *Alkylating agents.* The mechanism of action is via the alkylation of the guanine base of DNA. Example agents include: cisplatin, carboplatin, oxaliplatin, chlorambucil, and cyclophosphamide.
2. *Antimetabolites.* This class of chemotherapy drugs is chemically similar to purines or pyrimidines and interferes with DNA replication and RNA synthesis. Antifolate metabolites are also included in this chemotherapy drug class. Example agents include: fludarabine (purine), 5-fluorouracil (pyrimidine), and pemetrexed (antifolate).
3. *Cytotoxic antibiotics.* A class of antibiotic drugs that interfere with DNA replication and protein synthesis. Examples include: epirubicin, doxorubicin, bleomycin, and mitoxantrone.
4. *Alkaloids.* Plant-based drugs that interfere with cell division by preventing microtubule formation (vinca alkaloids—vincristine, vinblastine, and vinorelbine), stabilizing microtubules (taxanes, creating anaphase arrest, e.g., taxol, docetaxel), or by initiating G1/S cell arrest (podophyllotoxin).
5. *Topoisomerase inhibitors.* This class of chemotherapy drug is DNA topology inhibitors that interfere with both the transcription and replication of DNA by disruption of appropriate DNA coiling. Examples include: topotecan and etoposide.

Side Effects

The side-effect profile for patients will depend on the particular chemotherapy class or regimen used as well as factors inherent to the patients themselves. Common chemotherapy-related side effects are listed below:

Myelosuppression/Immunosuppression. Reduction of red cells, white cells, and platelets can occur, which may necessitate the use of blood transfusion and/or synthetic granulocyte colony-stimulating factor. Severe suppression can lead to febrile neutropenia, which can be life-threatening.

1. *Organ damage.* Various organ systems can be affected including: heart, liver, kidney, lung, brain, and peripheral nerves.
2. *General acute effects.* Fatigue, nausea, vomiting, diarrhea/constipation, dehydration, tumor lysis syndrome, and hair loss.
3. *General long-term effects.* Secondary cancer, infertility, impotency, cognitive impairment, and teratogenic potential.

11.4. HORMONAL THERAPY

Overview

Hormonal therapy is a form of anticancer treatment that involves the inhibition of steroid hormone production within the human body. Steroid hormones (including sex hormones such as estrogen and testosterone) are significant inducers of gene expression and cell growth in some cancers (e.g., breast and prostate). Interference of these specific endocrine system functions can lead to important anticancer clinical effects (Figure 11.2).

Hormonal Therapy Classes

1. *Aromatase inhibitors.* An inhibitor of the steroid enzyme aromatase that can reduce estrogen levels in postmenopausal women leading to cell arrest and programmed death in hormone responsive cells. Examples include: letrozole, anastrozole, and exemestane.
2. *Gonadotropin-releasing hormone (GnRH) analogs/antagonists.* A drug that causes chemical castration because of the downregulation of GnRH receptors (analogs) or direct blockage (antagonists) in the pituitary gland. Examples include leuprolide and goserelin (analogs) and degarelix (antagonist).
3. *Antiandrogens.* This class of drugs can either bind to androgen receptors (non-steroidal antiandrogens) or block the peripheral conversion of steroid hormone metabolites into testosterone (5-alpha reductase inhibitors). Examples include bicalutamide/flutamide (non-steroidal antiandrogen) and dutasteride/finasteride (5-alpha reductase inhibitors).
4. *Estrogen receptor modulators.* This class of drug serves as an antagonist of the estrogen receptor. Various drugs are in clinical use and include tamoxifen and raloxifene.

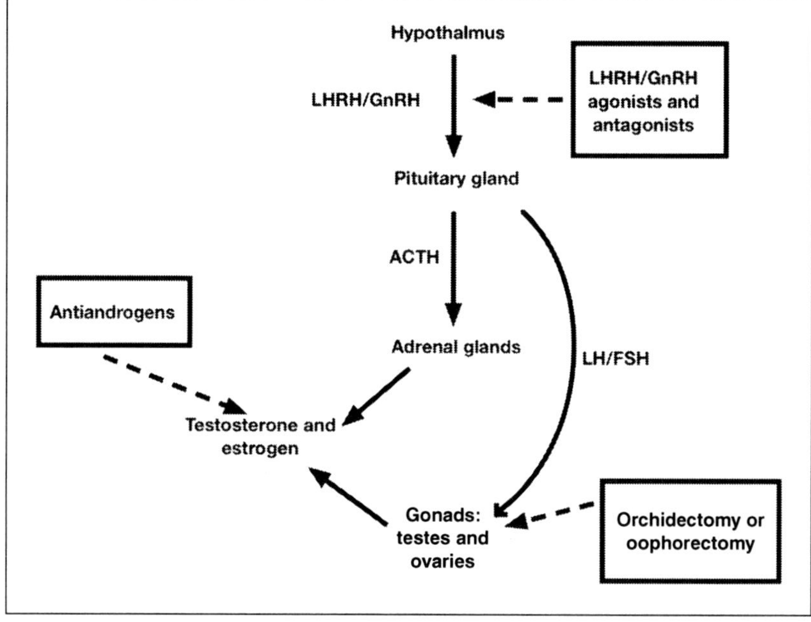

FIGURE 11.2 Hormonal therapy mechanism of action

11.5. TARGETED THERAPY

Overview

Targeted therapy refers to a drug class that interferes with cancer cell growth by direct inhibition of cellular processes instead of DNA replication of dividing cells (Figure 11.3). Two main classes of targeted therapy exist and include monoclonal antibodies and small molecules.

Monoclonal Antibodies

A monoclonal antibody is a highly specific cloned antibody that has been designed to bind to a specific epitope (determinant section of an antigen). In the context of cancer, cellular antigen(s) known to be associated with the form of cancer to be treated will be the target of these medications. The antibody needs to be conjugated with another entity that will deliver the anticancer effect.

1. *Immunoliposomes.* Liposomes attached to monoclonal antibodies contain anticancer drugs or genes.

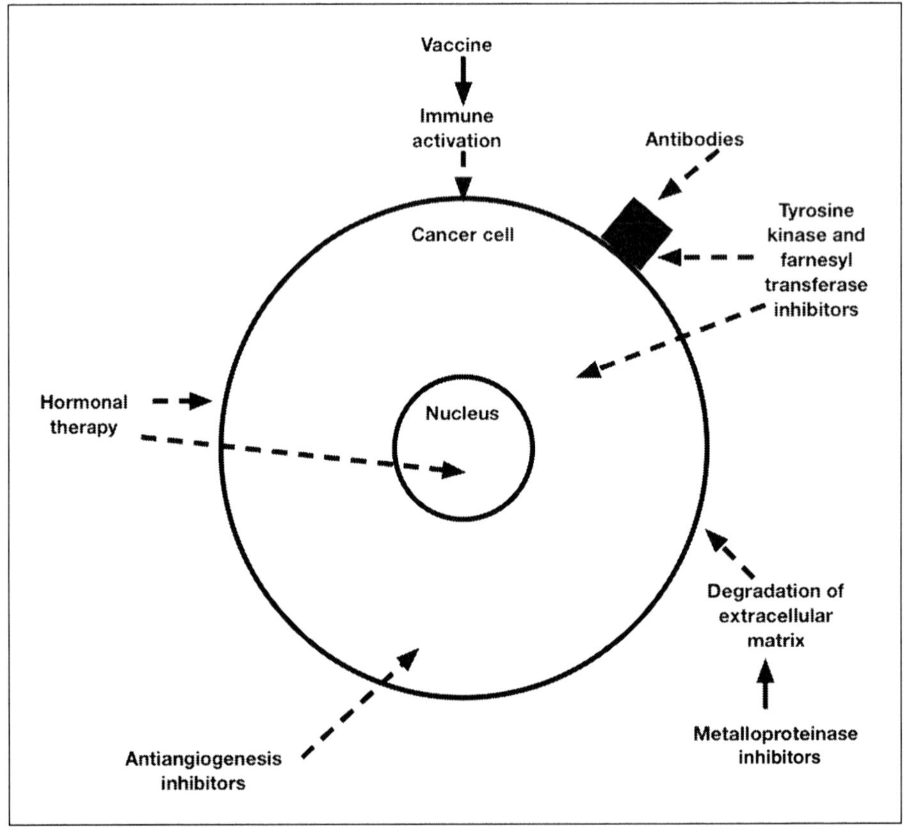

FIGURE 11.3 Targeted therapy mechanism of action

2. *Prodrug therapy.* Drug-activating enzyme is linked to the monoclonal antibody, which converts a generally non-toxic drug to an anticancer drug locally. This has the potential advantage of reducing systemic side effects.
3. *Radioimmunotherapy.* Radioactive compound is attached to the monoclonal antibody to have radiation-based anticancer impact. This approach has been utilized in lymphomas.

Small Molecules

Small molecules (low-molecular weight organic compound) have the desired mechanism of anticancer action by direct interference with critical cellular enzymatic pathways. Examples in clinical use include imatinib (chronic myeloid leukemia, GI stromal tumor tumors) and gefitinib/erlotinib (epidermal growth factor receptor tyrosine kinase inhibitor, lung cancer), and sunitinib (tyrosine kinase inhibitor, renal cancer).

11.6. PRIMARY RADIOTHERAPY

Radiotherapy Overview

Radiation therapy (radiotherapy) is defined as the therapeutic use of ionizing radiation to control or eradicate cancer cells to achieve clinically important goals such as cure, prolonged survival, local control, or palliation. Radiotherapy in the treatment of cancer can be given in different modes including: primary (radiotherapy treatment alone), neoadjuvant (before definitive treatment usually with surgery), adjuvant (after primary treatment usually with surgery), salvage (after recurrence), chemoradiation (sequential—chemotherapy before or after radiation, or concurrent—chemotherapy and radiation contemporaneously with each other), and palliative.

Radiotherapy can be delivered in multiple ways including external-beam radiation therapy, brachytherapy, and radionuclide therapy. External-beam radiation therapy can utilize various fundamental particles to underpin the therapeutic effect including: photons, electrons, and hadrons (e.g., protons and neutrons). Various forms of temporary or permanent brachytherapy systems are in clinical use. Radionuclide therapy involves the ingestion or injection of radioactive salts or chemical compounds to target cancerous tumors in a systemic fashion similar to other forms of drug therapy. Radiation can be combined with other treatment modalities including surgery, chemotherapy, targeted therapy, hormonal therapy, and immunotherapy depending on various pre-defined clinical indications.

Radiotherapy can be utilized for non-malignant conditions including: thyroid disease, gynecomastia, keloid scars, vascular restenosis, and heterotopic bone formation. Additionally, total body irradiation can be utilized for the preparation of bone marrow transplantation procedures for both oncological and non-oncological conditions.

Mechanism of Action

At the biological level, radiation therapy directly (or indirectly through intermediate-free radicals) damages cancer DNA to affect cell death (either by apoptosis or necrosis). Clinically, the goal of radiotherapy (which should be initially defined at time of consultation) is to define the cancer target(s) that require treatment to achieve the goal of treatment (simulation) and to institute the technical parameters to deliver radiotherapy to achieve this goal (planning). This is performed to optimize the therapeutic ratio between tumor control and normal tissue toxicity (Figure 11.4). Once radiotherapy is delivered, follow-up procedures are instituted to assess response, toxicity, and further salvage treatments as required by the clinical situation.

Primary Radiotherapy Clinical Scenarios

Radiation therapy alone for the primary treatment of cancer is a routine standard of care for several clinical scenarios such as: early stage larynx, prostate cancer, liver cancer, early stage lymphomas, and non-melanoma skin cancer. Radical radiotherapy can also be delivered to other clinical scenarios where standard of care multimodality treatment including chemotherapy and/or surgery are contraindicated. These scenarios include such situations as: central nervous system (CNS) tumors, head and neck cancers, lung cancer, gynecological cancer (e.g., cervix cancer), GI cancers (pancreas, anal canal), and bladder cancer.

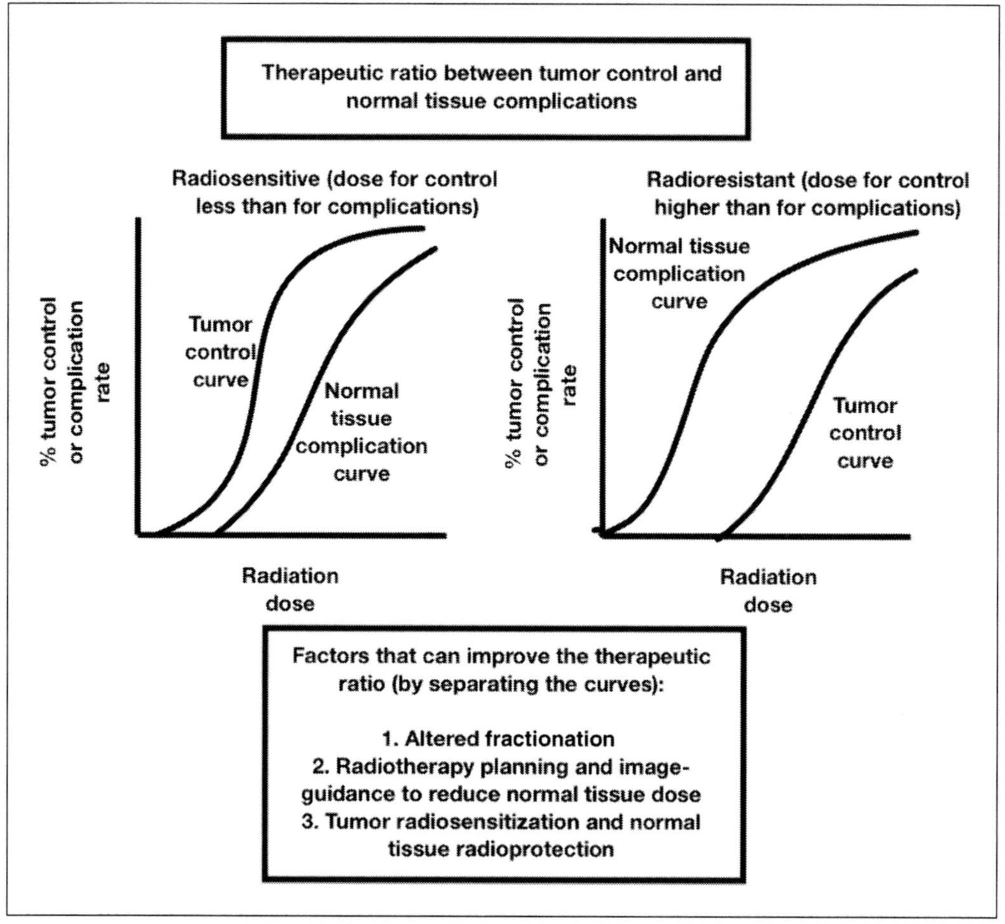

FIGURE 11.4 Radiation therapy therapeutic ratio

11.7. ADJUVANT/SALVAGE RADIOTHERAPY

Adjuvant Radiotherapy

Adjuvant radiation is a form of radiotherapy delivered prior to (neoadjuvant) or following (adjuvant) definitive primary therapy (usually surgery). The goal of such treatment depends on whether the radiation treatment is given neoadjuvantly or adjuvantly (see below). Additionally, radiation can be given concurrently with other treatments such as chemotherapy (neoadjuvant or adjuvant chemoradiation) to improve the effects of the treatment by additive (or supra-additive) effects of the treatment combination. Although external-beam radiation therapy is commonly used to deliver adjuvant therapy to the site of primary disease ± microscopic coverage of lymphatics/nodes, other radiotherapy approaches can be utilized including brachytherapy (e.g., post-operative treatment of the vaginal vault in endometrial cancer).

The use of radiation therapy in the neoadjuvant (pre-operative) setting has multiple benefits. These include: treating microscopic disease that may exist beyond anticipated surgical margins, improved resectability, treatment of nodal areas at risk, and improved surgical margins. The main disadvantage of pre-operative therapy is impaired surgical healing that can occur because of normal tissue effects of radiation therapy. The issue of impaired healing limits radiotherapy doses to < 50 Gy/25 fractions or 25 Gy/5 fractions (in hypofractionated pre-operative rectal cancer treatment). Common clinical indications for pre-operative radiotherapy include: Pancoast (superior sulcus) lung tumors, esophageal cancer, rectal cancer, and extremity sarcomas.

The post-operative adjuvant radiation therapy approach also has various benefits including: knowledge of pathological factors that can guide use and volumes for radiotherapy, and generally higher radiotherapy doses that can be delivered after surgical healing is complete. The main disadvantages of post-operative adjuvant radiation can include possible over-treatment in patients that are already cured, delayed management until healing is complete, and potential for tissue hypoxia. Common scenarios for the use of adjuvant radiation include: head and neck cancer, lung cancer, rectal cancer, gynecological cancers (cervix and endometrium), breast cancer, and prostate cancer.

Salvage Radiotherapy

Salvage radiotherapy refers to a clinical situation where radiotherapy is employed (either alone or in conjunction with other therapies) to radically treat recurrent disease after primary treatment failure. Often this is the case in situations where the patient has not received previous radiotherapy (e.g., surgery alone) and radical radiotherapy (or chemoradiotherapy) can be considered. However, sometimes local and/or regional failure can occur in a patient that has previously received either radical or adjuvant radiotherapy. If repeat radiotherapy (also known as radiotherapy re-treatment) is to be attempted, previous radiation dose/volume to critical structures, current disease stage, elapsed time between initial and salvage radiotherapy, and goal(s) of salvage treatment need to be considered prior to initiation of such therapy. Ideally, such treatment should be discussed in a multidisciplinary forum and a literature search of medical evidence elaborating on the benefits and risks of such treatment should be reviewed. Salvage radiotherapy is commonly considered in prostate cancer (post-prostatectomy prostate-specific antigen failure), although other salvage scenarios can occur (i.e., local or nodal relapse in lung and head and neck cancers).

11.8. CHEMORADIATION

Potential Mechanisms of Action

The combination of chemotherapy and radiation therapy has been used repeatedly in many tumor systems to optimize patient outcomes. The enhancement of anticancer effect can be additive (overall effect = chemo effect + radiotherapy effect) or supra-additive (overall effect > chemo effect + radiotherapy effect). The use of chemotherapy before radiation (neoadjuvant) is rationalized by the benefit of cell killing and tumor debulking prior to radiation therapy. In this scenario, fewer clonogenic cells may exist at the time of radiation therapy. However, accelerated repopulation of cancer cells may occur and can limit the effectiveness of this approach. Concurrent chemoradiotherapy may result in additive and supra-additive effects leading to improved local disease control (and subsequently reductions in distant metastatic failure); yet, this can come at the expense of additional normal tissue toxicities and related side effects.

Clinical Role of Chemoradiation

A significant clinical trial literature examining the combination of chemotherapy and radiation therapy to improve results for both primary/radical and neoadjuvant/adjuvant (to surgery) treatment scenarios exists. Several examples (not exhaustive) of the clinical role of chemoradiotherapy that are established in the medical literature are listed below:

1. *CNS high-grade gliomas.* Temozolamide plus radical concurrent radiation have been shown to provide improved survival.
2. *Head and neck cancers.* Platinum-based chemotherapy plus concurrent radiation as primary treatment or post-operatively in high-risk recurrence situations.
3. *Lung cancer.* Concurrent and adjuvant platinum-based chemotherapy with radiation as primary treatment for locally advanced tumors (both small cell and non-small cell types).
4. *Esophageal cancer.* Concurrent chemoradiation as primary or neoadjuvant treatment depending on surgical resectability and medical operability.
5. *Stomach and rectal cancer.* Various combinations of chemoradiotherapy integrated with surgical resection.
6. *Anal canal cancer.* Combined chemotherapy and radiation therapy have been shown to be curative and can assist in avoiding major surgery (including defunctioning colostomy) in the majority of cases.
7. *Bladder cancer.* Combined concurrent platinum-based chemoradiation as a treatment alternative to surgery (with surgical salvage) or as definitive treatment for medically inoperable patients.
8. *Cervical cancer.* Combined concurrent platinum-based chemoradiation therapy has been shown to be associated with survival benefits both in the primary and post-operative setting.

11.9. PALLIATIVE RADIOTHERAPY

Radiotherapy can also be used for the palliation of cancer-related issues. Palliative radiation therapy can be given alone or in conjunction with anticancer interventions such as surgery, chemotherapy, targeted therapy, and hormonal therapy. However, other medical interventions need to be considered for optimal patient management. These, depending on the clinical scenario, can include: optimal pain management, antinauseants, steroids, and anticonvulsants.

Indications for palliative radiotherapy can include treatment to alleviate a present symptom or treatment to prevent the development of future symptom(s). Although the mainstay for palliative radiation therapy is the use of external-beam radiation therapy, indications exist for the use of palliative brachytherapy (bronchial or esophageal obstruction) or palliative radiopharmaceuticals (strontium or samarium therapy for widespread metastatic disease in the skeleton).

Common clinical scenarios requiring palliative radiotherapy treatment include the following:

1. *CNS.* Brain metastases, intramedullary spinal cord metastases, orbital metastases.
2. *Head and neck.* Bleeding head and neck tumor, tracheal compression from anaplastic thyroid cancer.
3. *Thorax.* Superior vena cava obstruction, bronchial obstruction, esophageal obstruction, chest wall invasion, shortness of breath from a lung lesion.
4. *Abdominal.* Liver metastasis, pancreatic metastases, bleeding GI tumor, painful adrenal metastases.
5. *Pelvic.* Bleeding bladder cancer, gynecological bleeding tumor.
6. *Musculoskeletal.* Bone metastasis, spine metastases, spinal cord compression.

11.10. RADIATION ONCOLOGY DOCUMENTATION

Documentation of radiation oncology interactions with patients is a critical exercise to optimize patient care and communication with other health-care professionals. The main patient encounter interactions occur at initial consultation, on-treatment, end of radiotherapy treatment, and post-treatment follow-up. A full guideline regarding the ideal documentation of radiation oncology patient encounters can be found on the American College of Radiology website (www.acr.org). The contents of an initial consultation radiation oncology note and treatment summary are listed and expanded below.

Initial Consultation

1. *History of present illness.* Chief complaint(s) leading to cancer diagnosis.
2. *Diagnostic/staging tests.* Results of pre- or post-pathological diagnosis serum testing, imaging studies, or other clinical findings/consultations.
3. *Pathology results.* Results of biopsies and/or surgical interventions. Note of findings on the operative note should also be documented.
4. *Medications and allergies.* With particular attention to medications that can sensitize radiotherapy (e.g., targeted therapies) or may have important port-treatment effects (e.g., anticoagulants in prostate cancer radiotherapy).
5. *Patient and family history.* With attention to previous cancers and previous radiotherapy.
6. *Review of systems.* Relevant review of organ-specific symptoms that can be related to the cancer should be documented. Additionally, other generic issues such as performance status, weight loss, and fatigue should be assessed. Contraindications to radiotherapy (previous radiation, inflammatory bowel disease, connective tissue disorders, and DNA repair disorders) as well as the presence of implanted medical devices (e.g., Pacemaker or hip replacement) should be clearly documented.
7. *Physical examination.* Vitals, global assessment of health, and cancer-specific physical examination findings (and pertinent negatives) should be documented.
8. *Overall summary.* Overall summary of the clinical situation with overall tumor, nodes, and metastases stage and grouping should be documented.
9. *Treatment options.* Treatment options and approaches discussed with the patient should be listed. Alternative treatments and approaches discussed should also be documented.
10. *Plan of care.* Plan of treatment should be outlined. Radiation therapy dose, volume, and goal of treatment should be documented with reference to relevant clinical trials and/or practice guidelines, if applicable. Additional diagnostic tests and other simulation procedures should be documented as well. Acute and late side effects should be listed in the consultation note.

Radiation Treatment Summary

1. Cancer diagnosis and stage (opportunity to update if changed from consultation).
2. Treatment dates, response (tumor response if any and patient response including performance status and toxicities), and status (completed as planned, adapted, and reason for change in initial plan).

3. Clinical course (side effects, new medications prescribed, alterations of medications, use of ancillary services).
4. Radiotherapy details (details of external-beam or brachytherapy dose and treated volume).
5. Cancer management details (details of other cancer treatment including surgery, hormonal therapy, and chemotherapy, planned follow-up visits and interventions should also be listed).

Chapter 12

General Radiotherapy Considerations

KEY POINTS

- Comfortable and reproducible patient immobilization for radiotherapy are important for successful treatment. Various devices exist for this purpose and can include: thermoplastic masks/meshes, modular devices, stereotactic devices, cradles, and virtual immobilization techniques.
- Simulation of treatment is a process by which all relevant anatomical and geometrical information is obtained to plan treatment. Forms of simulation include: conventional simulation, virtual simulation, computed tomography (CT) simulation, and other forms of advanced simulation (fusion, four-dimensional [4D] techniques).
- Similar to other fields in medicine and science, radiation oncology has a series of documents defining standard nomenclature to define radiation units, procedures, reporting, and safety [the International Commission of Radiation Units and Measurements (ICRU) system]. With regards to the planning of external-beam radiation therapy, ICRU reports #29, 50, and 62 are highly relevant documents to be reviewed.
- Radiotherapy planning is a set of procedures to define all the degrees of freedom related to the delivery of radiotherapy (beam direction, angle, modulation, etc., for external-beam radiation therapy). In the context of external-beam radiation therapy, various forms of treatment planning and delivery exist and include: conventional radiation therapy, three-dimensional conformal radiation therapy (3DCRT), intensity-modulated radiation therapy (IMRT), arc therapy, and stereotactic body radiation therapy. Radiation therapy planning is also relevant for brachytherapy treatments.
- Image-guided radiation therapy (IGRT) refers to a set of kilovoltage (kV) and/or megavoltage (MV) two-dimensional/three-dimensional (2D/3D) imaging procedures implemented to confirm accurate and precise delivery of external-beam radiation therapy. Various options can be utilized and include: skin marks/patient anatomy, portal imaging, electronic portal imaging, tumor tracking, and adaptive radiation therapy.
- Particle therapy relates to the use of particles other than photons and electrons for therapeutic cancer treatment. Various types of such therapy include: proton therapy, neutron therapy, and heavy ion therapy.
- Brachytherapy refers to a form of radiation treatment that places a radioactive source in close proximity to a cancer target. This form of therapy can be classified by treatment duration, treatment intensity, and source placement. Examples of clinical applications include: prostate cancer, cervical/endometrial cancer, lung/esophageal cancer, breast cancer, and skin cancer.

- Radioisotope therapy utilizes radioactive agents conjugated with other chemicals/agents to direct therapy to a certain body/organ system. Examples of radioisotope therapies include: iodine-131 (thyroid cancer, lymphoma), strontium-89/samarium-153/radium-223 (bone metastases), and yttrium-90 (neuroendocrine tumors and lymphomas).
- Optimization of radiation treatment can involve the alteration of multiple factors usually under the control of radiation oncology personnel. These can include: treatment intent, consideration of alternatives, fractionation, critical structure volumes, immobilization, simulation, planning procedures, delivery procedures, modification of chemoradiation, and optimization of medical management.

12.1. PATIENT IMMOBILIZATION

Overview

Adequate patient immobilization is required for effective simulation and treatment of patients. Ideally, immobilization should support the patient in a comfortable and stable treatment position for as long as a treatment fraction is expected to last (which can range from a few minutes to an hour or more for stereotactic procedures). The immobilization device must be compatible with CT/MRI machines and should not obstruct expected radiation beams. Other considerations regarding immobilization devices include: cost, claustrophobic potential, anatomical appropriateness, maintenance of shape/position, and the ability to place reference marks on the device.

Specific Devices

1. *Thermoplastic mask/mesh.* Use of a polymer mesh that can change shape when heated by warm water to conform to patient anatomy. This type of immobilization device is used in the head and neck area but other locations can be immobilized using this technology.
2. *Modular devices.* Various immobilization devices can be created to secure almost any body site in the either supine or prone position. These systems are called modular because of the potential for adjusting the device to the anatomy of the patient.
3. *Stereotactic devices.* Invasive stereotactic systems exist for the treatment of cranial radiosurgery. Non-invasive body immobilization devices for stereotactic body radiation therapy (e.g., vacuum locking system with abdominal compression system) are also in clinical use.
4. *Cradles.* A cradle device consists of a mold or vacuum locking system placed between the patient and the treatment bed to immobilize large (or small) parts of the body. This approach is commonly used to treat chest, abdominal, and pelvic malignancies.
5. *Virtual immobilization.* Various technologies exist for "virtual" immobilization of radiotherapy targets that move due to physiological motion. This includes treatment gating systems (beam turned on or off based on anatomical motion or surrogate) and other breath control systems (automated breathing control via a valve approach).

12.2. SIMULATION

Overview

Treatment simulation is a process by which a radiation oncologist in concert with the radiotherapy team consisting of radiation therapists, dosimetrists, and physicists obtain the anatomical and geometrical information necessary to commence radiation planning. A prerequisite to patient simulation is patient assessment, definition of the goal of treatment, and adequate and comfortable patient immobilization.

The general goals of simulation include the definition and localization of targets and normal tissues and definition of normal patient anatomy including the external contour of the patient. These general goals support the ultimate goal of obtaining enough information to plan radiotherapy by specifying all clinical radiation beams in terms of location, size, and angle as well as final expected target/normal tissue dosimetry (see Section 12.4).

Conventional Simulation

Traditionally, a fluoroscopic unit calibrated similarly to a linear accelerator was utilized to define radiotherapy beam size, location, and angle to support both palliative and radical radiotherapy planning. The conventional simulator has a laser system identical to that found in the linear accelerator room to ensure that both coordinate systems match with regards to the various degrees of freedom possible (e.g., couch position and angle, gantry angle, and collimator-beam size and angle). Patients have tattoo marks placed on their skin referenced back to this laser system to ensure accurate treatment delivery. After the simulation procedure is completed, films are taken that define the beam and the radiation oncologist can draw shielding [poured or multi-leaf collimator (MLC)-based] to reduce radiotherapy exposure to areas not needing treatment.

Virtual Simulation

Virtual simulation is a set of simulation procedures similar to conventional simulation; yet, a CT-based system is used instead of a fluoroscopy unit. Radiation beams can be placed to direct therapy in a manner similar to conventional simulation; however, the radiation oncologist can review and utilize the 3D information available in the CT to help define beam direction, size, and shielding. The CT information provides superior soft tissue contrast that is not available in fluoroscopy imaging. Virtual simulation is particularly helpful in defining targets where bony landmarks are not available or are not reliable.

Computed Tomography Simulation

The mainstay of modern radiotherapy planning is the CT simulator. Similar to the conventional simulator, a laser system is used to support a consistent coordinate system. Use of CT information greatly assists in the definition of targets and normal tissue structures for radiotherapy planning. Use of a CT simulator is a prerequisite for modern treatment planning approaches including 3DCRT, IMRT, and stereotactic radiation therapy. CT simulation not only provides anatomical information regarding targets, normal tissues, and the external patient contour for treatment planning but also provides voxel-based Hounsfield unit information for dose calculation, to support isodose generation for planning optimization, review, and acceptance.

Advanced Forms of Simulation

Other imaging modalities can be fused with CT simulation information to better define targets for radiotherapy. MRI fusion is commonly used for CNS, head and neck, gynecological, and prostate treatment planning. Positron emission tomography (PET)–CT fusion is also used for head and neck and lung cancer planning. Also, in the context of lung cancer and liver cancer planning, newer 4D CT simulation techniques exist to take account of physiological motion to better define targets.

12.3. RADIOTHERAPY NOMENCLATURE

The ICRU

The ICRU is charged with the development of standard recommendations and nomenclature regarding units of radiation/radioactivity, radiotherapy procedures, uniform reporting, and radiation safety. Several reports are relevant to the planning of external-beam radiation therapy (reports #29, #50, and #62) and brachytherapy (reports #38 and #58). Nomenclature related to the routine use of external-beam radiation therapy is reviewed herein (Figures 12.1–12.3). Interested readers on the topic of gynecological (ICRU38) and interstitial brachytherapy (ICRU58) should review the respective reports for more information (www.icru.org).

ICRU29 Nomenclature

1. *Target volume.* The volume that the radiation oncologist has defined to receive the prescribed dosage of radiotherapy. This concept has been replaced by the planning target volume (PTV, see ICRU50 Nomenclature).
2. *Treated volume.* A volume that is encompassed by a clinically significant isodose surface/line (usually 95%). If a perfect radiation plan was created, the treated volume should exactly conform to the target volume. However, this is practically never the case because of planning imperfections (see conformity index below).
3. *Irradiated volume.* A volume that corresponds to a dose relevant to the normal tissues that surround the target volume. For example, in the treatment of radical lung cancer the volume that receives 20 Gy or greater is clinically significant for the prediction of subsequent radiation lung injury.

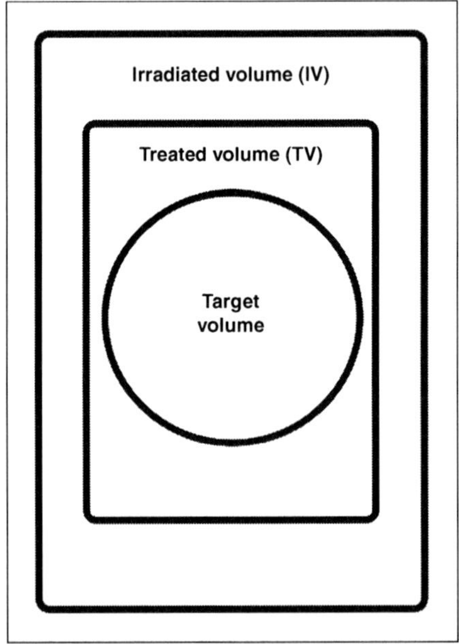

FIGURE 12.1 ICRU 29

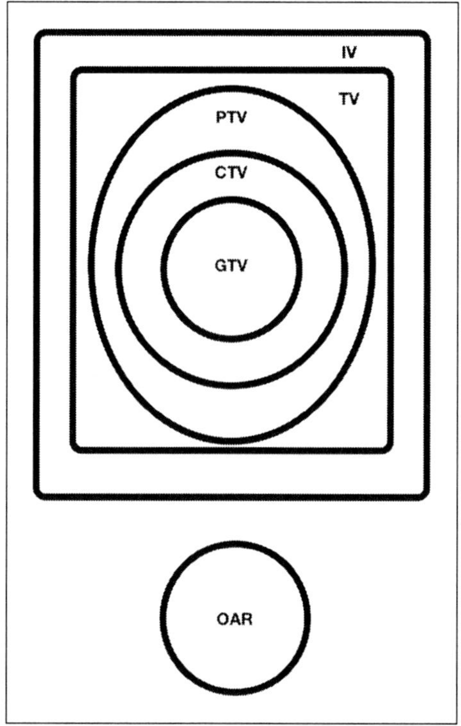

FIGURE 12.2 ICRU 50

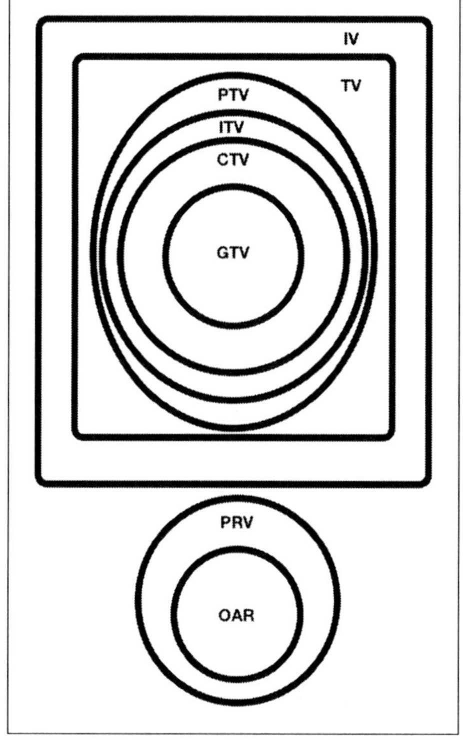

FIGURE 12.3 ICRU 62

ICRU50 Nomenclature

1. *Gross tumor volume (GTV).* Extent of disease based on visual inspection, palpation, and imaging.
2. *Clinical target volume (CTV).* This is an anatomical concept, which defines a volume containing the GTV as well as any patient anatomy that contains (or may contain) microscopic disease, which requires treatment. The CTV is independent of treatment modality, beam selection, or radiotherapy approach.
3. *Planning target volume (PTV).* This is a geometrical concept, which not only defines a new volume containing the CTV (and hence the GTV) but also includes a 3D margin to take into account any set-up, organ, patient, or beam inaccuracies. This volume will define the "target" for radiotherapy planning.
4. *Organs at risk (OAR).* Clinically relevant normal tissues near to radiotherapy targets that can express radiotherapy toxicity.
5. *ICRU reference point.* This defines a point in space and within the patient that the radiation treatment will be prescribed in reference to. This point is usually within the PTV, on or near the intersection of beam axes, and should be anatomically definable in a clear manner. The dose at the ICRU reference point is called the ICRU reference dose.
6. *Dose specification.* Various other dose points can be specified as well. The maximum dose is the highest dose within the PTV. This dose can be a point dose or on a clinically relevant volume (1.5 cm diameter). Other dose-points include minimum dose, average dose, and median dose within the PTV (or other structure listed above).
7. *Hot spot.* This refers to a volume outside the PTV that receives dosage higher than the prescription dose (100% of PTV dose). Usually considered significant for volumes with > 1.5 cm diameter (rule not used for small organs, e.g., orbit).

ICRU62 Nomenclature

1. *Internal margin (IM).* A component of the PTV concept relating to organ motion. Usually used for organs such as bladder, rectum, liver, and lungs that have physiological changes that can occur during the timespan of a radiotherapy fraction.
2. *Internal target volume (ITV).* A subcomponent of the PTV that contains the CTV and IM. All components of the ITV are tumor-related and patient-related. Uncertainty because of treatment-related factors are contained within the set-up margin (see below).
3. *Set-up margin (SM).* This component of the PTV contains margins associated with technical factors such as patient positioning, equipment uncertainty, and dosimetric uncertainty. The addition of SM to the ITV results in the traditional ICRU50 PTV concept.
4. *Conformity index (CI).* The conformity index describes the mathematical ratio between the treated volume and the PTV. For a perfect treatment, the CI is 1. Practically, assuming adequate coverage of the PTV volume, clinical CI usually is > 1.
5. *Planning organ at risk volume (PRV).* This is an extension of the OAR concept, which is similar to the PTV for target specification. The PRV includes physiological (IM) and technical (SM) uncertainty margins around the OAR to provide a final avoidance volume for radiotherapy planning.

12.4. TREATMENT PLANNING

Overview

Radiation treatment planning is a set of procedures whereby external-beam radiation therapy or brachytherapy treatment specifications (external beam: beam direction/weight/modulation, total dose, dose fractionation, dose–volume histograms; brachytherapy: high-dose rate (HDR) catheter position and source dwell times or LDR seed position and strengths) are set for treatment delivery. Using treatment simulation and target/normal tissue volumes, an iterative procedure of dosimetric simulation and optimization is performed until an acceptable isodose distribution is achieved that satisfies all treatment goals (i.e., predefined target and normal tissue dose parameters). Evaluation of radiation plans involves both the assessment of 2D/3D isodose distributions as well as target and normal tissue dose–volume histograms. Other considerations that need to be considered prior to plan acceptance include treatment feasibility and overall treatment time.

Various commercially available treatment planning systems are available for the planning of both external-beam radiotherapy and/or brachytherapy. Various mathematical algorithms (e.g., convolution–superposition method) are used to calculate the deposition of radiation dose in tissue. All algorithms require a CT simulation to generate a radiation therapy plan because CT Hounsfield units are directly related to electron density, which in turn is related to radiation dose deposition.

External-Beam Treatment Approaches

1. *Conventional radiation therapy.* Conventional external-beam radiation therapy is a 2D-based approach to treatment planning utilizing a calibrated fluoroscopy machine that "simulates" the beam characteristics of a linear accelerator (Figure 12.4). Conventional radiation therapy can also be utilized on 3D CT simulation machines using a procedure called virtual simulation. Virtual simulation is defined as the placement of 2D beams using the 3D CT simulation dataset, which allows the user to take advantage of the 3D target and normal tissue information. The advantage of these approaches includes the efficient nature and the longstanding historical (and successful) use of this approach. However, significant limitations exist which include: limited dose escalation leading to lower local control rates as well as uncertain dosimetry to normal tissues and targets.
2. *3D conformal radiation therapy (3DCRT).* This form of radiation planning uses the information from the CT simulation and target/normal tissue volumes to define multiple radiation beams that converge on the target (Figure 12.5). These beams are modified either with poured shielding (historical) or by MLC (computer controlled linear shields) to conform to the shape of the target of interest (i.e., PTV).
3. *Intensity-modulated radiation therapy (IMRT).* This form of external-beam radiation therapy uses computer optimization of radiation beam number and angle with modulation of each beam profile using MLC. This modulation can occur in sequential "step and shoot" MLC segments (subfields) or in continuous MLC motion during the treatment of each beam (Figure 12.6). The ultimate result is the production of highly conformal target treatments with high levels of normal tissue avoidance. Important disadvantages of IMRT can include extended treatment time, integral dose to distant tissue, and treatment overconfidence (highly conformal treatment with inappropriately tight margins). Plan optimization can be performed in a forward (place beams first followed by dose calculation) or inverse (definition of target and normal tissue dose priorities and dose limits, which is

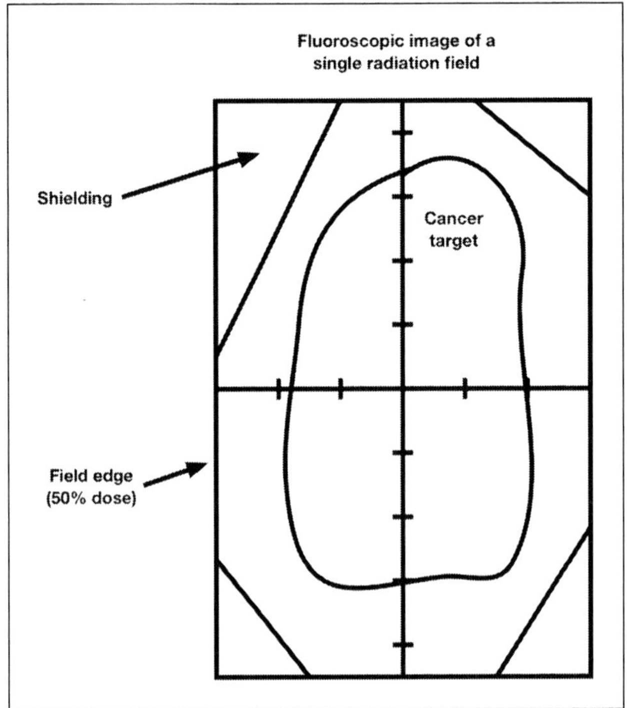

FIGURE 12.4 Conventional radiation therapy

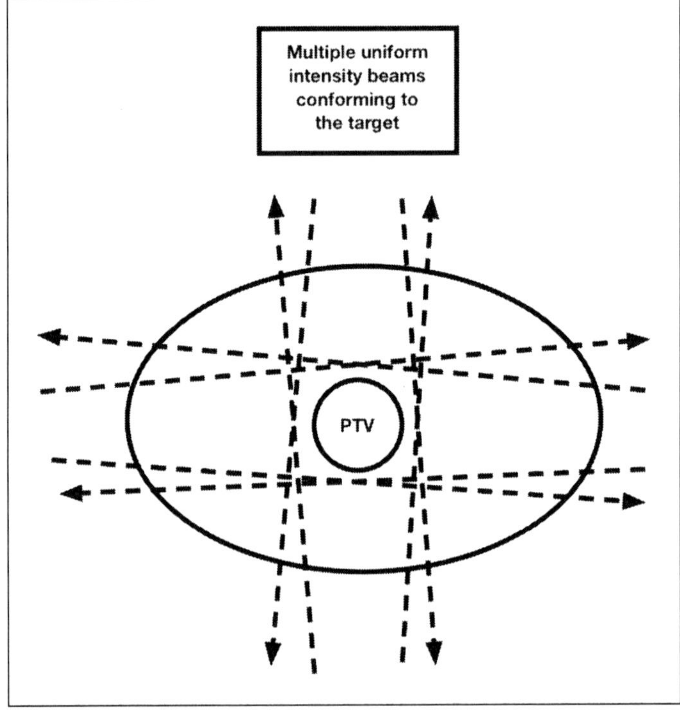

FIGURE 12.5 Three-dimensional conformal radiation therapy

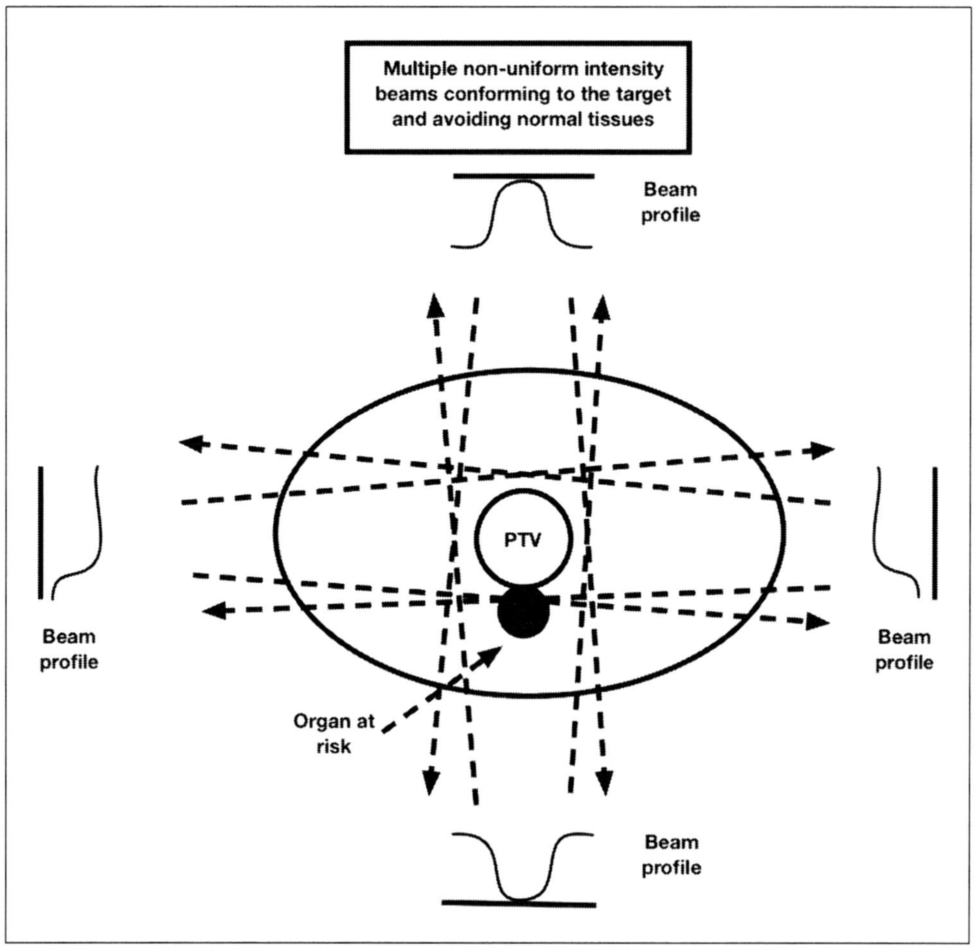

FIGURE 12.6 Intensity-modulated radiation therapy

then followed by computer optimization to provide the "best match" radiotherapy plan) method.

4. *Arc therapy.* Arc therapy is a form of IMRT treatment that uses arcs (radiation delivery while the linear accelerator gantry is moving in an arc) of radiotherapy instead of a fixed beam approach common with traditional IMRT approaches (Figure 12.7). Various systems are available to deliver arc treatment and include: intensity-modulated arc therapy, simplified intensity-modulated arc therapy, serial and helical tomotherapy, and volumetric-modulated arc therapy.
5. *Stereotactic radiosurgery.* This approach uses highly focused radiotherapy beams guided by pretreatment and on-treatment imaging (IGRT) to treat brain and spine tumors (Figure 12.8). This approach is usually combined with invasive fixation of the cranium (for brain tumors) to achieve high levels of immobilization to support the high dose of radiotherapy delivered to usually small target volumes. Commonly single fractions of radiotherapy are delivered; however, multiple fractions of radiotherapy can also be used particularly for larger tumors where normal tissue toxicity is a concern.
6. *Stereotactic body radiation therapy or stereotactic ablative radiation therapy.* This radiotherapy approach is similar to stereotactic radiosurgery but is directed to other areas of the body (e.g., small lung tumors). This approach uses highly conformal 3DCRT, arc therapy, or IMRT combined with patient immobilization (body immobilization or other non-invasive

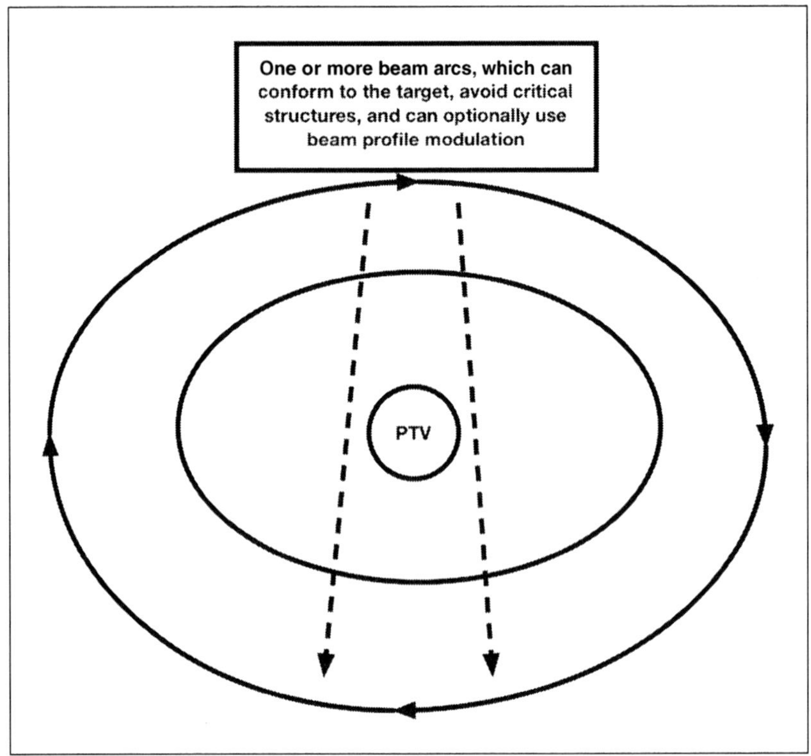

FIGURE 12.7 Arc-based radiation therapy

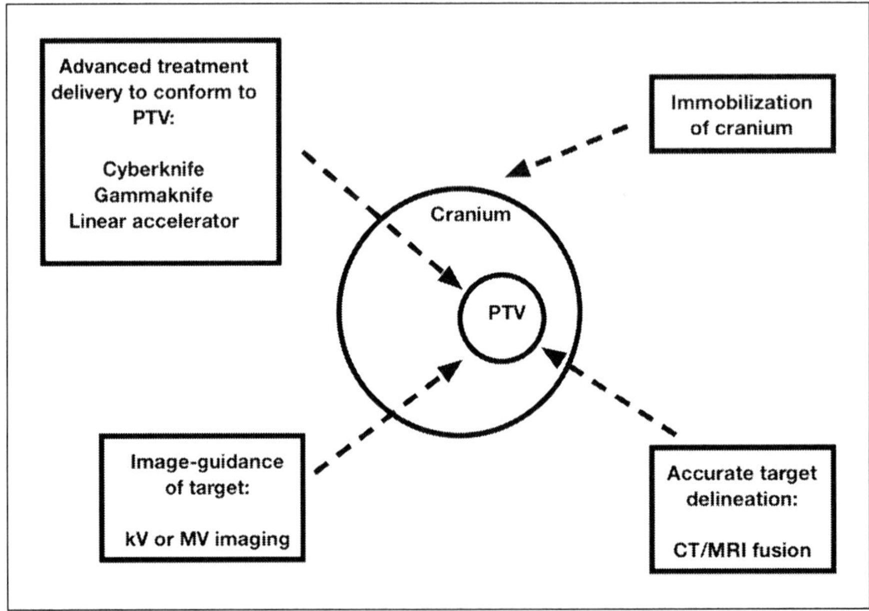

FIGURE 12.8 Stereotactic radiosurgery

devices) and IGRT (imaging to confirm location of tumor before and during the radiation procedure) to deliver highly accurate and precise hypofractionated radiotherapy to generally small (<5 cm) targets (Figure 12.9).

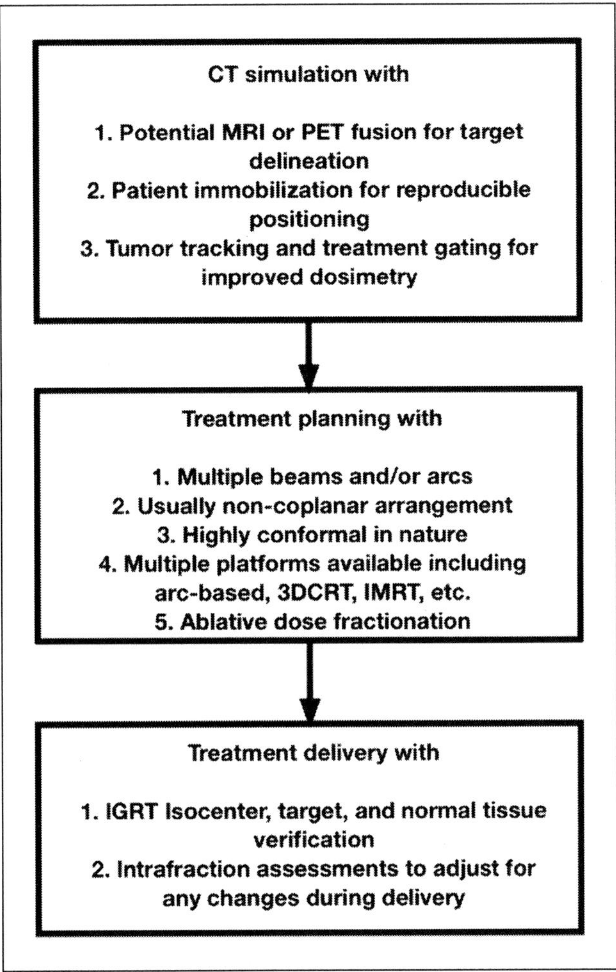

FIGURE 12.9 Stereotactic body radiation therapy

12.5. IMAGE-GUIDANCE

Image-Guided Radiation Therapy

Image-guided radiation therapy (IGRT) is a method by which repeated 2D and/or 3D imaging is utilized to direct radiation therapy back to the appropriate coordinate system as defined during radiation therapy simulation (Figure 12.10). These imaging sessions occur immediately prior to radiation delivery to define shifts and/or rotations in patient position prior to starting a "beam-on" radiation procedure. IGRT is separate from the use of imaging (such as CT, MRI, PET, or ultrasound) during simulation procedures as the former relates to treatment imaging to adapt patient position, whereas the latter deals with obtaining information to define cancer targets and normal tissue avoidance structures. Modern IGRT utilizes either kV diagnostic quality on-board imaging (e.g., fluoroscopy or kV cone-beam CT) or MV treatment energy on-board imaging (e.g., 2D kV planar portal image or a 3D MV cone-beam CT).

The ultimate rationale of IGRT is to improve both the accuracy (i.e., reduction of systematic error) and precision (i.e., reduction of random variance) of radiation delivery. Through these reductions of systematic and random errors, an improvement in tumor control and reduction of treatment toxicity is expected. IGRT is usually combined with IMRT treatment planning to combine the accuracy and precision of IGRT with the conformal target treatment and normal tissue avoidance of IMRT to further improve the therapeutic ratio.

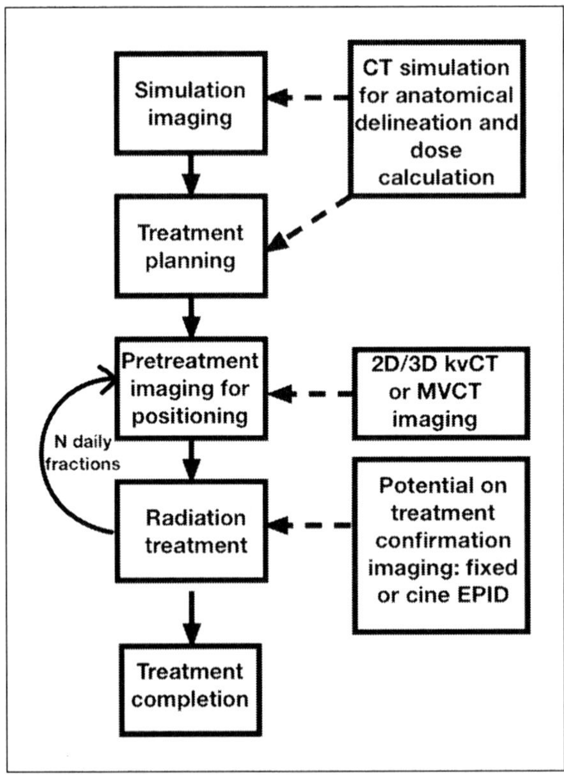

FIGURE 12.10 Image-guided radiation therapy

IGRT Options

Various IGRT options for improving radiotherapy delivery exist.

1. *Skin marks and surface anatomy.* Classically, the use of skin marks (e.g., tattoo or marker) and/or surface anatomy (e.g., field borders defined by anatomy) have been used to guide radiation treatment. When marks are utilized, they are cross-referenced to both documented field locations (e.g., center, corner, etc.) and the 3D coordinate system for the treatment unit (e.g., laser system). In this way, treatment that has been planned on the computer system is in alignment with the patient and the treatment unit.
2. *Portal imaging.* In this IGRT system, MV x-rays that pass through a patient during the treatment of a particular field are captured on radiographic film for inspection. The radiation oncologist would then have the option of accepting the film (and the set-up), shifting the patient to re-align for the next fraction of radiation treatment, or order a repeat port film to reassess the situation. Depending on the nature of the treatment, port films can be formed daily, weekly, or just on day one of treatment. This form of treatment delivery adaptation is usually used in an off-line imaging mode—IGRT imaging can impact future treatments but is not designed to impact the immediate treatment. This is because of the time required to obtain, process, and assess portal images on radiographic film.
3. *Electronic portal imaging.* These modern systems use on-board detectors to gather and then process information to provide 2D (kV or MV portal images) or 3D (kV or MV cone-beam images) gathered either immediately prior to, during, or after a radiation treatment beam is delivered. The advantage of this system is the fact that images can be reconstructed more quickly to provide 2D or 3D images that can be used to alter patient position or rotation immediately prior to treatment delivery. This "on-line" correction process can attempt to further improve the precision and accuracy of treatment delivery.
4. *Tumor tracking.* Systems have been developed whereby implantable objects (e.g., metal fiducial markers or radiofrequency beacon) or other external surrogates (e.g., infrared markers) can be tracked by computer systems to adapt treatment based on tumor and patient position. These integrated systems can be used to deliver gated radiotherapy whereby the radiation therapy beam can be controlled (i.e., shut on and off) depending on the location of the fiducial marker compared to acceptable variances allowed by the radiation oncology team.
5. *Adaptive radiation therapy.* This technology utilizes on-treatment imaging to identify significant changes in tumor target and/or normal tissue anatomy to warrant a reassessment of the treatment planning given the new realities of the cancer at the current time. The on-board imaging can be re-integrated with a treatment planning system and new contours and a modified radiation plan (including composite plan of delivered dose and expected new dose) can be generated (Figure 12.11). The goal of such adaptive treatment is to ensure that the therapeutic ratio of treatment is maintained—achieving effective target dose delivery while minimizing dose to normal tissue.

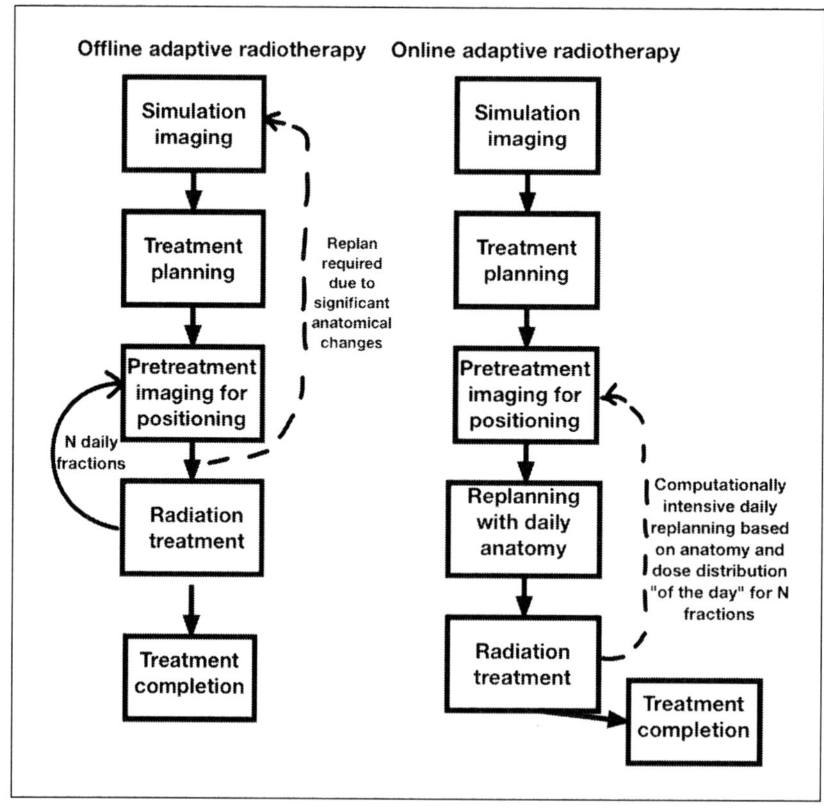

FIGURE 12.11 Adaptive radiation therapy

12.6. PARTICLE THERAPY

Overview

Particle therapy is a type of external-beam radiation therapy that is not based on traditional photon or electron particles (Figure 12.12). Particle therapy is otherwise known as hadron therapy (particles made of quarks), which are commonly found within the nucleus of atoms. Examples of hadron particles include protons, neutrons, and heavy ions (e.g., carbon ions), and all these particles have been exploited for therapeutic purposes.

Creation and Mechanism of Action

Particle therapy beams are created by accelerating positive ions (protons or heavy ions) in a cyclotron accelerator. Neutron beams are secondarily created by bombardment of an energetic proton beam into a beryllium target. In contrast to photon and electron beams where deposited dose degrades with depth, particle therapy beams demonstrate an increase of deposited dose until the maximum particle range is reached (i.e., the Bragg peak). Virtually no dose is deposited past this point, which can be therapeutically exploited to deliver target dose near critical structures. As opposed to photon/electron beam radiotherapy approaches, particle therapy deposits less dose to surrounding tissues and can be modulated to deliver

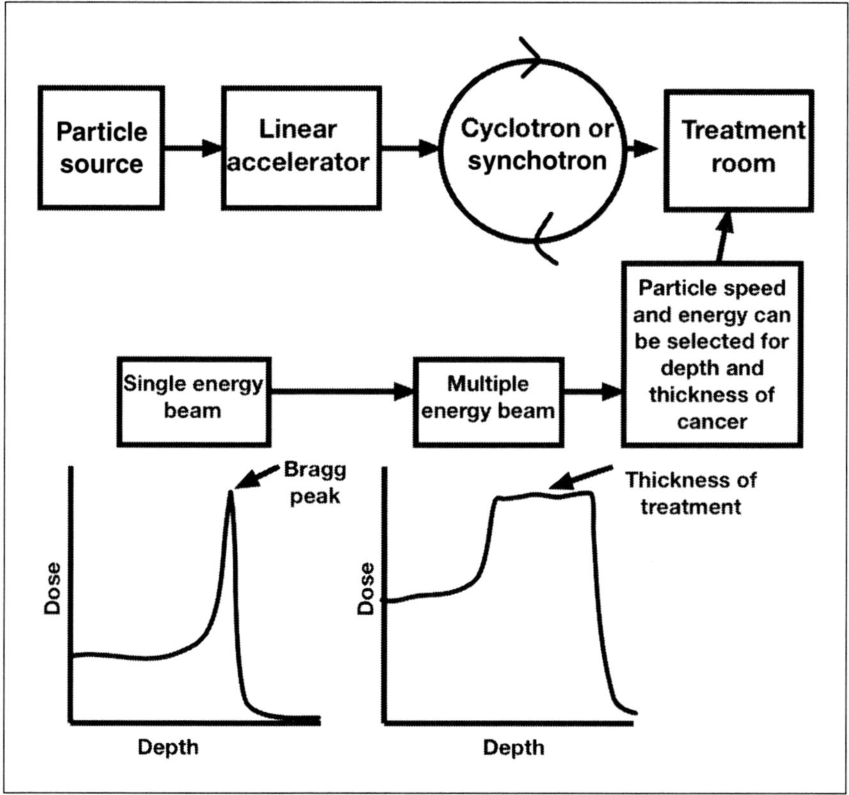

FIGURE 12.12 Particle therapy

highly conformal therapy. In order to deliver a clinical beam of particle radiotherapy, the pencil beam of particle therapy needs to be modulated using an electromagnetic approach (i.e., raster scan method).

Forms of Particle Therapy

1. *Proton therapy.* Compared to photon and electron therapy, proton beam therapy has the advantages of sharp range (i.e., Bragg peak), limited side scatter, and limited dose to normal tissue proximate to the target. Disadvantages include increased cost, space requirement, and increased skin dose (when compared to an equivalent photon beam).
2. *Neutron therapy.* Compared to protons, neutron therapy has the advantage of high linear energy transfer (LET, about 50× compared to photons) and oxygen independence (oxygen not required for DNA damage—useful for hypoxic tumors).
3. *Heavy ion therapy.* Carbon ion therapy has been clinically used to treat cancers. Compared to proton therapy, heavy ion therapy deposits a larger proportion of its energy near the Bragg peak but has the disadvantage of non-zero dose deposition past the peak because of nuclear reactions between the heavy ions and the underlying matter.

12.7. BRACHYTHERAPY

Overview

Brachytherapy is a form of radiation therapy that places a radionuclide source in physical proximity to a cancer target to deliver anticancer treatment. It has been used clinically since the beginning of the twentieth century after various proponents (Pierre Curie, Henri-Alexandre Danlos, and Alexander Graham Bell) suggested their use as anticancer treatment.

These brachytherapy sources are enclosed within a protective system (e.g., capsule, wire, seed) to prevent dissemination and absorption into the body. Advantages related to brachytherapy techniques include: localized delivery, low to minimal normal tissue radiotherapy, efficient delivery (short time and number of fractions), and acceptable toxicity profile. Additionally, any possible motion of targets and normal tissue are mitigated by the fact that radiotherapy sources typically remain in the same relative position. However, given the invasive nature of many brachytherapy procedures, patients do need to be eligible for various anesthetic procedures to facilitate the required procedure(s). Brachytherapy can be delivered alone or in conjunction with other therapies such as chemotherapy and/or external-beam radiation therapy.

Brachytherapy Radionuclides

Various radionuclides are utilized in brachytherapy procedures. A list of common radioisotopes including type of radioactive decay, decay energy, and half-life are depicted in Table 12.1.

Classification

Available forms of brachytherapy are classified by one of several methods:

1. *Duration.* Brachytherapy implants can be temporary or permanent in treatment duration. A temporary implant involves the placement of a radiation source for a preplanned time period followed by source removal usually on the order of minutes to hours. This preplanned time period depends on the radionuclide used, source strength, total dose to be prescribed, as well as various local anatomical factors. Remote after-loading systems

TABLE 12.1 Common Radionuclides in Brachytherapy

Radionuclide	Decay	Energy	Half-Life
Cesium-137	Gamma	0.66 MeV	30 years
Iodine-125	Gamma	27–36 kV	60 d
Iridium-192	Beta	380 kV	74 d
Palladium-103	Beta	21 kV	17 d

are commonly employed to temporarily deliver radiation dosage and store the radioactive source in a shielded housing when not in use. Manual after-loading can also be performed by the radiation oncologist depending on the radioactive source used (e.g., wire, needles). Permanent brachytherapy involves the manual placement of various encapsulated radioactive sources (such as seeds or pellet grains) in the treatment target. The radiotherapy dosage is typically delivered over weeks to months until the radioactive seeds have virtually zero activity and remain in the treatment location.

2. *Treatment intensity.* Various systems can deliver different rates of radiotherapy dosage (i.e., dose rate). These include low-dose rate (LDR, < 2 Gy/h, e.g., prostate seed implant), medium-dose rate (2–12 Gy/h), and HDR (> 12 Gy/h, e.g., prostate, lung, esophagus, and cervix). An intermittent treatment intensity system called pulsed-dose rate (PDR, intermittent dose given once per hour, e.g., gynecological) can be used to deliver LDR-like treatment.
3. *Source placement.* Placement of radioactive sources can either be interstitial (sources placed within the target tissue) or contact (source placed in a space next to the target tissue) in nature. Various contact approaches exist and include: intra-vascular (within blood vessels, e.g., coronary vessels), intra-luminal (in a lumen, e.g., esophagus), and intra-cavitary (in a body cavity, e.g., cervix).

Treatment Planning

Various classical systems have been developed for the planning of brachytherapy implant including the Paterson–Parker/Manchester system (uniform delivery of dose to a plane or volume), Quimby system (uniform distribution of equal linear activity sources), Memorial system (adapted Quimby system based on 1-cm lattices), and the Paris system (uniform activity line source implant performed in parallel). Modern brachytherapy planning is performed using a computer-based system, integrating pretreatment target and applicator imaging with a treatment planning system that can optimize source/seed placement, dwell time, and strength to plan optimal treatment. Once optimized, treatment is delivered according to the system to be used (e.g., LDR seeds, HDR temporary after-loading source).

Clinical Examples

Various cancer-specific clinical examples of brachytherapy treatment routinely utilized are listed below.

1. *Prostate cancer.* Prostate cancer can be treated with a permanent LDR seed implant or a temporary HDR implant either alone or in combination with external-beam radiation therapy. External-beam radiotherapy is utilized in cases where extracapsular, seminal vesicle, and/or nodal disease is known to exist or is suspected to exist. The side-effect profile and cancer control statistics of both permanent LDR and temporary HDR prostate brachytherapy implants compare favorably with other modalities of treatment including radical prostatectomy.
2. *Cervical/endometrial cancer.* Various forms of brachytherapy (LDR, PDR, HDR) can be used in either the primary or post-surgical treatment of cervical and uterine cancers. This form of brachytherapy is commonly combined with external-beam radiotherapy to cover parametrial and nodal microscopic/macroscopic disease depending on the clinical scenario.

3. *Lung/esophageal cancer.* Locally advanced lung, tracheal, and esophageal cancers can obstruct the underlying lumen leading to palliative issues such as shortness of breath, stridor, and obstruction. Intra-luminal HDR brachytherapy can be utilized to palliate lesions to reverse and/or prevent obstructive symptoms.
4. *Breast cancer.* HDR brachytherapy can be used to deliver localized radiotherapy in the post-lumpectomy situation to prevent local recurrence of disease. Compared to external-beam approaches, a smaller volume of radiation therapy (lumpectomy cavity vs. entire breast) can be delivered in a shorter period of time (e.g., 1 week vs. several weeks). Treatment can be planned and delivered either using an intracavitary (balloon catheter) or an interstitial (traditional catheter) system.
5. *Skin cancer.* Skin cancers can be treated using contact and interstitial approaches to avoid surgery with its potential cosmetic issues (e.g., eyes, ears, nose, and mouth). Treatment is usually delivered using HDR brachytherapy; however, LDR approaches using grains and needles are also available.

12.8. RADIOISOTOPE THERAPY

Overview

Radioisotope therapy is a form of radiation therapy that utilizes radioactive agents either alone (or as a salt) or conjugated with another chemical (antibody) to target treatment to a specific organ system (e.g., iodine 131 and thyroid). This form of therapy can be given in various modes including: oral, intravenous, and intra-cavitary. Because radioisotopes are not stable and will undergo radioactive decay, radiation dose can be delivered in proximity to where the radioisotope agents are deposited. The prototypical radioisotope utilized for clinical use is a short range beta emitter (to deposit dosage to nearby cancer cells) with a short to medium half-life (to clear radioactivity from the patient in a timely fashion).

Radioisotopes are also utilized for the treatment of cancer in ways that do not involve the physical absorption of the agent into the body. Teletherapy radiation treatment machines utilize cobalt-60 to deliver a 1.25-MV photon beam. Despite this technology being more than 50 years old, it is still in clinical use around the world. Additionally, brachytherapy techniques utilize many radioisotopes in their systems. These include iodine-125 (seeds), pallidium-103 (seeds), gold-198 (grains), iridium-192 (wires, HDR after-loading), as well as traditional brachytherapy radioisotopes for needle/tube-based treatment (radium-226, cesium-137, and cobalt-60).

Radioisotope Examples

1. *Iodine-131.* The primary mode of radioactivity of iodine-131 is beta decay (half-life 8.02 days). This agent is used for the diagnosis and the treatment (in iodine salt form) of thyroid cancer. Additionally, iodine-131-*meta*iodobenzylguanidine (^{131}I-MIBG) can be used for the treatment of other cancers (pheochromocytoma and neuroblastoma). Patients receiving iodine-131 therapy will receive post-treatment isolation information regarding pregnancy, home decontamination, and familial contact. The majority of iodine-131 is usually eliminated within 3 to 5 days (depending on initial dose). Iodine-131 has also been combined with an anti-CD monoclonal antibody for the treatment of refractory non-Hodgkin lymphoma.
2. *Strontium-89.* This agent (half-life of about 50 days, beta decay) is used for the treatment of bone metastases. The radioactive agent selectively binds to areas of affected bone (because of bone destruction).
3. *Samarium-153 lexidronam.* Also used for treatment of bone metastases in a similar manner to strontium-89.
4. *Radium-223 chloride.* A new agent for bone metastases treatment demonstrating a survival benefit of 2.8 months in phase III randomized controlled trial testing. Radium-223 has a half-life of 11.4 days and is a beta emitter with a short range equivalent to 10 cell diameters or less.
5. *Yttrium-90.* This radioisotope (half-life of 64 hours and beta decay) is clinically used in the treatment of neuroendocrine tumors and lymphomas.

12.9. THE RADIATION ONCOLOGISTS' TOOLBOX

Challenging clinical scenarios can exist that are difficult to safely manage the balance of the therapeutic ratio between the tumor/treatment effect and normal tissue toxicity. These scenarios can occur because of large treatment volumes, conformality of targets around normal tissues, as well as other clinical factors such as expected patient treatment tolerability because of performance status and/or comorbidity concerns, absolute/relative contraindications to radiotherapy, and reduced organ function (i.e., pulmonary function in lung cancer).

The following considerations can be assessed and altered as necessary to optimize treatment on a case-by-case basis.

1. *Alteration of treatment intent.* Examples include: radical, adjuvant, neoadjuvant, salvage, and palliative. If radical therapy is not feasible or safe, use of palliative intent treatment with palliative radiotherapy dose fractionations are appropriate.
2. *Consideration of alternative therapies.* Examples of such alternatives include: surgery, chemotherapy, hormonal therapy, and targeted therapy.
3. *Fractionation considerations.* Alteration of various parameters such as total dose, dose/fraction, overall treatment time, altered fractionation, and hypofractionation.
4. *Critical structure volume.* Consideration of using an altered margin around treatment targets or reduction or removal of various treatment volumes (e.g., exclusion of elective nodal treatment volumes).
5. *Patient immobilization.* Ensure that patient immobilization is adequate to properly target local and regional targets while minimizing OAR volumes. Various levels of immobilization exist ranging from none to invasive stereotactic techniques.
6. *Radiotherapy simulation.* Consideration of various simulation techniques: CT simulation, MRI fusion, and PET fusion.
7. *Radiotherapy planning.* Various factors can be adjusted to optimize target and normal tissue dosimetry including: beam type (photons, electrons, protons, brachytherapy), beam energy, beam arrangement/weighting, field matching, beam modification (wedges, MLC, compensators), and isodose and dose–volume histogram assessment. Advanced planning paradigms such as IMRT, stereotactic ablative radiotherapy, and adaptive planning strategies can also be considered.
8. *Radiotherapy delivery.* Various on-treatment factors can influence accuracy of delivery including: IGRT (2D/3D kV or MV) to reduce margins, treatment gating (beam on and off depending on a physiological marker, e.g., breathing trace), and tumor tracking.
9. *Modification of chemoradiation.* Various modification options exist and include: chemotherapy dose reduction, chemotherapy agent selection, and decoupling of chemotherapy and radiation (non-concurrent approach).
10. *Medical management.* Management of comorbidities and treatment-related toxicities can have equal or greater impact on patient survival than treatment directed toward the cancer itself (depending on the cancer involved). Assessment of relative/absolute contraindications to radiotherapy (connective tissue disorders, inflammatory bowel disease, multiple sclerosis, and DNA repair disorders) and other radiotherapy considerations (hip replacements, pacemakers, and implantable defibrillators) should be performed during the initial patient assessment.

PART III: TREATMENT PLANNING PROTOCOLS AND CONCEPTS

Chapter 13

Palliative Radiotherapy

13.1. BRAIN METS

Therapeutic Considerations

Patient population. Brain metastasis—single or multiple.

Dose Specification

Whole brain radiotherapy:

- 40 Gy in 20 fractions (2 Gy/fraction)
- 37.5 Gy in 15 fractions (2.5 Gy/fraction)
- 30 Gy in 10 fractions (3 Gy/fraction)
- 20 Gy in five fractions (4 Gy/fraction)

Single Brain Metastasis, Good Prognosis

- Expected survival > 3 months
- < 3 to 4 cm and amenable to safe complete resection
  - Radiosurgery alone (level 1)
  - Whole brain radiotherapy and radiosurgery (level 1)
  - Surgery and whole brain radiotherapy (level 1)
  - Surgery and radiosurgery/radiation boost to the resection cavity (level 3)
- > 3 to 4 cm and amenable to safe complete resection
  - Surgery and whole brain radiotherapy (level 1)
  - Surgery and radiosurgery/radiation boost to the resection cavity (level 3)
- < 3 to 4 cm, not resectable or incompletely resected
  - Whole brain radiotherapy and radiosurgery (level 1)
  - Radiosurgery alone
- > 3 to 4 cm, not resectable or incompletely resected
  - Whole brain radiotherapy (level 3)

Multiple Brain Metastases, Good Prognosis

- Expected survival > 3 months
- Limited number of brain metastases (all < 3–4 cm)
  - Radiosurgery alone (level 1)
  - Whole brain radiotherapy and radiosurgery (level 1)
  - Whole brain radiotherapy alone (level 1)
  - Safe resection for metastases causing significant mass effect and post-operative whole brain radiotherapy (level 3)

Poor Prognosis

- Expected survival < 3 months, any number of metastases
  - Palliative care with or without whole brain radiotherapy (level 3)

RTOG Recursive Partitioning Analysis

- Class I: KPS ≥ 70, < 65 years old, controlled primary, no extracranial metastasis
  - Median survival: 7.1 months
- Class II: all others
  - Median survival: 4.2 months
- Class III: KPS < 70
  - Median survival: 2.3 months

Simulation

- *Imaging.* Conventional or CT simulation
- *Position.* Supine, neck neutral
- *Immobilization.* Immobilization device (i.e., thermoplastic mask)
- *Scanning limits.* Clearing skull to bottom of C3

Target Volume(s)

- Whole brain radiotherapy (Figure 13.1)
  - Clearing skull superior, anterior, posterior
  - Inferior: bottom of foramen magnum or inferior to C1 or inferior to C2
  - Block eyes, nasal cavity, oral cavity with a margin on the skull

Treatment Planning

- Ensure adequate coverage of entire brain

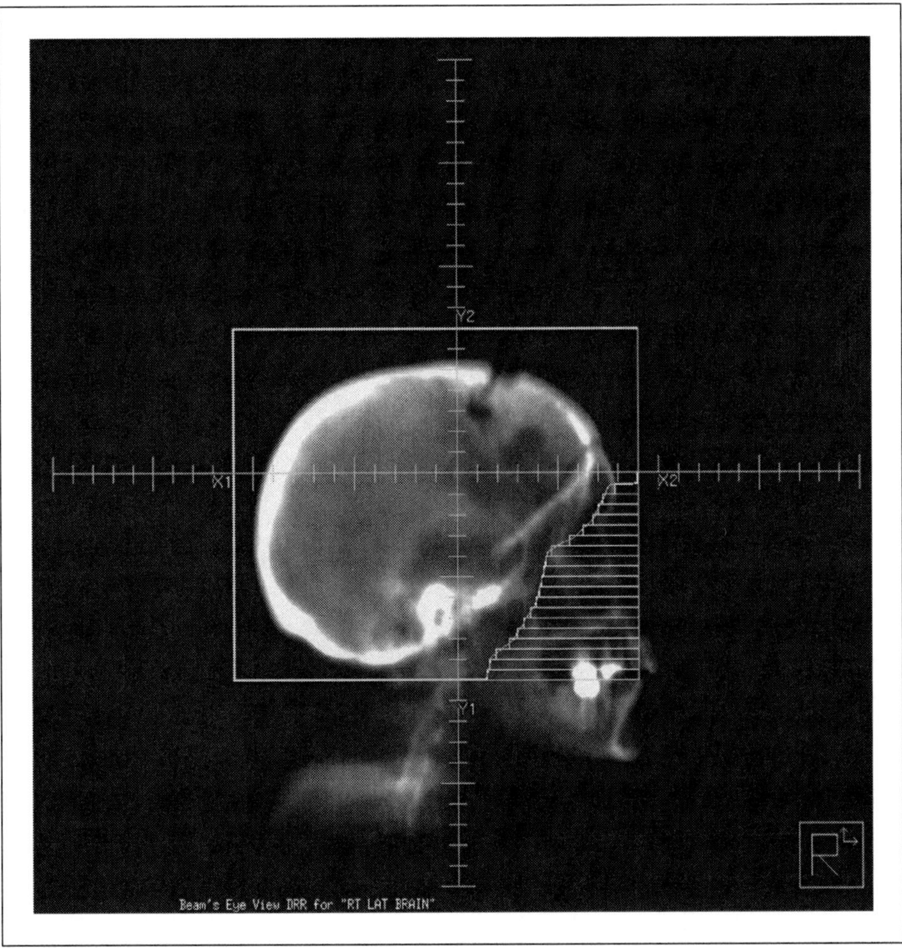

FIGURE 13.1 Right lateral whole brain digitally reconstructed radiograph (DRR)

Treatment Delivery

- *Technique.* Pair of opposed laterals
- *Image-guidance.* Onboard imaging if required

Toxicity

Acute:

- Fatigue, skin erythema, epilation/alopecia
- Otitis externa
- Headache, exacerbation of neurological symptoms
- Nausea, vomiting, altered taste

Late:

- Tanning of the scalp, fatigue, somnolence
- Memory loss, neurocognitive decline, behavioral change

- Radiation necrosis
- Sensorineural hearing loss, cataracts

Clinical Protocol References

Tsao MN, et al. Radiotherapeutic and surgical management for brain metastasis(es): an ASTRO evidence-based guideline. *Pract. Radiat. Oncol.* 2012;2(3):210–225.

Sperduto PW, et al. Diagnosis-specific prognostic factors, indexes, and treatment outcomes for patients with newly diagnosed brain metastases: a multi-institutional analysis of 4,259 patients. *Int. J. Radiat. Oncol. Biol. Phys.* 2010; 77(3): 655–661.

Gaspar LE, et al. Validation of the RTOG recursive partitioning analysis (RPA) classification for brain metastases. *Int. J. Radiat. Oncol. Biol. Phys.* 2000;47(4):1001–1006.

13.2. BONE METS

Therapeutic Considerations

- *Patient population.* Metastatic bone cancer
- *Concurrent treatments.* ±bisphosphonates, ±radionuclides, ±kyphoplasty, ±vertebroplasty, ±surgical decompression or stabilization

Treatment Goals

- Decrease pain and/or prevention of the morbidity caused by bony metastases

Dose Specification

- 30 Gy in 10 fractions (3 Gy/fraction)
- 24 Gy in six fractions (4 Gy/fraction)
- 20 Gy in five fractions (4 Gy/fraction)
- 8 Gy in one fraction

Treatment Considerations

- 8 Gy in one fraction
  - More convenient
  - 20% re-treatment rate
- Longer course treatment
  - 8% re-treatment rate
- No difference in side effects between the treatment fractionation schedules
- Re-treatment close to the spinal cord
  - Consider summing the biological equivalent dose from the initial and repeat treatment regimens
  - Estimate the risk of radiation myelopathy
- Surgery does not obviate the need for post-operative radiotherapy

Simulation

- *Imaging.* CT or conventional simulation
- *Position.* Supine for most situations
- *Immobilization.* To allow for consistent set-up

Target Volume(s)

Spine:

- Include at least one vertebral body above and below the painful vertebra(e)
- Treatment length should not exceed 20 cm

Long bones:

- Minimum margin should be 2 cm

Other sites:

- At discretion of treating physician

Treatment Planning

- *Spine.* Dose prescribed to mid-vertebral body for single posterior field
- *Other sites.* Should be prescribed to D_{max} for single incident fields
- Prescribe to mid-plane dose for opposed fields
    - Extremities, sacrum, pelvis: anterior–posterior (AP)/posterior–anterior (PA) fields
    - Thoracic, lumbar spine: PA field (AP/PA can be used if target more central)
    - Skull, scapula, sternum, clavicle: opposed electron field
    - Cervical spine: opposed lateral and oblique fields
    - Rib, superficial lesions: consider wedged pair fields or electrons

Treatment Delivery and Image-Guidance

Technique: photons; orthovoltage or electrons may be used at superficial sites
Image-guidance: simulation fields required to document target localization

Toxicity

Acute:

- Skin erythema, pain flare

Clinical Protocol References

NCIC SC23: a phase III double-blind study of dexamethasone versus placebo in the prophylaxis of radiation-induced pain flare following palliative radiotherapy for bone metastases.

Lutz, *et al.* Palliative radiotherapy for bone metastases: an ASTRO evidence-based guideline. *Int. J. Radiat. Oncol. Biol. Phys.* 2011;79(4):965–976.

Vassil AD, Videtic GMM. Handbook of treatment planning in radiation oncology. Chapter 13: palliative radiotherapy. New York: Demos Medical Publishing 2011:215–217.

13.3. LUNG/MEDIASTINAL

Therapeutic Considerations

- *Patient population.* Metastatic or select locally advanced non-small cell lung cancer who are not candidates for curative therapy
- *Concurrent treatments.* None, may consider sequential chemotherapy
- *Alternative treatments.* Palliative care, chemotherapy alone

Treatment Goals

- Relieve tumor-related symptoms
  - Hemoptysis, bronchial obstruction, cough, dyspnea, chest pain
  - Dysphagia related to esophageal compression
  - Superior vena cava syndrome, hoarseness, stridor
- Improve quality of life
- Symptoms not typically suitable for palliative radiotherapy
  - Malignant pleural effusion
  - Lymphangitic carcinomatosis
  - Multilobar parenchymal disease

Dose Specification

- All studies with external beam radiotherapy showed a beneficial effect.
  - No strong evidence favoring one schedule with respect to efficacy
  - No major differences with respect to improvement in quality of life between the schedules

Treatment Considerations

- High dose/fractionation external beam
  - 30 to 35 Gy in 10 fractions (3–3.5 Gy/fraction)
  - 36 to 45 Gy in 12 to 15 fractions (3 Gy/fraction)
  - 50 to 60 Gy in 25 to 30 fractions (2 Gy/fraction)

Advantages:

- Modest improvement in survival and symptom score, primarily in patients with good performance status (5% at 1 year, 3% at 2 years)

Disadvantages:

- Increased esophageal toxicity
- Low dose/fractionation external beam
  - 20 Gy in five fractions (4 Gy/fraction)
  - 16 to 17 Gy in two weekly fractions (8.5 Gy/fraction)
  - 10 Gy in one fraction

Advantages:
- Good symptom relief
- Fewer side effects

Disadvantages:
- Radiation myelopathy may be associated with 17 Gy in two fractions, thus requires appropriate planning
- Better for patients requesting shorter treatment course and/or poor performance status

Endobronchial Brachytherapy

- *Goal of therapy.* Relief of endobronchial symptoms
  - Cough, dyspnea, hemoptysis
- No defined role in routine initial palliative treatment of endobronchial obstruction
- Option for endobronchial brachytherapy after failure of external beam radiotherapy
  - Bronchial obstruction, hemoptysis, lung collapse

Chemotherapy

- No evidence to support use of concurrent chemotherapy and radiotherapy
  - Increased overall response rate (small)
  - Significant increased toxicity
  - No significant improvement in overall survival, progression free survival, or symptom palliation
- *Goal.* Sequence/integrate chemotherapy and radiotherapy in a non-concurrent fashion
  - Chemotherapy is a standard of care of metastatic/recurrent lung cancer

Clinical Protocol Reference

Rodrigues G, et al. Palliative thoracic radiotherapy in lung cancer: an American Society for Radiation Oncology evidence-based clinical practice guideline. *Pract Radiat Oncol* 2011;1:60–71.

Chapter 14

CNS Treatment Planning

14.1. LOW-GRADE GLIOMA

Therapeutic Considerations

- *Patient population.* Supratentorial, low-grade diffuse glioma (astrocytoma World Health Organization [WHO] grade II), oligoastrocytoma WHO grade II, or oligodendroglioma WHO grade II
- *Concurrent treatments.* None
- *Alternative treatments.* Temozolomide alone

Dose Specification

- 50.4 Gy in 28 fractions (1.8 Gy/fraction)

Simulation

- *Imaging.* Computed tomography (CT) simulation, maximum slice thickness 3 mm
- *Position.* Supine or prone
- *Immobilization.* Mask or frame with relocation accuracy < 5 mm
- *Other.* Image fusion with MRI and/or positron emission tomography (PET) for target definition

Target Volume(s)

- *Gross tumor volume (GTV).* Region of high signal intensity area on fluid attenuated inversion recovery (FLAIR) or T2-weighted MRI, corresponding to hypodense areas on CT images, include areas of enhancement on CT and/or tracer uptake on PET
- *If previous surgery.* Operative cavity and residual tumor
- *Clinical target volume (CTV).* CTV + 1 to 1.5 cm
  - Extension to contralateral hemisphere only when a midline structure is invaded by tumor

  - Tentorium and meninges considered anatomical borders (only 5 mm margin to encompass microscopic spread at these borders)
- *Planning target volume (PTV).* CTV + 0.5 to 0.7 cm

Treatment Planning

- *PTV.* Maximum dose homogeneity 95% to 107% prescription dose
- PTV should be encompassed by 95% isodose
  - 90% isodose is acceptable if close to organs at risk

Treatment Delivery

- *Technique.* Three-dimensional conformal radiation therapy (3DCRT)/intensity-modulated radiation therapy (IMRT)
- *Image-guidance.* At least weekly portal imaging or portal films

Organ(s) at risk

- *Brainstem.* $D_{max} < 55$ Gy
- *Globes (including retina, lens).* should not be included in any direct beam
- *Lens.* $D_{max} < 5$ Gy
- *Retina.* $D_{max} \leq 40$ Gy
- *Optic chiasm/nerves.* $D_{max} < 55$ Gy
- *Contralateral normal brain.* < 50% to 60% total dose

Toxicity

Acute:
- Fatigue, alopecia, skin reaction
- Headache, worsening neurological symptoms
- Mucositis (if nasopharynx included), reduced hearing, loss of taste, dry mouth

Late:
- Reduced hearing
- Mental slowing, memory disturbances, difficulty with concentrating
- Radiation necrosis

Clinical Protocol Reference

EORTC 22033, NCIC CE5, TROG 0601, MRC-BR13: primary chemotherapy with temozolomide versus radiotherapy in patients with low-grade gliomas after stratification for genetic 1p loss: a phase III study

14.2. ANAPLASTIC GLIOMA

Therapeutic Considerations

- *Patient population.* Anaplastic glioma
- *Concurrent treatments.* Surgery followed by radiation therapy and concomitant temozolomide and adjuvant temozolomide
- *Alternative treatments.* Temozolomide alone, radiotherapy alone

Dose Specification

- 59.4 Gy in 33 fractions (1.8 Gy/fraction)

Or

- 50.4 Gy in 28 fractions (1.8 Gy/fraction) + boost of 9 Gy in five fractions (1.8 Gy/fraction)
  - Total: 59.4 Gy in 33 fractions (1.8 Gy/fraction)

Simulation

- *Imaging.* CT simulation, maximum slice thickness of 3 mm, or MRI simulation
- *Position.* Supine or prone
- *Immobilization.* Immobilization device with relocation accuracy < 5 mm
- *Other.* MRI fusion of postoperative imaging, recommend contrast

Target Volume(s)

- *GTV.* Region of high signal intensity of T2-weighted or FLAIR MRI images and the region of enhancement on the postoperative CT/MRI (or region of enhancement on the preoperative CT/MRI) and the tumor resection cavity
- *CTV.* GTV + 1.5 to 2 cm
  - Extends to contralateral hemisphere only when midline structures (corpus callosum) and contralateral hemisphere are invaded by tumor
  - Tentorium and meninges are anatomical borders, thus a margin of 7 to 10 mm is sufficient at these borders
- *PTV.* CTV + 0.5 to 0.7 cm

Or

- *GTV1.* Region of high signal intensity of T2-weighted or FLAIR MRI and the region of enhancement on the postoperative MRI (or region of enhancement on the preoperative CT/MRI) and the tumor resection cavity
- *GTVboost.* Area of tumor enhancement and resection margin
- *CTV1.* GTV1 + 1.0 cm
  - Must not extend outside the brain
  - May be modified to meet organ at risk constraints
- *CTVboost.* GTVboost
  - If no GTVboost, then CTVboost = GTV1
- *PTV1.* CTV1 + 5 mm
- *PTVboost.* CTVboost + 5 mm

Treatment Planning

- *PTV.* D_{max} ≤ 107% of prescription dose
- *PTV.* D_{min} ≥ 95% of prescription dose
- > 95% of PTV to receive 100% of prescription dose

Treatment Delivery

- *Technique.* 3DCRT/IMRT
- *Image-guidance.* Verification fields at least weekly (electronic portal imaging device [EPID] or portal films)

Organ(s) at risk

- *Brainstem.* D_{max} ≤ 55 Gy
- *Lens.* D_{max} ≤ 5 Gy
- *Retina.* D_{max} ≤ 36 Gy
- *Optic chiasm, nerves.* D_{max} ≤ 54 Gy
- *Normal brain contralateral to tumor.* < 60% of total dose
- *Spinal cord.* D_{max} ≤ 45 Gy

Toxicity

Acute:

- Fatigue, alopecia, skin reaction
- Headache, nausea, altered taste, reduced hearing
- Mucositis (if nasopharynx included)

Late:

- Mental slowing, permanent hearing impairment, behavioral changes
- Cataracts, decreased vision
- Dry mouth, altered taste
- Hormonal deficiency
- Radionecrosis

Clinical Protocol References

RTOG0834, EORTC26053, NCIC CEC.1: phase III trial on concurrent and adjuvant temozolomide chemotherapy in non-1p/19q deleted anaplastic glioma: the CATNON intergroup trial.

RTOG1071/NCCTG N0577/CEC.2: phase III intergroup study of radiotherapy versus temozolomide alone versus radiotherapy with concomitant and adjuvant temozolomide for patients with 1p and 19q co-deleted anaplastic glioma. CODEL.

14.3. GLIOBLASTOMA MULTIFORME

Therapeutic Considerations

- *Patient population.* Glioblastoma multiforme, postresection, or biopsy
- *Concurrent treatments.* Daily temozolomide with radiotherapy followed by adjuvant temozolomide
- *Alternative treatments.* Radiotherapy alone, addition of novel agent

Dose Specification

- 60 Gy in 30 fractions (2 Gy/fraction)

Simulation

- *Imaging.* CT simulation
- *Position.* Supine
- *Immobilization.* Head immobilization
- *Other.* Recommend MRI fusion

Target Volume(s)

- *GTV1.* Gross tumor on T2-weighted or FLAIR on the postoperative MRI scan
  - Include all postoperative MRI enhancement, and surgical cavity
- *GTV2.* Contrast-enhanced T1-weighted abnormality of the postoperative MRI scan
  - Include surgical cavity margins
- *CTV1.* GTV1 + 2 cm
  - Can decrease margin to 0.5 cm around natural barriers (skull, ventricles, falx, allow sparing of optic nerve/chiasm)
- *CTV2.* GTV2 + 2 cm
  - Can decrease margin to 0.5 cm around natural barriers (skull, ventricles, falx, allow sparing of optic nerve/chiasm)
- *PTV1.* CTV1 + 0.3 to 0.5 cm
- *PTV2.* CTV2 + 0.3 to 0.5 cm

Treatment Planning

- *PTV1.* Treated to 46 Gy in 23 fractions
- *PTV2.* Boost volume/cone down to a total of 60 Gy (14 Gy in seven fractions)
- *PTV.* $D_{min} \geq 95\%$ of prescription dose
- *PTV.* $D_{max} \geq 105\%$ of prescription dose
- ≥ 95% of PTV to receive 100% of prescription dose
- 99% of PTV2 is covered by 54 Gy

Treatment Delivery

- *Technique.* IMRT/3DCRT
- *Image-guidance.* At least weekly image verification (EPID, cone-beam CT, megavoltage CT [MVCT])

Organ(s) at Risk

- *Brainstem.* $D_{max} \leq 60$ Gy
- *Lenses.* $D_{max} \leq 7$ Gy
- *Retinae.* $D_{max} \leq 50$ Gy
- *Optic chiasm.* $D_{max} \leq 56$ Gy
- *Optic nerves.* $D_{max} \leq 55$ Gy

Toxicity

Acute:

- Alopecia, fatigue, erythema, or soreness of the scalp
- Nausea, vomiting, dry mouth, altered taste
- Aggravation of brain tumor symptoms: headache, seizure, weakness
- Otitis externa, short-term hearing impairment

Late:

- Lethargy, transient worsening of neurological deficits in first 1 to 3 months
- Radiation necrosis, endocrine dysfunction
- Neurocognitive deficits, mental slowing, behavioral change
- Permanent hearing and visual impairment
- Radiation-induced neoplasms

Clinical Protocol Reference

RTOG 0825: phase III double-blind, placebo-controlled trial of conventional concurrent chemoradiation and adjuvant temozolomide, plus bevacizumab versus conventional concurrent chemoradiation and adjuvant temozolomide in patients with newly diagnosed glioblastoma.

14.4. MENINGIOMA

Therapeutic Considerations

- *Patient population:*
  - Intermediate risk: gross total resection of a WHO grade II meningioma or recurrent WHO grade I meningioma
  - High risk: WHO grade III meningioma, recurrent WHO grade II meningioma, newly diagnosed subtotally resected WHO grade II meningioma
- *Concurrent treatments.* Prior surgery or biopsy
- *Alternative treatments.* Observation until progression

Dose Specification

- *Intermediate risk.* 54 Gy in 30 fractions (1.8 Gy/fraction)
- *High risk.* 60 Gy in 30 fractions (2 Gy/fraction)

Simulation

- *Immobilization.* Non-invasive, stereotactic, re-locatable immobilization, reproduce setup to within 5 mm
- *Other.* Fuse postoperative MRI

Target Volume(s)

Intermediate risk:
- *GTV.* Tumor bed, include any residual nodular enhancement
  - Cerebral edema and a dural tail are not specifically included
- *CTV.* GTV + 1 cm
  - Can reduce margin to 0.5 mm around natural barriers (skull)
- *PTV.* CTV + 3 to 5 mm

High risk:
- *GTV.* Tumor bed and residual nodular enhancement
  - Cerebral edema and a dural tail are not specifically included
- *CTV60.* GTV + 1.0 cm
- *CTV54.* GTV + 2.0 cm
  - May be reduced to 1.0 cm around natural barriers
- *PTV60.* CTV + 3 to 5 mm
- *PTV54.* CTV + 3 to 5 mm

Treatment Planning

Intermediate risk:

- 54 Gy isodose line must cover ≥ 95% of PTV
- *PTV.* D_{min} ≥ 51 Gy
- *PTV.* D_{max} ≤ 62 Gy

High risk:

- 60 Gy isodose line must cover ≥ 95% of PTV60
  - PTV60: D_{min} ≥ 57 Gy
  - PTV60: D_{max} ≤ 69 Gy
- 54 Gy isodose line must cover ≥ 95% of PTV54
  - PTV54: D_{max} ≤ 62 Gy

Treatment Delivery

- *Technique.* 3DCRT/IMRT/tomotherapy
- *Image-guidance.* At least weekly portal imaging

Organ(s) at Risk

Intermediate risk:

- *Lens.* D_{max} ≤ 5 Gy
- *Retinae.* D_{max} ≤ 45 Gy
- *Optic nerves.* D_{max} ≤ 50 Gy
- *Optic chiasm.* D_{max} ≤ 54 Gy
- *Brainstem.* D_{max} ≤ 55 Gy

High risk:

- *Lens.* D_{max} ≤ 7 Gy
- *Retinae.* D_{max} ≤ 50 Gy
- *Optic nerves.* D_{max} ≤ 55 Gy
- *Optic chiasm.* D_{max} ≤ 56 Gy
- *Brainstem.* D_{max} ≤ 60 Gy

Toxicity

Acute:

- Fatigue, lethargy, scalp erythema and soreness, alopecia
- Otitis externa, reduced hearing
- Aggravation of neurological symptoms (headache, nausea, seizures, weakness)

Late:

- Mental slowing/cognitive defects, decreased memory, behavioral changes, flattened affect
- Hearing loss, cataracts, dry eyes, decreased sense of smell, decreased taste, dry mouth

- Decreased vision, visual field deficits, blindness
- Motor and/or sensory deficits, decreased balance
- Radiation necrosis

Clinical Protocol Reference

RTOG 0539: phase II trial of observation for low-risk meningiomas and of radiotherapy for intermediate and high-risk meningiomas.

14.5. CNS LYMPHOMA

Therapeutic Considerations

- *Patient population.* B-cell non-Hodgkin's lymphoma involving the brain
- *Concurrent treatments.* Chemotherapy containing methotrexate followed by whole brain radiotherapy (WBRT)
- *Alternative treatments.* Chemotherapy alone, palliative radiotherapy alone

Dose Specification

- 23.4 Gy in 13 fractions (1.8 Gy/fraction)

Simulation

- *Imaging.* CT or conventional simulation
- *Position.* Supine
- *Immobilization.* Thermoplastic mask or other immobilization device
- *Other.* Radio-opaque marker placed on right and left eye canthi

Target Volume(s)

- Pair of opposed lateral fields with field borders
- *Superior.* Clearing cranium + 1 to 2 cm
- *Inferior.* C2 to C3 interspace
- *Posterior.* Clearing cranium + 1 to 2 cm
- *Anterior.* Exclude anterior 2/3 of orbits (if orbital involvement: include entire orbit)
- Exclude oral cavity
- Anterior field edge made coplanar via gantry rotation to avoid contralateral ocular divergence
- Ensure inclusion of meninges

Treatment Planning

- Equal weighting of opposed lateral fields
- Dose prescribed to mid-separation of the beams

Treatment Delivery

- *Technique.* 3DCRT
- *Image-guidance.* First treatment and at least weekly verification using orthogonal images (film or EPID)

Organ(s) at Risk

- Not specified

Toxicity

Acute:
- Alopecia, erythema, dry desquamation, fatigue
- Headache, anorexia, nausea
- Middle ear congestion
- If eye treated: conjunctival irritation, dry eye

Late:
- Alopecia
- Persistent middle ear effusion, sensorineural hearing impairment
- Cataracts
- Neurocognitive dysfunction, radiation necrosis

Clinical Protocol Reference

RTOG 1114: phase II randomized study of rituximab, methotrexate, procarbazine, vincristine, and cytarabine with and without low-dose whole-brain radiotherapy for primary central nervous system lymphoma.

14.6. OLIGOMETASTATIC BRAIN

Therapeutic Considerations

- *Patient population.* Patients with one to three brain metastases, each < 3.0 cm and with good performance status
- *Concurrent treatments.* May give dexamethasone or other steroid at time of stereotactic radiosurgery (SRS)
- *Alternative treatments.* WBRT, radiosurgery alone, surgical resection, surgery followed by WBRT or radiosurgery, supportive care (steroid therapy)

Dose Specification

SRS component:
- Lesions < 2.0 cm: 22 Gy in one fraction
- Lesions 2 to 2.9 cm: 18 Gy in one fraction

WBRT component:
- 30 Gy in 12 fractions (2.5 Gy/fraction)

Simulation

- *Imaging.* Planning MRI (SRS), CT acceptable for WBRT
- *Position.* Supine
- *Immobilization:*
  - SRS: immobilization/patient localization system mandatory (head frame or thermoplastic mask)
  - WBRT: thermoplastic mask
- *Scanning limits.* Not specified

Target Volume(s)

SRS:
- *GTV.* Contrast-enhanced tumor on planning MRI (max diameter < 3.0 cm)
- *CTV.* GTV

WBRT:
- Entire brain and meninges, including frontal lobe, posterior halves of the eyes
- Extend ≥ 1 cm beyond the periphery of the scalp
- *Caudal.* Below the skull base at the top of C2 vertebral level

Treatment Planning

- *SRS.* Dose prescribed to the highest isodose line encompassing the CTV
  - Can range from 50% to 80%

- WBRT much start ≤ 14 days following SRS
  - Prescribed at the center of the cranial volume
  - Treated with two lateral, equally weighted photon beams
  - Dose uniformity variation: max +7%, and −5%

Treatment Delivery and Image-Guidance

- *Technique.* Gamma knife or linear accelerator with SRS capability for SRS
- *Image-guidance.* Gamma knife or linear accelerators with mini-multileaf technology or mounted on robotic arms utilizing skull tracking software for SRS

Organ(s) at risk

- *Optic chiasm.* $D_{max} < 8$ Gy

Toxicity

Acute:
- Skin erythema, alopecia, nausea, vomiting
- Headache, seizure, fatigue
- Cognitive disturbance, otitis externa, irritated eye

Late:
- Alopecia, radiation necrosis
- Cognitive disturbance, motor neuropathy, weakness, speech difficulty
- Decreasing hearing, otitis externa, cataracts, vision loss

Clinical Protocol Reference

ECOG, RTOG 0671, NCCTG N0574: phase III randomized trial of the role of whole brain radiation therapy in addition to radiosurgery in patients with one to three cerebral metastases.

Chapter 15

Head and Neck Treatment Planning

15.1. EARLY STAGE LARYNX

Therapeutic Considerations

- *Patient population.* T1/2 laryngeal cancer
- *Concurrent treatments.* None
- *Alternative treatments.* Trans-oral laser resection, open partial laryngectomy

Dose Specification

- 63 Gy in 28 fractions (2.25 Gy/fraction)

Simulation

- *Imaging.* CT simulation, 3-mm slice thickness
- *Position.* Supine
- *Immobilization.* Thermoplastic mask
- *Scanning limits.* Clearing the skull to lower neck
- *Other.* IV contrast for carotid delineation

Target Volume(s)

- *GTV.* Bilateral true vocal cords, gross disease
- *CTV.* Larynx (false and true vocal cords, anterior and posterior commissure, arytenoids, aryepiglottic folds), subglottic region
  - Extending from hyoid bone to bottom of the cricoid cartilage
- *PTV0.5.* CTV + 0.5 cm
- *PTV1.0.* CTV + 1.0 cm (used when greater uncertainty of patient set-up)

Treatment Planning

- *3DCRT:*
  - For anterior lesions: centrally placed 0.5 cm bolus on skin over treatment field
  - Right and left lateral treatment fields using wedge angles
  - Wedge angle: one which concentrated a dose of 102% to 105% anteriorly
  - Collimator angle chosen such that the posterior jaw was parallel to the cervical spine
  - Dose prescribed to isocenter
  - PTV $D_{95\%}$ = prescription dose

Or

- *IMRT:*
  - Three to four anterior fields
  - PTV maximum dose ≤ 105% of prescription dose
  - PTV $D_{95\%}$ = prescription dose

Treatment Delivery

- *Technique.* 3DCRT/IMRT

Organ(s) at Risk

IMRT:

- *Spinal cord.* D_{max} ≤ 45 Gy
- *Carotid arteries.* D_{max} ≤ 105% of prescription dose
- *Arytenoids.* Contoured for dose volume histograms (DVH) data

Toxicity

Acute:

- Fatigue, skin erythema, or desquamation
- Hoarseness, odynophagia, dysphagia, thick phlegm

Late:

- Carotid vascular disease, stroke
- Dysphagia

Clinical Protocol Reference

Gomez D, et al. An investigation of intensity-modulated radiation therapy versus conventional two-dimensional and 3D-conformal radiation therapy for early stage larynx cancer. *Rad Oncol* 2010;5:74.

15.2. NASOPHARYNX

Therapeutic Considerations

- *Patient population.* Nasopharyngeal cancer (WHO I–IIb/III, stage IIB–IVB), no head and neck surgery of the primary tumor or lymph nodes except biopsy
- *Concurrent treatments.* Concurrent cisplatin and adjuvant chemotherapy (cisplatin, 5-fluorouracil)
- *Alternative treatments.* Addition of a biological agent, palliative care

Dose Specification

- 70 Gy in 33 fractions (2.12 Gy/fraction) to macroscopic volume
- Optional 63 Gy in 33 fractions (1.9 Gy/fraction), see target volume(s) below
- 59.4 Gy in 33 fractions (1.8 Gy/fraction) to high-risk microscopic volume
- 54 Gy in 33 fractions (1.64 Gy/fraction) to lower risk microscopic volume

Simulation

- *Imaging.* CT simulation, scan thickness ≤ 3 mm
- *Position.* Supine
- *Immobilization.* Immobilization device to include at least the head and neck
  - Encourage shoulder immobilization
- *Scanning limits.* Include all areas to be irradiated
- *Other.* Consider fusion with magnetic resonance imaging (MRI)

Target Volume(s)

- *GTV.* Gross disease, grossly positive nodes (> 1 cm or necrotic center)
  - GTV-P: primary site
  - GTV-N: involved nodes
- *CTV70-P.* GTV-P + ≥ 5 mm (can be reduced to 1 mm close to critical structures)
- *CTV70-N.* GTV-N + ≥ 5 mm (can be reduced to 1 mm close to critical structures)
- *CTV63.* Small volume nodes—at discretion of treating physician
  - Small volume nodes in close proximity to critical structures
- *CTV59.4-P.* Include all potential routes of spread for gross disease
  - Includes CTV70-P and at least GTV-P + 10 mm
  - Include: entire nasopharynx, anterior 1/2 to 1/3 clivus (entire clivus if involved), skull base (including foramen ovale and rotundum), pterygoid fossae, parapharyngeal space, inferior sphenoid sinus (in T3–T4 disease including the entire sphenoid sinus), posterior 1/3 to 1/4 nasal cavity, and maxillary sinuses (ensure pterygopalatine fossae is covered)
  - Cavernous sinus should be included in high-risk patients (if T3–T4 or bulky disease involving the roof of the nasopharynx)
  - Outermost boundary should be at least 10 mm from GTV70-P

- *CTV59.4-N.* Include all potential routes of spread
  - Surrounding subclinical region in the low neck if gross nodes are present
  - Includes CTV70-N and at least GTV-N + 10 mm
  - Include bilateral: upper deep jugular (junctional, parapharyngeal), subdigastric (jugulodigastric, level II), midjugular (level III), low jugular and supraclavicular (level IV), posterior cervical (level V), retropharyngeal, submandibular (level IB; can be spared if N0)
  - As per the Radiation Therapy Oncology Group (RTOG) contouring atlas
  - Outermost boundary should be at least 10 mm from GTV70-N
- *CTV54.* Low neck if no involved lymph nodes in lower neck
- *PTV70.* CTV70 + 5 mm
- *PTV63.* CTV63 + 5 mm
- *PTV59.4.* CTV59.4 + 5 mm
- *PTV54.* CTV54 + 5 mm

Or

- Alternative—beam split technique
  - *GTV.* As above
  - *CTV70-P and N.* As above
  - *CTV 59.4.* As above
  - *Low neck.* Conventional anterior–posterior (AP) or AP/posterior–anterior (PA) field
    - Depth of 3 cm from anterior surface (AP field) or midline for AP/PA fields
    - No involved lower neck nodes: 50 Gy in 25 fractions (2 Gy/fraction)
    - Gross nodes: 70 Gy
    - Small volume nodes: 63 Gy

Treatment Planning

- *PTV70.* ≥ 95% of PTV70 covered by 70 Gy isodose line
  - $D_{99\%}$ ≥ 65.1 Gy
  - ≤ 20% to receive ≥ 77 Gy
  - ≤ 5% to receive ≥ 80 Gy
  - Mean dose ≤ 74 Gy
- *PTV63.* ≥ 95% of PTV63 covered by 63 Gy isodose line
  - $D_{99\%}$ ≥ 58.6 Gy
  - ≤ 20% to receive ≥ 77 Gy
  - ≤ 5% to receive ≥ 80 Gy
- *PTV59.4.* ≥ 95% of PTV59.4 covered by 59.4 Gy isodose line
  - $D_{99\%}$ ≥ 55.2 Gy
  - ≤ 20% to receive ≥ 77 Gy
  - ≤ 5% to receive ≥ 80 Gy
- *PTV54.* ≥ 95% of PTV54 covered by 54 Gy isodose line
  - $D_{99\%}$ ≥ 50.2 Gy
  - ≤ 20% to receive ≥ 65.3 Gy
  - ≤ 5% to receive ≥ 68.3 Gy

Treatment Delivery

- *Technique.* 3DCRT, IMRT
- *Image-guidance.* At least orthogonal films

Organ(s) at Risk

- *Brachial plexus.* $D_{max} \leq 66$ Gy
- *Brainstem.* $D_{max} \leq 54$ Gy
  - Planning organ and risk volume (PRV; brainstem +1 mm): $V_{60Gy} \leq 1\%$
- *Spinal cord.* $D_{max} \leq 45$ Gy
  - PRV (cord +5 mm): $V_{50Gy} \leq 1\%$
- *Optic nerves.* $D_{max} \leq 50$ Gy
  - PRV (nerve +1 mm): $D_{max} \leq 54$ Gy
- *Chiasm.* $D_{max} \leq 50$ Gy
  - PRV (chiasm +1 mm): $D_{max} \leq 54$ Gy
- *Temporomandibular joints.* $D_{max} \leq 70$ Gy
- *Mandible.* $D_{max} \leq 70$ Gy
- *Parotid glands.* One gland: mean dose < 26 Gy
  - Or: at least 20 mL of combined volume < 20 Gy
  - Or: at least 50% of one gland to receive < 30 Gy
- *Cochlea.* $V_{55Gy} \leq 5\%$
- *Oral cavity (excluding PTVs).* Mean dose < 40 Gy
- *Eyes.* $D_{max} < 50$ Gy
- *Lens.* $D_{max} < 25$ Gy
- *Esophagus (including postcricoid pharynx).* Mean dose < 45 Gy
- *Glottis larynx.* Mean dose < 45 Gy
- *Contour for DVH data.* Pituitary, temporal lobes

Toxicity

Acute:

- Tanning or erythema of skin, fatigue
- Change in taste and/or smell, xerostomia, thick saliva
- Dysphagia, odynophagia, weight loss, hoarseness
- Otitis
- Alopecia

Late:

- Change in taste and/or smell, xerostomia, thick saliva, dysphagia
- Alopecia, otitis, hearing loss, hoarseness
- Dental caries, hypersensitivity to teeth, loss of teeth
- Nerve damage, osteoradionecrosis, hypothyroidism
- Hoarseness

Clinical Protocol Reference

RTOG 0615: a phase II study of concurrent chemoradiotherapy using 3DCRT or IMRT + bevacizumab for locally or regionally advanced nasopharyngeal cancer.

15.3. NON-NASOPHARYNX HEAD AND NECK

Therapeutic Considerations

- *Patient population.* Squamous cell cancer of the head and neck (excluding the nasopharynx) with node positive and/or T3–T4 disease
- *Concurrent treatments.* High-dose cisplatin
- *Alternative treatments.* Accelerated radiotherapy with cisplatin or a monoclonal antibody, standard fractionation radiotherapy with a monoclonal antibody

Dose Specification

- 70 Gy in 35 fractions (2 Gy/fraction)

Simulation

- *Imaging.* CT simulation, maximum 3 mm thickness
- *Position.* Supine, arms at their sides
- *Immobilization.* Thermoplastic mask with shoulder immobilization
- *Scanning limits.* At least the orbits superiorly to 1 cm below the suprasternal notch inferiorly
- *Other.* IV contrast is permitted, fusion with MRI and positron emission tomography (PET) may be used

Target Volume(s)

- *GTV.* Grossly involved regions of primary tumor or nodes
  - Grossly involved nodes are those > 1 cm or evidence of necrosis
- *CTVs.* Limited by potential barriers of tumor spread
  - Exclude air cavities, external contour, bony/fascial planes
  - Neck nodal volumes are contoured as per the anatomic guidelines in the consensus documents (Gregoire 2003, 2006)
- *PTVs.* Constrained to 5 mm within the external contour (modPTV) unless the disease is near (3 mm) or at the skin surface (bolus required)
- *3DCRT:*
  - CTV70: GTV + 0.5 to 1 cm
    - Necrotic lymph nodes or lymph nodes immediately adjacent to obvious gross nodal disease should be encompassed by CTV70
  - CTV60: used in cases of uncertainty
    - May be used instead of a subclinical dose CTV expansion around the GTV
    - Nodes < 1 cm (+5 mm expansion) not thought to harbor gross disease but at risk of containing more than subclinical disease
    - May include those volumes adjacent to an ill-defined GTV or lymph nodes ≤ 1 cm
  - CTV50: CTV70 + 0.5 cm
    - Include neck nodal regions at risk of subclinical disease in relation to the primary site according to consensus documents (Gregoire 2003, 2006)

- Patients with ipsilateral N2a, N2b, or N3 disease must have the contralateral neck treated
- Patients with N0 or N1 disease may be considered for ipsilateral neck treatment only in the case of well-lateralized tonsil primaries
- PTV70: CTV70 + 5 mm
- PTV60: CTV60 + 5 mm
- PTV50: CTV50 + 5 mm

Or

- *IMRT:*
  - CTV70: GTV + 0.5 to 1 cm
    - Necrotic lymph nodes or lymph nodes immediately adjacent to obvious gross nodal disease should be included
  - CTV63: used in cases of uncertainty
    - May be used instead of a subclinical dose CTV expansion around the GTV
    - Nodes < 1 cm (+5 mm expansion) not thought to harbor gross disease but at risk of containing more than subclinical disease
    - May include those volumes adjacent to an ill-defined GTV or lymph nodes ≤ 1 cm
  - CTV56: CTV70 + 0.5 cm
    - Include neck nodal regions at risk of subclinical disease in relation to the primary site according to consensus documents (Gregoire 2003, 2006)
    - Patients with ipsilateral N2a, N2b, or N3 disease must have the contralateral neck treated
    - Patients with N0 or N1 disease may be considered for ipsilateral neck treatment only in the case of well-lateralized tonsil primaries
  - PTV70: CTV70 + ≥ 5 mm
  - PTV63: CTV63 + ≥ 5 mm
  - PTV56: CTV56 + ≥ 5 mm

Treatment Planning

- *Posterior neck volumes.* May be treated with electrons
- *Junctions between upper and lower neck fields.* Asymmetrically matched (nondivergent match), not placed over gross disease
  - Spinal cord must be shielded in regions of junctions
  - Anterior photon fields and posterior neck electron fields junctioned at the field edge and must contain an overlap of 5 mm over gross nodal disease
- *Oropharyngeal tumors undergoing IMRT.* May have low neck treated with non-IMRT techniques (AP/PA) junctioned to IMRT-treated volume above
  - As long as there is no gross nodal disease in the junction or lower neck
  - Midline shielding used in the low neck to cover spinal cord at the junction
  - 50 Gy in 25 fractions can be used
- *All PTVs.* ≤ 1% to receive ≤ 93% prescribed dose
- *PTV70.* V_{70Gy} ≥ 95%
  - D_{max} ≤ 115% prescribed dose
- *PTV60 and PTV63.* D_{max} ≤ 120% prescribed dose
- *PTV50 and PTV 56.* D_{max} ≤ 125% prescribed dose
- *3DCRT:*
  - Beam arrangements are discretionary, and defined to achieve dosimetric goals
  - Parallel opposed photon fields: dose prescribed to midplane in the central axis
  - Posterior neck electrons: prescribed to an isodose ≥ 95%
  - PTV70: 70 Gy in 35 fractions (2 Gy/fraction)

- PTV60: 60 Gy in 30 fractions (2 Gy/fraction)
- PTV50: 50 Gy in 25 fractions (2 Gy/fraction)

Or

- *IMRT:*
  - PTV70: 70 Gy in 35 fractions (2 Gy/fraction)
  - PTV63: 63 Gy in 35 fractions (1.8 Gy/fraction)
  - PTV56: 56 Gy in 35 fractions (1.6 Gy/fraction)

Treatment Delivery

- *Technique.* 3DCRT or IMRT
- *Image-guidance.* Portal imaging of all fields (3DCRT) or orthogonal fields (IMRT)
  - Can use kilovoltage (kV) or megavoltage (MV) conebeam CT
  - At least weekly, starting on the first day of treatment

Organ(s) at Risk

- *Brainstem.* D_{max} < 54 Gy, max dose to 0.1 mL < 50 Gy
  - Brainstem PRV (brainstem +5 mm): maximum dose to 0.1 mL < 60 Gy
- *Spinal cord.* D_{max} < 48 Gy, max dose to 0.1 mL < 45 Gy
  - Spinal cord PRV (cord +5 mm): maximum dose to 0.1 mL < 52 Gy
- *Brain.* Maximum dose to 0.1 mL < 70 Gy
- *Optic structures (chiasm, globes, optic nerves).* D_{max} < 45 Gy
- *Parotids.* Mean dose to at least one parotid < 26 Gy
  - Median dose to at least one parotid < 30 Gy
  - At least 20 mL of combined volume, both parotids < 20 Gy
- *Mandible.* Max dose to 0.1 mL within overlapping PTV70 < 73.5 Gy
  - Maximum dose to 0.1 mL outside of PTV70 < 70 Gy
- *Glottic larynx.* Maximum dose to 0.1 mL < 50 Gy
- *Skin and unspecified tissue outside PTVs/Organ(s) at Risk (OARs).* Maximum dose to 1% or 1 mL < 77 Gy
- *Brachial plexus.* D_{max} < 60 Gy (3DCRT) or 63 Gy (IMRT)
- *Normal midline structures and mucosal surfaces not included in PTVs.* D_{max} < 60 Gy
- Unspecified normal tissues (external to PTVs and excluding OARs):
  - Maximum dose to 1 mL < 77 Gy

Toxicity

Acute:

- Skin erythema, desquamation, epilation, fatigue
- Mucositis, dysphagia, odynophagia, esophagitis
- Requirement of feeding tube, weight loss
- Serous otitis, nasal congestion
- Loss of taste, xerostomia, sialadenitis, hoarseness

Late:

- Skin fibrosis, bone necrosis
- Xerostomia, dental caries, requirement of feeding tube, dysphagia, trismus

- Chronic otitis media, hearing loss
- Cranial nerve dysfunction, radiation myelitis

Clinical Protocol Reference

NCIC HN6: a phase III study of standard fractionation radiotherapy, with concurrent high-dose cisplatin versus accelerated fractionation radiotherapy, with panitumumab in patients with locally advanced stage III and IV squamous cell carcinoma of the head and neck.

15.4. HIGH-RISK POSTOPERATIVE HEAD AND NECK CANCER

Therapeutic Considerations

- *Patient population.* Squamous cell carcinoma of the head and neck (oral cavity, oropharynx, or larynx) with clinical stage T2–3N0–2 or T1N1–2
- *Concurrent treatments.* High-dose cisplatin
- *Alternative treatments.* Radiotherapy alone, radiotherapy with carboplatin, or a monoclonal antibody (cetuximab, panitumumab), active surveillance

Indications for Adjuvant Radiotherapy ± Chemotherapy

Chemoradiotherapy:
- Positive resection margins
- Extracapsular extension
- Multiple pathologically positive lymph nodes

Radiotherapy alone:
- Positive lymph nodes without extracapsular extension
- pT3–4N0 (except T3N0 larynx)
- Perineural and/or vascular invasion
- Oral/oropharynx cancer with lymph node involvement at level IV or V

Dose Specification

- 60 Gy in 30 fractions (2 Gy/fraction)

Simulation

- *Imaging.* CT simulation, maximum slice thickness ≤ 3 mm
- *Position.* Supine
- *Immobilization.* Immobilization device (aquaplast or thermoplast mask)
- *Scanning limits.* Not specified
- *Other.* IV contrast for delineation of major vessels
  - Fusion of preoperative imaging if available

Target Volume(s)

- *CTV60.* Primary tumor bed (as per preoperative imaging, physical exam/endoscopy, operative findings, pathologic findings)
  - Include region(s) of grossly involved lymphadenopathy
  - Should not extend to within 2 mm of the skin
  - May also map preoperative GTV (from preoperative CT scan) and add a margin for microscopic spread (1.5–2 cm)
  - Include ipsilateral pathologically positive hemi-neck (levels 2a, 3, 4); if both sides are positive, include both in CTV60

- Nodal levels 1, 2b, 5a, 5b are included in selected circumstances
- Level 1 must be included for oral cavity cancer
- Level 5a must be included for oropharynx cancer
- *CTV56.* All regions felt to be at risk for microscopic cancer not in CTV60
  - That is, contralateral hemi-neck for base of tongue
  - Volume should not be closer than 5 mm to the skin
- *CTV66.* Optional
  - Region(s) felt to be at especially high risk (very close/positive margin)
- *PTVs.* Without daily image-guidance: CTV + 5 to 10 mm
  - With daily image-guidance: CTV + 2.5 to 5 mm

Treatment Planning

- Management of the low neck/supraclavicular region
  - Dose to supraclavicular nodal region may be limited to 50 Gy if level 4 nodes were dissected and found to be negative, or in the case of oral cavity cancer with level 3 nodes dissected and found to be negative
  - Management of the lower neck: if using match, requires a midline spinal cord block in lower neck fields
- *PTV60.* $V_{60Gy} \geq 95\%$
  - $D_{min} \geq 56$ Gy (if more than 8 mm from the skin)
  - $D_{max} < 70$ Gy
- *PTV56.* 1.85 Gy/fraction
- *PTV66.* 2.2 Gy/fraction

Treatment Delivery

- *Technique.* IMRT
- *Image-guidance.* One of the following
  - Orthogonal kV images
  - Linear-accelerator mounted kV and MV conebeam CT images
  - Linear-accelerator mounted MV CT images (TomoTherapy)

Organ(s) at Risk

- *Spinal cord +5 mm.* Dose to 0.03 mL ≤ 48 Gy
- *Brainstem +3 mm.* Dose to 0.03 mL ≤ 52 Gy
- *Lips.* Mean dose < 20 Gy
  - For nonoral cavity cancers: $D_{max} < 30$ Gy
  - For oral cavity cancers: $D_{max} < 50$ Gy
- *Oral cavity.* Nonoral cavity cancers: mean dose < 30 Gy
  - Oral cavity cancers: mean dose < 50 Gy
  - Try to avoid hot spots (> 60 Gy) within the oral cavity
- *Parotids.* One parotid to mean dose < 26 Gy
  - At least 50% of one parotid to < 30 Gy
  - At least 20 mL of one parotid < 20 Gy
- *Pharynx.* Try to achieve $D_{33\%} \leq 50$ Gy
  - Mean dose < 45 Gy
  - $D_{15\%} < 60$ Gy

- *Cervical esophagus.* Attempt to reduce as much as possible
  - Oral and oropharynx cancer: $D_{33\%} < 45$ Gy, mean dose < 35 Gy, $D_{15\%} < 54$ Gy
  - Larynx: $D_{33\%} < 50$ Gy, mean dose < 45 Gy, $D_{15\%} < 60$ Gy
- *Glottic and supraglottic larynx.* $D_{max} < 45$ Gy when feasible
- *Mandible.* Reduce as much as possible, avoid hot spots
  - $D_{max} < 66$ Gy
- *Unspecified tissue outside the targets.* $D_{5\%} < 58$ Gy
  - $D_{1\%}$ (or 1 mL) < 64 Gy

Toxicity

Acute:

- Skin erythema and desquamation, fatigue, weight loss, local epilation
- Mucositis, dysphagia, odynophagia, xerostomia
- Altered taste or smell, thick saliva, hoarseness
- Otitis media
- Dental caries, hypersensitivity of teeth

Late:

- Neck fibrosis, trismus
- Altered taste or smell, otitis, hearing loss
- Dysphagia, requirement of a feeding tube, risk of aspiration
- Hypothyroidism
- Myelitis, damage to cranial and other head and neck nerves, nerve pain
- Spinal damage
- Breathing problems

Clinical Protocol Reference

RTOG 0920: a phase III study of postoperative radiation therapy (IMRT) ± cetuximab for locally advanced resected head and neck cancer.

15.5. RE-IRRADIATION HEAD AND NECK

Therapeutic Considerations

- *Patient population.* Squamous cell carcinoma of the oral cavity, oropharynx, hypopharynx, larynx, or recurrent neck metastases from unknown primary
- *Concurrent treatments.* Chemotherapy (cisplatin, paclitaxel)
- *Alternative treatments.* Chemotherapy alone (platinum containing), surgery ± chemo/radiation

Dose Specification

- 60 Gy in 40 fractions (1.5 Gy/fraction), given twice daily (BID, Monday–Friday on weeks 1, 3, 5, and 7)
- At least 4 hours between treatments

Simulation

- *Imaging.* CT simulation, scan thickness ≤ 5 mm
- *Position.* Supine
- *Immobilization.* Head and neck immobilization device must be used
  - Thermoplastic mask recommended
  - Should include shoulders if lower neck is treated
  - If target volume includes oral tongue, a tongue immobilizer is recommended
- *Other.* IV contrast recommended
  - Image fusion with MRI and/or PET with image fusion if available

Target Volume(s)

- *GTV.* Gross disease (based on CT, MRI, PET, endoscopy, physical examination)
- *PTV.* GTV + ≥ 5 mm; recommend: GTV + 15 mm (where possible)
  - May be decreased to 1 mm if near a critical structure (spinal cord)

Treatment Planning

- *IMRT:*
  - PTV: $D_{95\%} \geq 60$ Gy
    - $D_{max} \leq 110\%$ prescription dose
    - $D_{min} \geq 90\%$ prescription dose

Or

- *3DCRT:*
  - PTV: $D_{max} \leq 110\%$ isocenter dose

Treatment Delivery

- *Technique.* 3DCRT, IMRT, tomotherapy
- *Image-guidance.* Port films or portal images of each field on day 1
  - Orthogonal images on day 1
  - Weekly verification films or images

Organ(s) at Risk

- Need to consider previous doses to organs at risk
- These constraints are for lifetime doses:
  - Spinal cord PRV (cord +5 mm): $D_{max} \leq 54$ Gy
  - Brainstem PRV (brainstem +5 mm): $D_{max} \leq 60$ Gy
  - Larynx (top of thyroid cartilage to bottom of cricoid cartilage, not including PTV)
    - As low as possible

Toxicity

Acute:
- Fatigue, regional alopecia, skin erythema, and desquamation
- Mucositis, dysphagia, odynophagia weight loss, xerostomia, hoarseness
- Hypogeusia, dysgeusia, requirement for a feeding tube
- Otitis

Late:
- Regional alopecia, skin fibrosis
- Dysphagia, xerostomia, hoarseness, requirement for a feeding tube
- Hypothyroidism, loss of hearing
- Osteoradionecrosis, myelopathy, neuropathy
- Carotid stenosis or rupture

Clinical Protocol Reference

RTOG 0421: a phase III trial for locally recurrent, previously irradiated head and neck cancer: concurrent re-irradiation and chemotherapy versus chemotherapy alone

15.6. ANAPLASTIC THYROID

Therapeutic Considerations

- *Patient population.* Anaplastic thyroid cancer
- *Concurrent treatments.* Chemotherapy
- *Alternative treatments.* Hyperfractionated radiotherapy ± chemotherapy, palliative radiotherapy, radiotherapy with other chemotherapy agents or novel agents, surgery followed by radiation ± chemotherapy, clinical trial

Dose Specification

- 66 Gy in 33 fractions (2 Gy/fraction) to macroscopic volume
- 59.4 Gy in 33 fractions (1.8 Gy/fraction) to high-risk microscopic volume

Simulation

- *Imaging.* CT simulation, slice thickness ≤ 3 mm
- *Position.* Same position used for treatment
- *Immobilization.* An immobilization device to include at least the head and neck, recommend shoulder immobilization
- *Scanning limits.* Include entire lung volumes
- *Other.* Suggest fusion with diagnostic CT scan

Target Volume(s)

- *GTV-P.* All known gross disease from CT, clinical information and endoscopy
  - If postoperative: preoperative gross disease + surgical bed
- *GTV-N.* Lymph nodes > 1 cm or with a necrotic center
  - If postoperative: preoperative nodal disease
- *CTV66-P.* GTV-P + ≥ 5 mm
- *CTV66-N.* GTV-N + ≥ 5 mm
- *CTV59.4.* CTV66-P + 5 mm and areas at high risk for microscopic disease
  - Ensure coverage of tracheal-esophageal groove, levels II to VI, upper mediastinum to the level of the carina
  - May include level I and retropharyngeal nodes
  - Outer boundary should include GTV-P + GTV-N + ≥ 10 mm
- *PTV66-P.* CTV66-P + ≥ 5 mm
- *PTV66-N.* CTV66-N + ≥ 5 mm
- *PTV59.4.* CTV59.4 + ≥ 5 mm

Treatment Planning

- *PTV66.* $D_{95\%}$ covered by 66 Gy isodose line
  - $D_{99\%}$ ≥ 61.4 Gy

    - < 20% to receive ≥ 72.6 Gy
    - < 5% to receive ≥ 75.9 Gy
- *PTV59.4.* $D_{95\%}$ covered by 59.4 Gy isodose line
    - $D_{99\%}$ ≥ 55.2 Gy
    - < 20% to receive 71.8 Gy
    - < 5% to receive 75 Gy
- *Any PTV.* < 1% to receive ≤ 93% of its prescribed dose

Treatment Delivery

- *Technique.* IMRT

Organ(s) at Risk

- *Spinal cord.* D_{max} (0.03 mL) < 45 Gy
    - Spinal cord +5 mm: D_{max} (0.03 mL) < 50 Gy
- *Brachial plexus.* D_{max} (0.03 mL) < 66 Gy
- *Glottic larynx.* Mean dose < 60 Gy
- *Lung.* < 20% of total lung volume to receive > 20 Gy
- *Oral cavity.* Mean dose < 35 Gy
- *Parotids.* At least one gland: mean dose < 26 Gy
    - ≥ 20 mL of combined volume to receive < 20 Gy
    - ≥ 50% of one gland < 30 Gy
- *Submandibular glands.* Mean dose < 39 Gy
- *Unspecified tissue outside the targets.* < 8 mL to receive ≥ 59.4 Gy
    - < 1 mL to receive ≥ 65.3 Gy

Toxicity

Acute:

- Fatigue, skin erythema, and desquamation
- Mucositis, dysphagia, odynophagia, xerostomia, thick saliva, weight loss
- Hoarseness
- Otitis, local epilation
- Dental cavities, loss of teeth

Late:

- Dysphagia, requirement of a feeding tube, aspiration, xerostomia
- Hypothyroidism
- Myelitis, neuropathy, nerve pain
- Breathing problems
- Otitis, hearing loss, local epilation/hair loss

Clinical Protocol Reference

RTOG 0912: a randomized phase II study of concurrent intensity modulated radiation therapy (IMRT), paclitaxel and pazopanib (NSC737754)/placebo, for the treatment of anaplastic thyroid cancer.

Chapter 16

Breast Treatment Planning

16.1. DUCTAL CARCINOMA IN SITU

Therapeutic Considerations

- *Patient population.* Completely excised ductal carcinoma in situ (DCIS), postlumpectomy
- *Concurrent treatments.* None
- *Alternative treatments.* Mastectomy

Dose Specification

- 50 Gy in 25 fractions (2 Gy/fraction) or 42.5 Gy in 16 fractions (2.6 Gy/fraction)
  - ±Boost of 10 to 16 Gy in five to eight fractions (2 Gy/fraction)

Simulation

- *Imaging.* Computed tomography (CT) simulation, scan thickness ≤ 5 mm
- *Position.* Supine, with ipsilateral or bilateral arms extended about the head or the ipsilateral arm at a right angle to the torso
  - Prone positioning may be used
- *Immobilization.* Breast board or another form of immobilization
- *Scanning limits.* At least 5 cm above the superior border of the whole breast to at least 5 cm below the inferior border of the breast
- *Other.* Wire lumpectomy scar and clinical boundaries of the breast

Target Volume(s)

- If the whole breast target volume is not contoured:
  - Borders of the tangential fields set clinically to include the entire ipsilateral breast + 1 to 1.5 cm margin
    - *Superior.* Just below the clavicle

- *Inferior.* 1 to 1.5 cm below the infra-mammary fold or lowest part of the breast (whichever is lower)
- *Medial.* At or near midsternum to encompass the breast tissue with a 1- to 1.5-cm margin
- *Lateral.* Midaxillary line to include breast tissue with a 1- to 1.5-cm margin
- Axillary scar and drain sites outside of the breast volume are excluded

- If the whole breast target volume is contoured:
  - Clinical target volume (CTV): soft tissue of the whole breast down to the pectoralis fascia, excluding first 5 mm deep to skin and underlying muscle, ribs, lung, and heart
    - Surgical clips should be included
    - Planning target volume (PTV): CTV + 1 to 1.5 cm, excluding surface 5 mm deep to external skin contour
- Tumor bed boost
  - *CTVboost.* Seroma cavity (± surgical clips) + 1-cm margin
    - May decrease margin to 0.5 cm if all surgical margins ≥ 1 cm
    - Exclude first 5 mm deep to external skin contour, pectoralis muscle, ribs, lung, and heart
    - Used to determine aperture of treatment fields
  - *PTVboost.* CTVboost + 5 to 10 mm
  - *boostPTVeval.* PTV excluding lung, ribs, pectoralis major muscle, surface 5 mm deep to external skin contour
    - Used for generating dose volume histograms (DVHs)

Treatment Planning

- Bolus to the scar is not used
- Bolus over the whole breast may be used if photon energy > 10 megavolts is necessary
- Dose homogeneity on the central plane should be within +7%, and −5%
- Whole breast field arrangement: medial and lateral tangential opposing fields
  - Posterior beam edges may be aligned or angled anteriorly to minimize lung dose
  - Anterior border of the fields should be ≥ 1 cm anterior to the skin surface
- Tumor bed boost
  - Electrons: prescribed to D_{max}, boostPTVeval should be encompassed by ≥ 90% isodose line
  - Photons: normalized ≥ 90% isodose should encompass PTVboost

Treatment Delivery

- *Technique.* 3DCRT, IMRT
- *Image-guidance.* Portal films for the tangential fields should be imaged in the treatment position at least once during treatment

Organ(s) at Risk

- *Lung.* ≤ 2 cm at any point along the length of the tangent
- *Heart (left-sided lesions).* Exclude the heart in the high dose region without under-dosing the primary tumor bed
- *Recommend.* Max heart distance ≤ 1.5 cm

Toxicity

Acute:
- Skin erythema or desquamation, fatigue
- Breast discomfort and swelling

Late:
- Breast tanning, fibrosis, or change in contour
- Cough, dyspnea, lung fibrosis
- Rib fracture, myocardial infarction, heart failure
- Secondary malignancy
- Cardiomyopathy

Clinical Protocol Reference

TROG 0701, MA33, BIG 3–07: a randomized phase III study of radiation doses and fractionation schedules for DCIS of the breast.

16.2. PARTIAL BREAST IRRADIATION

Therapeutic Considerations

- *Patient population.* Stage 0, I, or II breast cancer postlumpectomy with tumor size ≤ 3 cm and ≤ 3 histologically positive nodes
- *Concurrent treatments.* Hormonal therapy as needed, chemotherapy after partial breast irradiation if needed
- *Alternative treatments.* Whole breast irradiation, mastectomy

Dose Specification

- 38.5 Gy in 10 fractions (3.85 Gy/fraction) twice daily (BID)
  - Daily BID treatments separated by ≥ 6 hours

Simulation

- *Imaging.* CT simulation, scan thickness ≤ 5 mm
- *Position.* Supine
- *Immobilization.* Not specified
- *Scanning limits.* At/above the mandible and extend several cm below the infra-mammary fold, include the entire lung

Target Volume(s)

- *Excision cavity.* Outlined using help of surgical clips
- *CTV.* Excision cavity +15 mm
  - Limited to 5 mm from skin surface
  - Exclude chest wall and pectoralis muscles
- *PTV.* CTV + 10 mm
- *PTVeval.* PTV, with exclusion of structures outside the ipsilateral breast (including chest wall, pectoralis muscles, and lung), the first 5 mm of tissue under the skin
  - Used for DVH constraints and analysis

Treatment Planning

- *PTVeval.* $D_{90\%}$ ≥ 90% prescribed dose
- D_{max} ≤ 120% prescribed dose

Treatment Delivery

- *Technique.* 3DCRT, usually three to five field noncoplanar beam arrangement
- *Image-guidance.* Before first treatment: port films of each beam and orthogonal pair
  - Orthogonal pair (anterior–posterior [AP] and lateral) prior to fraction 5

Organ(s) at Risk

- *Uninvolved normal breast.* < 60% whole breast to receive ≥ 50% prescribed dose
  - < 35% whole breast to receive prescribed dose
- *Contralateral breast.* D_{max} < 3% prescribed dose
- *Ipsilateral lung.* < 15% to receive 30% prescribed dose
- *Contralateral lung.* < 15% to receive 5% prescribed dose
- *Heart (right-sided lesions).* < 5% to receive 5% prescribed dose
- *Heart (left-sided lesions).* < 5% to receive 40% prescribed dose
- *Thyroid.* D_{max} ≤ 3% prescribed dose

Toxicity

Acute:
- Skin erythema or desquamation, breast swelling, fatigue
- Sore chest wall muscles, pain
- Cough, dyspnea

Late:
- Skin tanning, change in breast contour
- Pericarditis, rib fracture
- Second malignancy

Clinical Protocol Reference

RTOG 0413, NSABP B-39: A randomized phase III study of conventional whole breast irradiation versus partial breast irradiation for women with stage 0, I, or II breast cancer.

16.3. LOCAL BREAST

Therapeutic Considerations

- *Patient population.* Stage 0 to II breast cancer treated with lumpectomy or neoadjuvant chemotherapy followed by lumpectomy
- *Concurrent treatments.* None
- *Alternative treatments.* Mastectomy, brachytherapy

Dose Specification

- 50 Gy in 25 fractions (2 Gy/fraction) or 42.5 Gy in 16 fractions (2.67 Gy/fraction)
- Sequential boost to lumpectomy cavity: 12 Gy in 6 fractions (2 Gy/fraction) or 14 Gy in seven fractions (2 Gy/fraction)

Simulation

- *Imaging.* CT simulation, scan thickness ≤ 5 mm
- *Position.* Supine or prone
- *Immobilization.* Alpha cradle, breast board, wing board, and/or other method used
- *Scanning limits.* At or above the mandible to at least below the infra-mammary fold
  - Ensure the entire lung volume to be encompassed
- *Other.* Radio-opaque markers: lumpectomy incision, outline of palpable breast tissue (at least from 2 to 10 o'clock), superior border of the breast

Target Volume(s)

- As per the RTOG breast contouring atlas (www.rtog.org)
- *Lumpectomy GTV.* Lumpectomy scar, seroma, excision cavity volume, architectural distortion and/or surgical clips
- *Lumpectomy CTV.* Lumpectomy GTV + 1 cm
  - Limit anterolaterally 5 mm from skin
  - Do not cross midline
  - Pectoralis and/or serratus anterior are excluded unless clinically indicated
- *Lumpectomy PTV.* Lumpectomy CTV + 7 mm (exclude heart)
- *Lumpectomy PTVeval.* Lumpectomy PTV
  - Exclude parts outside the ipsilateral breast and the first 5 mm of tissue under the skin
  - Exclude expansion beyond the posterior extent of breast tissue (chest wall, pectoralis muscle, lung)
  - Do not cross midline
- *Breast CTV.* All palpable breast tissue demarcated with radio-opaque markers
  - Should include lumpectomy CTV
  - Limits: First 5 mm under the skin, posteriorly at the anterior surface of pectoralis and serratus anterior muscle
  - Exclude chest wall, bony thorax, and lung

- *Breast PTV.* Breast CTV + 7 mm (exclude heart, do not cross midline)
- *Breast PTVeval.* Breast PTV
  - Exclude parts outside the ipsilateral breast and the first 5 mm of tissue under the skin
  - Posterior limit is the anterior surface of ribs
  - Do not cross midline

Treatment Planning

- *Lumpectomy boost.* Can be given as 3DCRT, IMRT, or with electrons
- *Breast PTVeval.* > 95% to receive ≥ 95% prescription dose
  - < 30% to receive ≥ 100% of boost prescribed dose
  - < 50% to receive ≥ 107% of prescribed dose
  - D_{max} ≥ 115% of prescribed dose
- *Lumpectomy PTVeval.* > 95% to receive ≥ 95% prescription dose
  - < 5% to receive ≥ 110% of boost prescribed dose
  - D_{max} ≤ 115% of boost prescribed dose

Treatment Delivery

- *Technique.* IMRT, 3DCRT
- *Image-guidance.* Port films or images for each 3DCRT beam and orthogonal pair
  - Minimum orthogonal films or treatment images every five fractions

Organ(s) at Risk

- *Contralateral breast.* D_{max} ≤ 3 Gy
- *Ipsilateral lung.* V_{20Gy} ≤ 15%
  - V_{10Gy} ≤ 35%
  - V_{5Gy} ≤ 50%
- *Contralateral lung.* V_{5Gy} ≤ 10%
- *Heart.* V_{25Gy} ≤ 5% (left-sided cancers), $V_{25\%}$ = 0% (right-sided cancers)

Toxicity

Acute:
- Skin erythema or desquamation, pain
- Soreness or tightness of chest wall or axillary muscles
- Cough, shortness of breath

Late:
- Skin discoloration, change in breast appearance, breast swelling
- Cardiomegaly, coronary artery disease, rib fracture
- Second malignancy

Clinical Protocol Reference

RTOG 1005: a phase III trial of accelerated whole breast irradiation, with hypofractionation plus concurrent boost versus standard whole breast irradiation plus sequential boost for early stage breast cancer.

16.4. REGIONAL BREAST

Therapeutic Considerations

- *Patient population.* Node positive breast cancer
- *Concurrent treatments.* ±adjuvant chemotherapy, ±hormonal therapy
- *Alternative treatments.* Mastectomy and axillary lymph node dissection or sentinel lymph node biopsy ± chemotherapy, ±hormonal therapy

Dose Specification

- 50 Gy in 25 fractions (2 Gy/fraction)
- ±10 Gy in five fractions (2 Gy/fraction) boost to lumpectomy site for positive or close margins

Simulation

- *Imaging.* Fluoroscopy or CT simulation
- *Position.* Supine with ipsilateral arm raised above the head
- *Immobilization.* Breast board or other immobilization device
- *Other.* Suggest wire of lumpectomy scar

Target Volume(s)

- *Breast:*
  - POP fields tangentially arranged across the breast
  - Central axis of the medial and lateral fields should lie along the same line
  - Medial border: line at or near the midsternum, ensure inclusion of breast and 1- to 1.5-cm margin
  - Lateral border: midaxillary line, ensure inclusion of breast and 1- to 1.5-cm margin
  - Superior border: at or above sternal angle
  - Inferior border: 1 to 1.5 cm below the infra-mammary crease or lowest part of the breast, whichever is lower
- *Supraclavicular/axillary field:*
  - Superior border: include the entire supraclavicular fossa (usually C5/6)
  - Inferior border: at or above sternal angle
  - Medial border: pedicles of the vertebrae
  - Lateral border: include the coracoid process (just medial to the humeral head)
  - Humeral head block: medially at the acromioclavicular joint and inferiorly to include part of the inferior portion of the humeral head

Treatment Planning

- Coplanar match between the breast tangents and supraclavicular/axillary fields using asymmetric collimation or half beam block

- Wedges or compensators should be used to ensure uniform dose distribution throughout the target volume, or IMRT
  - Dose homogeneity of ±7%
- Bolus to the scar should be avoided
- Boost to the lumpectomy site allowed (10 Gy in five fractions [2 Gy/fraction])
  - For positive resection margin
- Supraclavicular/axillary field can be treated with a single anterior field or AP/posterior-anterior (PA) fields
  - *Single anterior field.* Dose prescribed at 3 cm
  - *AP/PA.* Dose prescribed to mid-separation
- The anterior supraclavicular field may be angled 5° to 10° medially to avoid the trachea, esophagus, and spinal cord

Treatment Delivery

- *Technique.* 3DCRT (or IMRT)
- *Image-guidance.* Portal imaging recommended

Organ(s) at Risk

- Amount of lung tissue at the central axis of the breast fields should be ≤ 2 cm

Toxicity

Acute:

- Fatigue, skin erythema, or desquamation
- Breast tenderness or swelling

Late:

- Skin fibrosis, telangiectasias, lymphedema
- Radiation pneumonitis or fibrosis
- Coronary artery disease, pericarditis, cardiac failure
- Rib fracture
- Brachial plexopathy
- Secondary malignancy

Clinical Protocol Reference

NCIC MA20: a phase III study of regional radiation therapy in early breast cancer.

Chapter 17

Thoracic Treatment Planning

17.1. EARLY STAGE NON-SMALL CELL LUNG CANCER

Therapeutic Considerations

- *Patient population.* T1, T2 (≤ 5 cm), T3 (≤ 5 cm, chest wall primary tumors only), N0, M0 non-small cell lung cancer (NSCLC). Tumor must not be within 2 cm of proximal bronchial tree
- *Concurrent treatments.* None
- *Alternative treatments.* Surgical resection, standard external beam radiotherapy ± chemotherapy

Dose Specification

- 60 Gy (54 Gy with modern treatment planning system in homogeneity corrections) in three fractions (20 Gy/fraction), over 1.5 to 2 weeks
- Can potentially use risk-adapted approach of five to eight (55 Gy/5 fractions or 60 Gy/8 fractions) fractions for tumors near critical structures such as chest wall, brachial plexus

Simulation

- *Imaging.* CT simulation, maximum 3-mm slice thickness
- *Position.* Stable position allowing accurate reproducibility
- *Immobilization.* Stereotactic frame that surrounds patient on three sides, with reference to stereotactic coordinate system
- *Other.* IV contrast
  - *Inhibition of internal organ motion.* Reliable abdominal compression, accelerator beam gating with respiratory cycle, tumor tracking, or active breath-holding technique

Target Volume(s)

- *GTV.* Gross tumor volume (on pulmonary windows) unless atelectasis, adjacent vessels, mediastinal, or chest wall structures close by
- *CTV.* GTV
- *PTV.* CTV + 1.0 cm craniocaudal, 0.5 cm axially

Treatment Planning

- All treatment must be completed within 16 days
  - Minimum 40 hours, and maximum 8 days between each treatment
  - Usually no more than two fractions per week
- Minimum field dimension: 3.5 cm
- Three-dimensional (3D) coplanar or non-coplanar beam arrangements
  - Non-opposing, non-coplanar are preferable
  - Typically ≥ 10 beams used
  - For arc rotation: minimum 340°
- Prescription lines covering PTV typically 60% to 90% line
- Treatment normalized such that 100% corresponds to the center of the PTV
- Prescription isodose surface chosen such that 95% of the PTV is covered by the prescription isodose
  - 99% of PTV receives ≥ 90% of the prescription dose
- Dose > 105% prescription should occur within the PTV
  - Cumulative volume of tissue outside PTV receiving > 105% prescription dose should be ≤ 15% of the PTV volume

Treatment Delivery

- *Technique.* Three-dimensional conformal radiation therapy (3DCRT), intensity-modulated radiation therapy (IMRT), cyberknife, tomotherapy
- *Image-guidance.* Isocenter or reference point port films (anti/post and lateral) for each treatment
  - Verification CT scans and portal films at treating physician's discretion

Organ(s) at Risk

- *Spinal cord.* D_{max} < 18 Gy (6 Gy/fraction)
- *Esophagus.* D_{max} < 27 Gy (9 Gy/fraction)
- *Ipsilateral brachial plexus.* D_{max} < 24 Gy (8 Gy/fraction)
- *Heart/pericardium.* D_{max} < 30 Gy (10 Gy/fraction)
- *Trachea and ipsilateral bronchus.* D_{max} < 30 Gy (10 Gy/fraction)
- *Skin—any point.* D_{max} < 24 Gy (8 Gy/fraction)
- *Whole lung (right and left).* V_{20Gy} < 10%
  - Exclude GTV and tracheal/ipsilateral bronchus.

Toxicity

Acute:

- Fatigue, skin erythema, or desquamation
- Radiation pneumonitis, cough, dyspnea
- Fever, chest wall discomfort

Late:

- Bronchial injury, focal collapse of lung, dyspnea, lung fibrosis, pneumonitis
- Requirement for permanent oxygen therapy
- Pericarditis, chest pain, arrhythmia, myocardial infarction, heart failure
- Myelitis, brachial plexopathy
- Esophageal stricture, dysphagia
- Hemoptysis

Clinical Protocol Reference

RTOG 0618: a phase II trial of stereotactic body radiation therapy in the treatment of patients with operable stage I/II NSCLC.

17.2. LOCALLY ADVANCED NSCLC

Therapeutic Considerations

- *Patient population.* Unresectable stage IIIA/B NSCLC, N2, or N3 disease with an undetectable primary tumor, no supraclavicular or contralateral hilar adenopathy
- *Concurrent treatments.* Carboplatin and paclitaxel, other regimens include: vinca alkaloid (i.e., vinblastine, vinorelbine) and platinum agent (that is, cisplatin, carboplatin)

Dose Specification

- 60 Gy in 30 fractions (2 Gy/fraction)

Simulation

- *Imaging.* CT simulation, 3-mm slice thickness
- *Immobilization.* immobilization device in treatment position
- *Scanning limits.* level of the cricoid cartilage to include the entire liver volume
- *Other.* suggest a fluorodeoxyglucose positron emission tomography (PET)/CT fusion
  - Optional use of IV contrast
  - Encourage use of 4D treatment planning (gating, breath-hold, maximum intensity projection)

Target Volume(s)

- *GTV.* Primary tumor and clinically positive nodes (> 1 cm short axis) or pretreatment PET (SUV > 3), internal target volume (ITV) may be used instead of GTV to capture motion due to respiration
- *CTV.* GTV + 0.5 to 1 cm
  - If ITV used, CTV: ITV + 0.5 to 1 cm
- *PTV:*
  - Free breathing non-ITV: ≥ 1.5 cm (superior/inferior) and 1 cm in axial plane
  - Breath-hold, gating non-ITV: margin ≥ 1 cm in sup/in and 0.5 cm axially
  - ITV approach: 0.5 to 1 cm

Treatment Planning

- 95% of PTV covered by prescription dose
  - Minimum PTV dose ≥ 95% prescription dose

Treatment Delivery

- *Technique.* 3DCRT, IMRT
  - 3DCRT: use combination of coplanar or non-coplanar fields

- *Image-guidance*:
  - Day one portal or orthogonal images
  - Weekly verification or orthogonal images
  - Can use cone beam CT or other CT devices

Organ(s) at Risk

- *Spinal cord.* $D_{max} \leq 50.5$ Gy
- *Lungs.* volume of both lungs—$V_{20Gy} \leq 37\%$
  - Mean lung dose (lung minus CTV): ≤ 20 Gy
- *Brachial plexus.* $D_{max} < 66$ Gy
- *Esophagus.* Mean dose < 34 Gy
  - V_{60Gy} should be calculated
- *Heart.* $V_{60Gy} < 1/3$, $V_{45Gy} < 2/3$, $V_{40Gy} < 100\%$

Toxicity

Acute:

- Skin erythema or desquamation, local epilation
- Cough, dyspnea, fatigue
- Dysphagia, odynophagia
- Cytopenia

Late:

- Local epilation
- Dysphagia, esophageal stricture
- Tracheal or bronchial bleed, tracheal or bronchial stricture
- Pericarditis, myocarditis, pneumonitis
- Transverse myelitis, brachial plexopathy

Clinical Protocol Reference

RTOG 0617, NCCTG N0628, CALGB 30609, ECOG R0617: a randomized phase III comparison of standard-dose (60 Gy) versus high-dose (74 Gy) conformal radiotherapy with concurrent and consolidation carboplatin/paclitaxel ± cetuximab (IND #103444) in patients with stage IIIA/IIIB NSCLC.

17.3. LIMITED STAGE SCLC

Therapeutic Considerations

- *Patient population.* Limited stage SCLC
- *Concurrent treatments.* Cisplatin, etoposide
  - Prophylactic cranial irradiation if at least stable disease after treatment

Dose Specification

- 45 Gy in 30 fractions (1.5 Gy/fraction), given twice daily (BID)

Or

- 60 to 66 Gy in 30 to 33 fractions (2 Gy/fraction), given once daily

Simulation

- *Imaging.* CT simulation, ≤ 5-mm slice thickness
- *Position.* Supine, arms above head
- *Immobilization.* Chest board and fixed arm position
- *Scanning limits.* Cricoid to L2
- *Other.* Optional PET scan

Target Volume(s)

- *GTV.* As seen on the mediastinal and lung windows
  - Involved nodes: ≥ 1 cm in short axis
  - Include PET positive nodes
- *CTV.* GTV + 0.5 cm
- *PTV.* CTV + 1 cm superior/inferior and 0.8 cm laterally

Treatment Planning

- Prophylactic nodal irradiation is not employed
- *PTV.* ±5% of prescribed dose ideally, and no more than ±7%
- For BID treatment: each treatment must be 6 to 8 hours apart

Treatment Delivery

- *Technique.* 3DCRT, IMRT
- *Image-guidance.* Recommend daily verifications (orthogonal images) for the first 3 days, then weekly
  - Cone-beam CT can be used

Organ(s) at Risk

- *BID treatment:*
  - Total lung (minus PTV): $V_{20Gy} \leq 35\%$
  - Spinal cord: $D_{max} \leq 42$ Gy
  - Heart: total dose to < 30%
    - 50% total dose to < 50%
- *Daily treatment:*
  - Total lung (minus PTV): $V_{20} \leq 35\%$
  - Spinal cord: $D_{max} \leq 48$ Gy
  - Heart: total dose to < 30%
    - 50% total dose to < 50%.

Toxicity

Acute:

- Fatigue, pneumonitis, skin erythema, or desquamation
- Esophagitis, anorexia, nausea
- Anemia, leukopenia, thrombocytopenia

Late:

- Pulmonary fibrosis, dyspnea, fatigue

Clinical Protocol Reference

NCIC BR28, CONVERT: concurrent once-daily versus twice-daily radiotherapy: a two-arm randomized controlled trial of concurrent chemoradiotherapy comparing twice-daily and once-daily radiotherapy schedules in patients with limited stage SCLC and good performance status.

17.4. PROPHYLACTIC CRANIAL IRRADIATION

Therapeutic Considerations

- *Patient population.* Limited stage SCLC with complete/partial response to treatment (can consider therapy for good performance status and any response extensive stage SCLC)
- *Concurrent treatments.* Previous induction chemotherapy ± thoracic radiotherapy

Dose Specification

- 25 Gy in 10 fractions (2.5 Gy/fraction)
- 30 Gy in 15 fractions (2 Gy/fraction)

Simulation

- *Imaging.* CT or fluoroscopic simulation
- *Position.* Supine
- *Immobilization.* Head immobilization
- *Scanning limits.* Clearing skull to below C3

Target Volume(s)

- Two opposed lateral beams, equally weighted
  - Include entire cranial contents
  - ≥ 1 cm around bony skull superiorly, inferiorly, anteriorly, posteriorly
  - Ensure blocking of the lens, oral cavity, nasal cavity

Treatment Planning

- Treat using two opposed coaxial equally weighted beams
  - On central ray at mid-separation of beams

Treatment Delivery

- *Technique.* 3DCRT, 4 or 6 MV
- *Image-guidance.* Not specified

Toxicity

Acute:

- Alopecia, scalp erythema
- Headache, nausea, vomiting

- Dry mouth, change in taste
- Otitis media, decreased hearing
- Lethargy, worsening of pre-existing neurological deficits

Late:

- Radiation necrosis, cognitive dysfunction, accelerated atherosclerosis
- Memory loss, behavioral change, fatigue
- Cataracts, blindness
- Radiation-induced neoplasm

Clinical Protocol Reference

RTOG 0212, PCI 01: a phase II/III randomized trial of two doses (phase III—standard vs. high) and two high dose schedules (phase II—once vs. BID) for delivering prophylactic cranial irradiation for patients with limited disease SCLC.

Chapter 18

Gastrointestinal Treatment Planning

18.1. ESOPHAGUS (RESECTABLE)

Therapeutic Considerations

- *Patient population.* Nonmetastatic adenocarcinoma of the esophagus involving the mid, distal, and/or gastroesophageal junction (GEJ)
- *Concurrent treatments.* Paclitaxel, carboplatin with radiation followed by surgery
- *Alternative treatments.* Neoadjuvant radiotherapy with 5-fluorouracil (5FU) and cisplatin followed by surgery, surgery alone, surgery with adjuvant chemoradiotherapy

Dose Specification

- 45 Gy in 25 fractions with a boost of 5.4 Gy in three fractions (1.8 Gy/fraction)

Simulation

- *Imaging.* Computed tomography (CT) simulation, 3- to 5-mm slice thickness
- *Position.* Supine or prone
- *Immobilization.* Individualized immobilization device
- *Scanning limits.* Entire thoracic cavity and abdomen to the bottom of the kidneys
- *Other.* Esophageal contrast may be used
- Recommend fusion of diagnostic CT scan and/or positron emmision tomography/CT

Target Volume(s)

- *GTVp.* Primary tumor in the esophagus
- *GTVn.* Grossly involved regional lymph nodes
- *CTVp.* GTVp + 4 cm expansion superior and inferior, following the contours of the esophagus and proximal stomach; and 1.0 to 1.5 cm radial expansion

- *CTVn.* GTVn + 1.0 to 1.5 cm
  - Can be expanded to cover the para-esophageal and celiac nodal regions
  - CA should be covered for tumors of the distal esophagus and GEJ
- *PTV.* CTVn + CTVp + 0.5 to 1.0 cm (does not need to be uniform)
  - 4DCT is allowed to customize the PTV expansion
- *PTVboost.* GTVp + GTVn with a 0.5 to 1.0 cm expansion
  - 4DCT is allowed to customize the PTV expansion

Treatment Planning

- 45 Gy in 25 fractions (1.8 Gy/fraction)
  - PTV: $V_{45Gy} \geq 95\%$
  - PTV: $V_{50Gy} \leq 10\%$
  - D_{max} (to lung > 2 cm outside PTV) < 40 Gy

- Boost of 5.4 Gy
  - PTV: $V_{5.4Gy} \geq 95\%$
  - PTV: $V_{6Gy} \leq 10\%$

Treatment Delivery

- *Technique.* Three-dimensional conformal radiation therapy (3DCRT)
- *Image-guidance.* 4DCT allowed, first day port films or portal images of each field, twice weekly verification films/images of orthogonal views (anterior or posterior and lateral projection)
  - Daily image-guidance is encouraged

Organ(s) at Risk

- *Lungs.* Lung—(PTV + 2 cm) ≤ 40 Gy
  - Total lung volume: $V_{30Gy} < 20\%$
  - $V_{20Gy} < 30\%$ (ideally $V_{20Gy} < 25\%$)
  - $V_{10Gy} < 40\%$, $V_{5Gy} < 60\%$
  - Mean lung dose < 20 Gy
- *Heart.* $D_{100\%} < 30$ Gy, $D_{50\%} < 40$ Gy
- *Liver.* $V_{30Gy} \leq 60\%$, mean dose ≤ 25 Gy
- *Combined kidneys.* $D_{70\%} \leq 20$ Gy
- *Only one functioning kidney.* $D_{80\%} \leq 20$ Gy
- *Spinal cord.* $D_{max} \leq 45$ Gy

Toxicity

Acute:

- Dysphagia, esophagitis, nausea, vomiting, diarrhea, weight loss
- Fatigue, skin erythema
- Radiation pneumonitis

Late:

- Esophageal stricture, dysphagia, esophageal, or gastric bleeding
- Carditis, myelitis
- Subcutaneous fibrosis
- Pulmonary fibrosis
- Esophageal fistula

Clinical Protocol Reference

RTOG 1010: a phase III trial evaluating the addition of trastuzumab to trimodality treatment of HER2-overexpressing esophageal adenocarcinoma.

18.2. ESOPHAGUS (UNRESECTABLE)

Therapeutic Considerations

- *Patient population.* Unresectable squamous cell or adenocarcinoma of the esophagus or GEJ that is unresectable
- *Concurrent treatments.* Cisplatin, paclitaxel
- *Alternative treatments.* Palliative care, other chemotherapy regimens, palliative radiotherapy

Dose Specification

- 50.4 Gy in 28 fractions (1.8 Gy/fraction)

Simulation

- *Imaging.* CT simulation, 3- to 5-mm slice thickness
- *Position.* Supine or prone
- *Immobilization.* Immobilization device in treatment position
- *Scanning limits.* Cricoid cartilage and extending through the liver
- *Other.* Barium swallow is optional, recommend fusion with diagnostic CT scan

Target Volume(s)

- *Gross tumor volume (GTV).* Gross disease (tumor only)
- *Clinical target volume (CTV).* GTV + 4 cm proximal/distal, 1 cm lateral, clinically involved nodes, locoregional nodes
  - Cervical primary: include supraclavicular fossae
  - Mid-esophagus: include paraesophageal nodes
  - Distal esophagus: include celiac nodes
- *PTV.* CTV + 1 to 2 cm.

Treatment Planning

- *PTV.* $D_{100\%} \geq 93\%$ of prescription dose. $D_{max} \leq 107\%$ of prescription dose
- Cervical primary
  - Three-field technique is preferable (two anterior obliques and a posterior field)
  - Acceptable to treat with an anterior-posterior (AP)/posterior-anterior (PA) to 39.6 Gy, then switch to obliques to exclude the spinal cord
  - Supraclavicular field is treated separately, and can be supplemented with electrons

Treatment Delivery

- *Technique.* 3DCRT
- *Image-guidance.* Port films/images on day 1 and at least twice per week

Organ(s) at Risk

- *Lung.* $V_{20Gy} < 30\%$
- *Spinal cord.* $V_{50Gy} < 5$ cm (length)
  - $V_{47Gy} < 20$ cm (length)
- *Heart.* $V_{50Gy} < 1/3$
  - $V_{45Gy} < 2/3$
  - $V_{40Gy} < 100\%$
- *Liver.* $V_{35Gy} < 50\%$
  - $V_{30Gy} < 100\%$
- *Kidney.* $V_{50Gy} < 1/3$
  - $V_{30Gy} < 2/3$
  - $V_{23Gy} < 100\%$

Toxicity

Acute:

- Fatigue, skin erythema, and desquamation
- Nausea, vomiting, diarrhea, weight loss, esophagitis, abdominal discomfort
- Myelosuppression
- Radiation pneumonitis

Late:

- Subcutaneous fibrosis
- Esophageal stricture or fistula
- Carditis, myelitis
- Pulmonary fibrosis

Clinical Protocol Reference

RTOG 0436: a phase III trial evaluating the addition of cetuximab to paclitaxel, cisplatin, and radiation for patients with esophageal cancer who are treated without surgery.

18.3. ADJUVANT GASTRIC

Therapeutic Considerations

- *Patient population.* Surgically resected adenocarcinoma of the stomach or GEJ with T3/4 or node positive disease
- *Concurrent treatments.* One cycle of 5FU followed by radiotherapy with 5FU then two cycles of 5FU

Dose Specification

- 45 Gy in 25 fractions (1.8 Gy/fraction)

Simulation

- *Imaging.* CT simulation
- *Position.* Not specified, as long as position is reproducible
- *Immobilization.* Strongly encouraged
- *Other.* Recommend fusion of preoperative CT scan

Target Volume(s)

- *Tumor bed.* Tumor based on preoperative imaging and pathologic findings.
  - Include areas of involved adenopathy
- *CTV.* According to description and Tables 18.1–18.4 (based on location on primary tumor and T and N stage).

TABLE 18.1 Gastroesophageal Junction Fields

Stage	Clinical Target Volumes
General Principles	Cover stomach if can exclude 2/3 of one kidney. If > 5cm margins pathologically, treatment of residual stomach is optional for node negative. OARs are heart, lung, spinal cord, kidneys, liver.
T2-T3 Node Negative	Extend to include medial left hemi-diaphragm and adjacent body of pancreas (inclusion of pancreatic tail discretionary) Lymph nodes: May omit or include peri-gastric nodes. If T3, consider also including peri-esophageal, mediastinal, and celiac nodes. Can consider excluding nodes if D1/D2 resection and more than 10–15 examined lymph nodes.
T4 Node Negative	Stomach inclusion preferable (unless wide margins as above). Extend to include medial left hemi-diaphragm and adjacent body of pancreas (inclusion of pancreatic tail discretionary), as well as sites of adherence using 3–5 cm margins. Lymph nodes: Include nodes related to sites of adherence. Consider peri-gastric, peri-esophageal, and celiac nodes. If esophageal involvement, include mediastinal nodes.
Node Positive	Stomach inclusion preferable. Contour tumour bed as per respective T stage for node negative. Lymph nodes: Proximal peri-gastric, peri-esophageal, celiac and mediastinal nodes. Consider including pancreatico-duodenal and porta-hepatis nodes only if significant percentage node positivity.

*Adapted from Tepper and Gunderson, Semin Oncol 2002.

- N+: coverage of tumor bed, residual stomach, resection margins, nodal drainage regions
- N− and good surgical nodal resection (D1 + D2, with pathological evaluation of ≥ 10–15 nodes) and wide margin on the primary (≥ 5 cm), treatment of the nodal beds is not necessary
- Treatment of residual stomach depends on normal tissue morbidity and risk of relapse

- *PTV.* CTV + ≥ 1 cm (expansion does not need to be uniform)

TABLE 18.2 Cardia and Proximal Third of Stomach Fields

Stage	Clinical Target Volumes
General Principles	Cover stomach preferable for most if can exclude 2/3 of one kidney. If > 5cm margins pathologically, treatment of residual stomach is optional for node negative. OARs are heart, lung, spinal cord, kidneys, liver.
T2-T3 Node Negative	Extend to include medial left hemi-diaphragm and adjacent body of pancreas (inclusion of pancreatic tail discretionary) Lymph nodes: May omit or include peri-gastric nodes. If T3, consider also including peri-esophageal, mediastinal, and celiac nodes. Can consider excluding nodes if D1/D2 resection and more than 10–15 examined lymph nodes.
T4 Node Negative	Stomach inclusion preferable (unless wide margins as above). Extend to include medial left hemi-diaphragm and adjacent body of pancreas (inclusion of pancreatic tail discretionary), as well as sites of adherence using 3–5 cm margins. Lymph nodes: Include nodes related to sites of adherence. Consider peri-gastric and celiac nodes. If esophageal involvement, include peri-esophageal and mediastinal nodes.
Node Positive	Stomach inclusion preferable. Contour tumour bed as per respective T stage for node negative. Lymph nodes: Peri-gastric, celiac, splenic, and supra-pancreatic nodes. Consider including peri-esophageal and mediastinal nodes, especially if esophageal involvement. Consider including pancreatico-duodenal and porta-hepatis nodes if significant percentage node positivity.

*Adapted from Tepper and Gunderson, Semin Oncol 2002.

TABLE 18.3 Body and Middle Third of Stomach Fields

Stage	Clinical Target Volumes
General Principles	Include stomach for all stages, and attempt to exclude 2/3 of one kidney OARs are spinal cord, kidneys, liver, heart, and lungs.
T2-T3 Node Negative	Include the body of the pancreas (inclusion of pancreatic tail discretionary) Lymph nodes: May omit or include peri-gastric nodes. Consider including splenic, celiac, supra-pancreatic, pancreatico-duodenal and porta-hepatis nodes. May consider excluding nodes if D1/D2 resection and more than 10–15 examined lymph nodes.
T4 Node Negative	Include body of pancreas (inclusion of pancreatic tail discretionary), as well as sites of adherence using 3–5 cm margins. Lymph nodes: Include nodes related to sites of adherence. Consider inclusion of the peri-gastric, splenic, celiac, supra-pancreatic, pancreatico-duodenal and porta-hepatis nodes
Node Positive	Contour tumour bed as per respective T stage for node negative. Lymph nodes: Cover the peri-gastric, splenic, celiac, supra-pancreatic, pancreatico-duodenal and porta-hepatis nodes. May consider also including the splenic hilum.

*Adapted from Tepper and Gunderson, Semin Oncol 2002.

TABLE 18.4 Antrum, Pylorus, Distal Stomach Fields

Stage	Clinical Target Volumes
General Principles	Include stomach for most, and attempt to exclude 2/3 of one kidney. If > 5 cm margins pathologically, treatment of residual stomach is optional for node negative if inclusion would result in significant morbidity due to volume of irradiated normal tissue OARs are spinal cord, kidneys, liver, heart, and lungs.
T2-T3 Node Negative	Include the head of pancreas (inclusion of pancreatic tail discretionary), and 1st and 2nd parts of duodenum. Lymph nodes: May omit or include peri-gastric nodes. Consider including supra-pancreatic, pancreatico-duodenal, porta-hepatis and celiac nodes. May consider excluding these nodes if D1/D2 resection and more than 10–15 examined lymph nodes, and 0–2 lymph nodes positive.
T4 Node Negative	Stomach inclusion preferable. Include the head of pancreas (inclusion of pancreatic tail discretionary), 1st and 2nd parts of duodenum as well as sites of adherence using 3–5 cm margins. Lymph nodes: Include nodes related to sites of adherence. Consider inclusion of the peri-gastric, supra-pancreatic, pancreatico-duodenal, porta-hepatis and celiac nodes.
Node Positive	Stomach inclusion preferable, otherwise contour tumour bed as per respective T stage for node negative. Lymph nodes: Cover the peri-gastric, supra-pancreatic, pancreatico-duodenal, porta-hepatis and celiac nodes. Consider splenic hilum (may exclude if D1/D2 resection and more than 10–15 examined lymph nodes, and 0–2 lymph nodes positive)

*Adapted from Tepper and Gunderson, Semin Oncol 2002.

Treatment Planning

- *Dose uniformity variation.* 95% to 107% of prescription dose

Treatment Delivery

- *Technique.* 3DCRT, AP-PA techniques are acceptable
- *Image-guidance.* Set of orthogonal films and portal films day 1

Organ(s) at Risk

- *Heart.* $D_{50\%} < 25$ Gy (combined left and right ventricles)
- *Kidney.* $D_{50\%} < 20$ Gy (combined volume)
  - $\geq 2/3$ of one kidney not irradiated
- *Liver.* $D_{30\%} < 30$ Gy
- *Spinal cord.* $D_{max} < 45$ Gy

Toxicity

Acute:

- Fatigue, skin erythema
- Loss of appetite, nausea, vomiting, weight loss, diarrhea
- Decreased blood counts

Late:

- Skin changes including localized hair loss
- Decreased kidney function, decreased liver function
- Spinal cord myelopathy

Clinical Protocol Reference

CALGB 80101 and RTOG 0571: phase III intergroup trial of adjuvant chemoradiation after resection of gastric or gastroesophageal adenocarcinoma.

18.4. UNRESECTABLE PANCREAS

Therapeutic Considerations

- *Patient population.* Locally advanced, unresectable pancreatic cancer
- *Concurrent treatments.* Gemcitabine prior to radiotherapy, capecitabine during radiotherapy
- *Alternative treatments.* Chemotherapy alone, addition of biological agent, continuation of concurrent chemotherapy until progression, supportive care

Dose Specification

- 54 Gy in 30 fractions (1.8 Gy/fraction)

Simulation

- *Imaging.* CT simulation, slice thickness ≤ 3 mm
- *Position.* Not specified
- *Immobilization.* Not specified
- *Scanning limits.* Diaphragm to pubic symphysis
- *Other.* Recommended intravenous (IV) contrast
  - Suggest fusion with diagnostic CT scan

Target Volume(s)

- *GTV.* Lymph nodes > 1 cm
  - Not necessary to include entire pancreas
- *CTV.* Not defined as regional lymph nodes are not included
- *PTV.* GTV + 2 cm (anterior and posterior) and 3 cm (superior and inferior)

Treatment Planning

- Completion of radiotherapy within 49 days
- Require 3 to 5 beams
- PTV dose homogeneity: maximum ±5% prescribed dose

Treatment Delivery

- *Technique.* 3DCRT
- *Image-guidance.* Weekly films and/or portal images

Organ(s) at Risk

- *Spinal cord.* $D_{max} \leq 45$ Gy
- *Liver.* $D_{60\%} < 30$ Gy, $D_{33\%} < 20$ Gy
- *Kidneys.* One kidney ≤ 18 Gy
    - Or 2/3 of one kidney spared

Toxicity

Acute:
- Fatigue, skin reaction
- Nausea, vomiting, loss of appetite, weight loss
- Stress ulcers
- Diarrhea, liver, and renal dysfunction

Late:
- Fatigue, skin discoloration
- Liver and renal dysfunction, change in bowel habits

Clinical Protocol Reference

LAP07, GERCOR, ECOG E4201: randomized multicenter phase III study in patients with locally advanced adenocarcinoma of the pancreas: gemcitabine with or without chemoradiotherapy and with or without erlotinib.

18.5. POSTOPERATIVE PANCREAS

Therapeutic Considerations

- *Patient population.* Resected head of pancreas adenocarcinoma
- *Concurrent treatments.* Surgery, adjuvant chemotherapy (five cycles gemcitabine), then 5FU with radiation if no progression on gemcitabine
- *Alternative treatments.* Surgery alone, surgery and adjuvant chemotherapy, chemoradiotherapy alone, chemotherapy alone

Dose Specification

- 50.4 Gy in 28 fractions (1.8 Gy/fraction)

Simulation

- *Imaging.* CT simulation, slice thickness ≤ 3 mm
- *Position.* Supine, arms up
- *Immobilization.* Alpha cradle or vacuum bag
- *Scanning limits.* Not specified
- *Other.* IV contrast recommended, or fuse diagnostic CT with contrast, also can fuse preoperative CT scan

Target Volume(s)

- *CTV.* As per the RTOG contouring atlas (www.rtog.org)
  - CA: most proximal 1.0 to 1.5 cm + 1.0 to 1.5 cm expansion
  - Superior mesenteric artery (SMA): proximal 2.5 to 3.0 cm + 1.0 to 1.5 cm expansion
  - PV: from bifurcation of the PV to the PV confluence with either the SMV or splenic vein + 1.0 to 1.5 cm expansion
  - Pancreaticojejunostomy (PJ): follow the pancreatic remnant medial and anterior to the junction with the jejunal loop + 0.5 to 1.0 cm
  - Aorta: from the CA/PV/PJ (whichever is most superior) to the bottom of L2 or to the inferior portion of the preoperative tumor volume + 2.5 to 3.0 cm to the right, 1.0 cm to the left, 2.0 to 2.5 cm anteriorly, 0.2 cm posteriorly (ensure coverage of paravertebral nodes laterally, but avoid the kidneys)
  - Resected GTV: preoperative gross tumor mass
  - May include surgical clips (if placed for tumor-related or radiation planning purposes) + 0.5 to 1.0 cm expansion (or no expansion)
  - Include maximum 0.1 cm of vertebral body
  - If pancreaticogastrostomy done, do not include in CTV
  - Merge all the above to create CTV
- *PTV.* CTV + 0.5 cm

Treatment Planning

- 90% of PTV receives 95% of prescribed dose
- 99% of CTV receives 95% of prescribed dose
- $D_{max} \leq 55.9$ Gy
- $V_{52.9Gy} \leq 5.0$ cm^3
- $D_{min} \geq 45.4$ Gy

Treatment Delivery

- *Technique.* 3DCRT/intensity-modulated radiation therapy (IMRT)/tomotherapy
- *Image-guidance.* Daily image guided radiation therapy is permitted, motion management permitted

Organ(s) at Risk

- *Kidneys.* $D_{50\%} < 18$ Gy for each kidney
  - Mean dose < 18 Gy
  - If only one kidney: $D_{15\%} \leq 18$ Gy
- *Liver.* Mean dose ≤ 25 Gy
- *Stomach.* $D_{max} \leq 54$ Gy, $D_{15\%} < 45$ Gy
- *Small bowel.* $D_{max} \leq 54$ Gy, $D_{15\%} < 45$ Gy
- *Spinal canal.* $D_{max} \leq 45$ Gy

Toxicity

Acute:
- Abdominal discomfort, nausea, vomiting, diarrhea
- Loss of appetite, weight loss
- Fatigue, skin erythema, local epilation, pancytopenia
- Muscle aches in treated area

Late:
- Change in liver or kidney function
- Bowel obstruction, gastric, duodenal, or small bowel ulceration
- Dry skin

Clinical Protocol Reference

EORTC 40884–22084, NCIC, SWOG, RTOG 0848: a phase III trial evaluating both erlotinib and chemoradiation as adjuvant treatment for patients with resected head of pancreas adenocarcinoma.

18.6. RECTUM

Therapeutic Considerations

- *Patient population.* Adenocarcinoma of the rectum (T3–4, N0–2, and M0)
- *Concurrent treatments.* Neoadjuvant capecitabine (5FU) and oxaliplatin with radiation and adjuvant 5FU, leucovorin and oxaliplatin (FOLFOX)
- *Alternative treatments.* Neoadjuvant radiotherapy alone (25 Gy in five fractions), postoperative chemoradiation

Dose Specification

- 45 Gy in 25 fractions plus a 5.4 Gy in three fractions boost (1.8 Gy/fraction)

Simulation

- *Imaging.* CT simulation, max 5-mm slice thickness
- *Position.* Supine or prone, arms up
- *Immobilization.* Custom immobilization device (alpha cradle, vacuum lock bag) if supine
    - Belly board if prone
- *Other.* Full bladder, bowel exclusion techniques when feasible

Target Volume(s)

- *GTVrectal.* All known gross disease
- *GTVnodal.* Grossly involved lymph nodes
- *CTVrectal.* GTVrectal + 1.5 cm radially, 2.5 cm craniocaudally
- *CTVnodal.* GTVnodal + 1.5 cm
- *CTVa.* Mesorectum (peri-rectal fat and presacral space)
    - T3: include the internal iliac lymph nodes
    - T4: include the internal and external iliac lymph nodes
    - As per the RTOG contouring atlas
- *CTVboost.* GTVrectal with associated mesorectum and presacral region + 2 cm superior, anterior and 2 cm around GTVrectal
- *PTVpelvis.* CTVrectal + CTVnodal + CTVa + 0.5 cm
- *PTVboost.* CTVboost + 0.5 to 1.0 cm

Treatment Planning

- *Phase 1.* IMRT treatment to PTVpelvis: 45 Gy in 25 fractions
- *Phase 2.* 3DCRT boost to PTVboost: 5.4 Gy in 3 fractions
- *PTV.* $V_{93\%}$ prescribed dose ≥ 98%
    - $V_{105\%}$ prescribed dose ≤ 10%
    - $V_{115\%}$ prescribed dose ≤ 5%

Treatment Delivery

- *Technique.* IMRT (pelvis), 3DCRT (boost)
- *Image-guidance.* Orthogonal films or images

Organ(s) at Risk

- *Bladder.* $D_{40\%} \leq 40$ Gy, $D_{25\%} \leq 45$ Gy, $D_{max} < 50$ Gy
- *Femoral heads.* $D_{40\%} \leq 40$ Gy, $D_{25\%} \leq 45$ Gy, $D_{max} < 50$ Gy
- *Small bowel.* $V_{35Gy} \leq 180$ mL, $V_{40Gy} \leq 100$ mL, $V_{45Gy} \leq 65$ mL

Toxicity

Acute:

- Rectal frequency, diarrhea, rectal discomfort
- Skin irritation and desquamation, fatigue, local epilation
- Urinary frequency, dysuria
- Loss of pubic hair

Late:

- Bowel stricture, obstruction, perforation or fistula formation, rectal bleeding
- Sterility, urethral obstruction
- Hip fracture, skin discoloration

Clinical Protocol Reference

RTOG 0822: a phase II evaluation of preoperative chemoradiotherapy utilizing IMRT in combination with capecitabine and oxaliplatin for patients with locally advanced rectal cancer.

18.7. ANAL CANAL

Therapeutic Considerations

- *Patient population.* Invasive primary carcinoma of the anal canal, T2–4, N0–3
- *Concurrent treatments.* 5FU, mitomycin-C
- *Alternative treatments.* Radiation alone, surgery

Dose Specification

- *T2N0.* 50.4 Gy in 28 fractions (1.8 Gy/fraction)
- *T3–4, N+.* 54 Gy in 30 fractions (1.8 Gy/fraction)

Simulation

- *Imaging.* CT simulation, slice thickness ≤ 5 mm
- *Position.* Supine or prone, arms up
- *Immobilization.* Custom immobilization device (that is, alpha cradle)
- *Scanning limits.* All tissues to be irradiated must be included
- *Other.* Oral and IV contrast recommended, air in the rectum, anal marker at verge or at the inferior extend of the tumor

Target Volume(s)

- As per the RTOG anorectal contouring atlas (www.rtog.org) excluding uninvolved bone, genitourinary structures, muscle, and bowel
- *T2N0:*
  - GTVA: all known gross primary anal tumor volume
  - CTVA: GTV and anal canal + 2.5 cm (exclude bone and air)
  - CTV42: lymph node areas: mesorectal (peri-rectal, presacral), inguinals, external and internal iliacs + 1.0 cm
  - PTVA: CTVA + ≥ 1.0 cm
  - PTV42: CTV42 + ≥ 1.0 cm
- *T3–4N0:*
  - GTV: all known gross disease
  - CTVA: GTV and anal canal + 2.5 cm (exclude bone and air)
  - CTV45: lymph node areas: mesorectal (peri-rectal, presacral), inguinals, external and internal iliacs + 1.0 cm
  - PTVA: CTVA + ≥ 1.0 cm
  - PTV45: CTV45 + ≥ 1.0 cm
- *N+:*
  - GTV: all known gross disease
  - GTVN50.4: involved nodal regions with gross lymph node involvement ≤ 3 cm
  - GTV54: involved nodal regions with gross lymph node involvement > 3 cm
  - CTVA: GTV and anal canal + 2.5 cm (exclude bone and air)
  - CTV45: Lymph node areas: mesorectal (peri-rectal, presacral), inguinals, external and internal iliacs) + 1.0 cm

- CTV50.4: GTV50.4 + 1.0 cm
- CTV54: GTV54 + 1.0 cm
- PTVA: CTVA + ≥ 1.0 cm
- PTV45: CTV45 + ≥ 1.0 cm
- PTV50.4: CTV50.4 + ≥ 1.0 cm
- PTV54: CTV54 + ≥ 1.0 cm

Treatment Planning

- *T2N0:*
  - PTVA: to receive 50.4 Gy in 28 fractions (1.8 Gy/fraction)
  - PTV42: to receive 42 Gy in 28 fractions (1.5 Gy/fraction)
- *T3–4N0:*
  - PTVA: to receive 54 Gy in 30 fractions (1.8 Gy/fraction)
  - PTV45: to receive 45 Gy in 30 fractions (1.5 Gy/fraction)
- *N+:*
  - PTVA: to receive 54 Gy in 30 fractions (1.8 Gy/fraction)
  - PTV45: to receive 45 Gy in 30 fractions (1.5 Gy/fraction)
  - PTV50.4: to receive 50.4 Gy in 30 fractions (1.68 Gy/fraction)
  - PTV54: to receive 54 Gy in 30 fractions (1.8 Gy/fraction)

- Prescription isodose surface will encompass ≥ 90% of PTVs (for the primary tumor and involved lymph nodes)
- Prescription isodose surface will encompass ≥ 85% of uninvolved nodal PTVs
- ≤ 5% of any PTV to receive < 90% of the prescription dose
- ≤ 2% of any PTV will receive < 80% of the prescription dose
- ≤ 2% of the primary tumor PTV will receive > 115% of the prescription dose

Treatment Delivery

- *Technique.* IMRT, tomotherapy
- *Image-guidance.* Recommend daily portal imaging (especially for prone patients using a bowel displacement device)
  - For tomotherapy: require axial CT images (≥ 5 cm length)
  - Recommend setup verification images for cephalocaudad and transverse position verification

Organ(s) at Risk

- *Bladder.* $D_{50\%} \leq 35$ Gy, $D_{35\%} \leq 40$ Gy, $D_{5\%} < 50$ Gy
- *External genitalia.* $D_{50\%} \leq 20$ Gy, $D_{35\%} \leq 40$ Gy, $D_{5\%} \leq 50$ Gy
- *Femoral heads.* $D_{50\%} \leq 30$ Gy, $D_{35\%} \leq 40$ Gy, $D_{5\%} \leq 44$ Gy
- *Iliac crest.* $D_{50\%} \leq 30$ Gy, $D_{35\%} \leq 40$ Gy, $D_{5\%} \leq 5.0$ Gy
- *Small bowel.* $V_{30Gy} \leq 200$ mL, $V_{35Gy} \leq 150$ mL, $V_{45Gy} \leq 20$ mL, $D_{max} \leq 50$ Gy
- *Large bowel.* $V_{30Gy} \leq 200$ mL, $V_{35Gy} \leq 150$ mL, $V_{45Gy} \leq 20$ mL
- *Peri-anal skin.* Contoured

Toxicity

Acute:

- Dermatitis, ulceration, local epilation
- Nausea, vomiting, diarrhea, rectal bleeding, anal discomfort/pain
- Fatigue, sterility

Late:

- Anal canal fibrosis, decreased anal function, anal fistula formation
- Vaginal dryness, bleeding or narrowing, dyspareunia
- Skin dryness, skin necrosis
- Difficulty with urination
- Sterility/infertility

Clinical Protocol Reference

RTOG 0529: a phase II evaluation of dose-painted IMRT in combination with 5FU and mitomycin-c for reduction of acute morbidity in carcinoma of the anal canal.

Chapter 19

Genitourinary Treatment Planning

19.1. LOW-RISK PROSTATE CANCER

EXTERNAL-BEAM APPROACH

Therapeutic Considerations

- *Patient population.* T1c–T2c and PSA < 10 ng/mL and Gleason score ≤ 6
- *Concurrent treatments.* May consider neoadjuvant hormonal therapy for a bulky prostate gland
- *Alternative treatments.* Active surveillance, brachytherapy, radical prostatectomy

Dose Specification

- 73.8 Gy in 41 fractions (1.8 Gy/fraction)

Simulation

- *Imaging.* Computed tomographic (CT) simulation, slice thickness ≤ 0.5 cm
- *Position.* Supine
- *Immobilization.* Daily image-guidance required, no specific device
- *Scanning limits.* At/above iliac crest to the perineum
- *Other.* Empty rectum, full bladder, urethrogram recommended

Target Volume(s)

- *GTV.* Prostate gland including all known disease
- *CTV.* GTV
- *PTV.* CTV + 0.4 to 1.0 cm

Treatment Planning

- *Maximum PTV homogeneity.* ±7%
- *Minimum PTV dose (encompassing ≥ 98% of PTV).* 73.8 Gy
- *Minimum CTV dose (encompassing ≥ 100% CTV).* 73.8 Gy

Treatment Delivery

- *Technique.* Intensity-modulated radiation therapy (IMRT)/three-dimensional conformal radiation therapy (3DCRT)
- *Image-guidance.* Daily localization with fiducial markers, transabdominal ultrasound, or other modality is required

Organ(s) at Risk

- *Bladder.* $V_{80Gy} < 15\%$, $V_{75Gy} < 25\%$, $V_{70Gy} < 35\%$, $V_{65Gy} < 50\%$
- *Rectum.* $V_{75Gy} < 15\%$, $V_{70Gy} < 25\%$, $V_{65Gy} < 35\%$, $V_{60Gy} < 50\%$
- *Penile bulb.* Mean dose ≤ 52.5 Gy

Toxicity

Acute:

- Abdominal cramping, diarrhea, rectal urgency, proctitis, hematochezia
- Urinary frequency/urgency, dysuria, hematuria, urinary tract infection (UTI), incontinence
- Radiation dermatitis

Late:

- Injury to bowel or bladder including obstruction or bleeding
- Erectile dysfunction, second malignancy

Clinical Protocol Reference

RTOG0415: a phase III randomized study of hypofractionated 3DCRT/IMRT versus conventionally fractionated 3DCRT/IMRT in patients with favorable-risk prostate cancer.

LOW-DOSE RATE BRACHYTHERAPY APPROACH

Therapeutic Considerations

- *Patient population.* T1b–2b, Gleason score ≤ 6, PSA ≤ 10 ng/mL (with appropriate prostate volume to avoid pubic arch interference)
- *Alternative treatments.* Active surveillance, prostatectomy, external-beam radiation
- *Dose specification.* 145 Gy (125-I) or 125 Gy (103-Pd)

Simulation

- *Pre-implant:*
  - Imaging: TRUS
- *Post-implant:*
  - Imaging: CT, 3- to 5-mm slice thickness

Target Volume(s)

- *CTV.* Prostate (as per pre-implant TRUS)
- *PTV.* CTV + 3 mm circumferentially; 5 mm to base and apex; posterior border can have 0 mm expansion

Treatment Planning

- *103Pd.* Minimum peripheral dose to PTV: 125 Gy
- *125I.* Minimum peripheral dose to PTV: 145 Gy
- Entire gland to receive at least 80% of planned dose
- $D_{90\%}$ > 90% of prescription dose
- $D_{90\%}$ < 130% of prescription dose

Treatment Delivery

- *Technique.* Interstitial brachytherapy
- *Image-guidance.* TRUS

Organ(s) at Risk

- Not specified

Toxicity

Acute:
- Urinary irritation

Late:
- Urinary irritation, incontinence

Clinical Protocol Reference

NCIC PR11, CALBG 140602, ECOG JPR11, RTOG 0873, SWOG PR11, ICR-CTSU ProSTART: a phase II study of active surveillance therapy against radical treatment in patients diagnosed with favorable-risk prostate cancer.

19.2. INTERMEDIATE-RISK PROSTATE CANCER

EXTERNAL-BEAM APPROACH

Therapeutic Considerations

- *Patient population.* T2b–T2c and/or PSA 10 to 20 ng/mL and/or Gleason score 7, if all three are present then it requires ≤ 50% of biopsy cores to be positive
- *Concurrent treatments.* Consider up to 6 months luteinizing hormone-releasing hormone (LHRH) agonist + antiandrogen for 10 days
- *Alternative treatments.* External-beam radiation with brachytherapy boost, radical prostatectomy

Dose Specification

- 79.2 Gy in 44 fractions (1.8 Gy/fraction)

Simulation

- *Imaging.* CT simulation, slice thickness ≤ 3 mm
- *Position.* Supine
- *Immobilization.* Thermoplastic immobilization cast or molded foam cradle for stabilization
- *Scanning limits.* Top of iliac crests to perineum
- *Other.* Full bladder, consider intravascular (IV) contrast

Target Volume(s)

- *GTV.* Prostate gland including all known disease
- *CTV.* GTV + proximal 1.0 cm of seminal vesicle tissue
- *PTV.* CTV + 0.5 to 1.0 cm

Treatment Planning

- 98% of PTV to receive prescription dose
- *Maximum PTV dose.* ≤ 84.7 Gy (107% prescription dose)
- *Minimum PTV dose.* > 75.2 Gy (95% prescription dose)

Treatment Delivery

- *Technique.* IMRT/3DCRT
- *Image-guidance.* Day 1 and weekly port films, transabdominal ultrasound, kilovoltage (kV), megavoltage (MV) imaging permitted

Organ(s) at Risk

- *Bladder.* $V_{80Gy} < 15\%$, $V_{75Gy} < 25\%$, $V_{70Gy} < 35\%$, $V_{65Gy} < 50\%$
- *Rectum.* $V_{75Gy} < 15\%$, $V_{70Gy} < 25\%$, $V_{65Gy} < 35\%$, $V_{60Gy} < 50\%$
- *Penile bulb.* Mean dose ≤ 52.5 Gy

Toxicity

Acute:
- Abdominal cramping, diarrhea, rectal urgency, proctitis, hematochezia
- Urinary frequency, urgency, dysuria, hematuria, urinary tract infection, incontinence
- Radiation dermatitis

Late:
- Injury to bowel or bladder including obstruction and bleeding
- Erectile dysfunction, secondary malignancy

Clinical Protocol Reference

RTOG 0815: a phase III prospective randomized trial of dose-escalated radiotherapy with or without short-term androgen deprivation therapy for patients with intermediate-risk prostate cancer.

COMBINATION HIGH-DOSE RATE (HDR) BRACHYTHERAPY AND EXTERNAL-BEAM APPROACH

Therapeutic Considerations

- *Patient population.* T1c–T2c, Gleason score 2 to 6, PSA 10 to 20 or T3a–T3b, Gleason score 2 to 6, PSA ≤ 20 or T1c–T3b, Gleason score 7 to 10, PSA ≤ 20
- *Concurrent treatments.* None
- *Alternative treatments.* External-beam radiation alone ± androgen deprivation, prostatectomy

Dose Specification

- *External beam.* 45 Gy in 25 fractions (1.8 Gy/fraction)
- *HDR brachytherapy.* 19 Gy in two fractions (9.5 Gy/fraction)

Simulation

- External beam:
  - *Imaging.* CT simulation
  - *Position.* Not specified

- *Immobilization.* Not specified
- *Scanning limits.* Not specified
- *Other.* Full bladder
- HDR brachytherapy (after catheter placement):
  - *Imaging.* CT simulation, slice thickness ≤ 3 mm
  - *Position.* Supine
- *Scanning limits.* All the CTV with at least 9-mm superior and inferior margin must include the tips of the catheters
- *Other.* Catheters in situ

Target Volume(s)

- External beam:
  - GTV
  - *CTV.* GTV + prostate, seminal vesicles ± whole pelvis depending on lymphatic risk
  - *PTV.* CTV + 1 to 1.5 cm
    - Include pelvic radiation if: 2/3 PSA + [(Gleason score – 6) × 10] is > 15%
  - Pelvic field borders
    - Superior: bottom of L5
    - Inferior: inferior border of ischial tuberosity, or 2 cm below prostate
    - Lateral: ≥ 2 cm lateral to pelvic brim
    - Anterior: anterior to pubic symphysis
    - Posterior: include the S2 vertebral body
- HDR brachytherapy:
  - CTV: T1c–T2b: prostate, T3a–T3b: prostate and extra-capsular extension
  - PTV: CTV

BRACHYTHERAPY PROCEDURE

- *Imaging.* TRUS guidance for after-loading catheter placement
- *Catheters.* CT compatible, ≥ 14 inserted
- *Anesthesia.* Epidural, spinal, or general
- *Immobilization.* Not specified
- *Other.* Urinary catheterization, cystoscopy after insertion of catheters, fiducial marker seeds placed under TRUS guidance at base and apex of prostate

Treatment Planning

- External beam:
  - Dose should be prescribed to the minimum target dose (highest isodose line which encompasses the PTV)
- HDR brachytherapy:
  - Dose prescribed to periphery of PTV
  - V_{19Gy} > 90% of PTV can be given before or after external-beam radiation therapy (EBRT)
  - Two fractions within 6 to 24 hours of each other

Treatment Delivery

- *Technique.* 3DCRT, minimum four fields
- *Image-guidance.* Not specified

Organ(s) at Risk

- HDR brachytherapy:
  - Bladder: $V_{75\% \text{ of prescription dose}} < 1$ mL
  - Rectum: $V_{75\% \text{ of prescription dose}} < 1$ mL
  - Urethra: $V_{75\% \text{ of prescription dose}} < 1$ mL

Toxicity

External beam:

Acute:

- Abdominal cramping, diarrhea, rectal urgency, proctitis, hematochezia
- Urinary frequency, urgency, dysuria, hematuria, urinary tract infection, incontinence
- Radiation dermatitis, epilation, fatigue

Late:

- Rectal urgency, proctitis, hematochezia
- Urinary frequency, urgency, hematuria, urinary tract infection, incontinence
- Impotence

HDR brachytherapy:

Acute:

- Infection, discomfort, fatigue, nausea
- Abdominal cramps, diarrhea
- Bladder irritation, hematuria, urinary tract infection, urinary obstruction, incontinence

Late:

- Rectal bleeding, intestinal obstruction
- Urinary obstruction, bladder irritation, urethral stricture, secondary malignancy

Clinical Protocol Reference

RTOG 0321: phase II trial of combined HDR brachytherapy and external-beam radiotherapy for adenocarcinoma of the prostate.

19.3. HIGH-RISK PROSTATE CANCER

Therapeutic Considerations

- *Patient population.* Gleason score 9 to 10 and PSA ≤ 150 and any T-stage or Gleason score 8 and PSA < 20 and ≥T2 or Gleason score 7 to 8 and PSA 20 to 150 and any T-stage
- *Concurrent treatments.* 24 months LHRH agonist (started 8 weeks before external-beam radiation) and antiandrogen (started 8 weeks before, and stopped after completion of, external-beam radiation)

Dose Specification

- 72.0 to 75.6 Gy in 40 to 42 fractions (1.8 Gy/fraction)
- *Pelvic fields.* 46.8 Gy in 26 fractions (1.8 Gy/fraction) followed by
- *Boost to PTV.* 25.2 to 28.8 Gy in 14 to 16 fractions (1.8 Gy/fraction)

Simulation

- *Imaging.* CT simulation, ≤ 0.5 cm thickness
- *Position.* As per the institutional standard
- *Immobilization.* Standard institutional immobilization
- *Scanning limits.* At or above the iliac crest to the perineum
- *Other.* Full bladder, empty rectum

Target Volume(s)

- *3DCRT pelvic fields.* Superior: L5–S1 interspace (minimum bottom of SI joints)
  - Lateral: ≥ 1 cm lateral to pelvic brim
  - Inferior: inferior border of ischial tuberosity
  - Posterior: approximately S2–3 interspace
  - Anterior: anterior to pubic symphysis
- *IMRT pelvic.* GTV: prostate (+entire seminal vesicles if T3b)
  - See RTOG contouring atlas (www.rtog.org)
  - CTVnodes: iliac vessels + 0.7 to 1.0 cm, excluding musculature, organs, bone, obturators, and presacral space
  - CTVpro: GTV + 1.0 cm proximal seminal vesicles (if not already included)
  - PTV nodes: CTVnodes + CTVpro + 5 mm
- *Boost.* GTV: prostate (+ entire seminal vesicles if T3b), all known gross disease
  - CTV: GTV + proximal 1.0 cm seminal vesicles (unless entire seminal vesicles included)
  - PTV: CTV + 0.5 to 1.5 cm

Treatment Planning

- *Pelvic dose.* < 5% deviation for 46.8 Gy
  - Minimum dose to ≥ 95% = 46.8 Gy
  - Maximum 7% in homogeneity (in ≤ 3% of the volume)

- *Boost*. Minimum dose encompassing ≥ 95% PTV: 25.2 Gy
  - PTV to receive minimum 95% of the prescription dose

Treatment Delivery

- *Technique*. IMRT/3DCRT
- *Image-guidance*. Not specified

Organ(s) at Risk

- Not specified

Toxicity

Acute:

- Alopecia, fatigue
- Abdominal cramping, diarrhea, rectal urgency, proctitis, hematochezia
- Urinary frequency/urgency, dysuria, hematuria, urinary tract infection, incontinence
- Radiation dermatitis, secondary malignancy

Late:

- Injury to bowel or bladder including obstruction, bleeding, incontinence
- Erectile dysfunction, infertility

Clinical Protocol Reference

RTOG 0521: a Phase III protocol of androgen suppression (AS) and 3DCRT/IMRT versus AS and 3DCRT/IMRT followed by chemotherapy with docetaxel and prednisone for localized, high-risk prostate cancer.

19.4. PROSTATE BED (ADJUVANT)

Therapeutic Considerations

- *Patient population.* T2–3N0M0 prostate cancer, post-prostatectomy, undetectable PSA
  - T2 patients: Gleason score ≥ 7, pre-operative PSA > 10 ng/mL, and positive surgical margins
  - T3 patients: Gleason score ≥ 7; and one or more of pre-operative PSA > 10 ng/mL, positive surgical margins, seminal vesicle invasion
  - If Gleason score is < 7, then requires two or more of the above factors
- *Concurrent treatments.* Consider LHRH agonist for 2 years starting with radiation and 1-month antiandrogen
- *Alternative treatments.* Active surveillance

Dose Specification

- 63 to 66 Gy in 35 to 37 fractions (1.8 Gy/fraction)

Simulation

- *Imaging.* CT or fluoroscopic simulation
- *Position.* Supine
- *Other.* Optional use of rectal marker, 30 mL of urinary contrast in empty bladder followed by retrograde urethrogram (demonstrate apex/beak of dye at the GU diaphragm); consider fusion of pre-operative CT scan

Target Volume(s)

Refer to RTOG prostate bed contouring atlas (www.rtog.org) for specific details

- *Anterior.* Posterior edge of pubic symphysis
  - Above the pubic symphysis: include the posterior 1 to 2 cm of bladder wall
- *Posterior.* Anterior wall of rectum and mesorectal fascia
  - May need to be concave laterally
- *Superior.* 3 to 4 cm above the pubic symphysis or at the level of the vas deferens
  - Include remnants of seminal vesicles if involved
- *Inferior.* 8 to 12 mm below vesicourethral anastomosis
  - May include further inferior if concern about apical margin: can extend to slice above the penile bulb
- *Lateral.* Levator ani muscles, obturator internus, sacrorectogenitopubic fascia (above the symphysis pubis)

Treatment Planning

- *Minimum CTV dose.* ≥ 95% of prescribed dose
- *Maximum CTV dose.* ≤ 105% of prescribed dose

Treatment Delivery

- *Technique.* 3DCRT (four-field box)
- *Image-guidance.* Simulation fields of each treatment field, port films of each treatment field

Organ(s) at Risk

- *Bladder.* Inferior portion will receive same dose as CTV
- Whole rectum < 55 Gy
- Femoral heads < 50 Gy

Toxicity

Acute:

- Abdominal cramping, diarrhea, rectal urgency, or hematochezia
- Urinary frequency, dysuria, hematuria, urinary tract infection, incontinence
- Erythema, epilation, fatigue

Late:

- Impotence
- Change in bowel habit, injury to bowel and pelvis area
- Urinary incontinence, hematuria, frequency, secondary malignancy

Clinical Protocol References

RTOG 0011 and NCIC PR9: phase III randomized study of adjuvant therapy for high-risk pT2–3N0 prostate cancer

Michalski JM, et al. Development of RTOG consensus guidelines for the definition of the clinical target volume for postoperative conformal radiation therapy for prostate cancer. *Int. J. Radiat. Oncol. Biol. Phys.* 2010;76(2):361–8.

19.5. PROSTATE BED (SALVAGE)

Therapeutic Considerations

- *Patient population.* Node negative prostate cancer, post-radical prostatectomy with PSA 0.1 to 2.0 ng/mL, pT3 or pT2 with or without a positive prostatectomy surgical margin, Gleason score ≤ 9
- *Concurrent treatments.* Consider short-term androgen deprivation (start 2 months before initiation of radiotherapy)
- *Alternative treatments.* Androgen deprivation, active surveillance

Dose Specification

- 64.8 to 70.2 Gy in 36 to 39 fractions (1.8 Gy/fraction) to prostate bed
- *Optional.* 45 Gy in 25 fractions (1.8 Gy/fraction) to pelvis + boost to prostate bed to total dose of 64.8 to 70.2 Gy in 36 to 39 fractions (1.8 Gy/fraction)

Simulation

- *Imaging.* CT simulation, slice thickness ≤ 0.5 cm
- *Position.* Supine
- *Immobilization.* Consider immobilization of hips and feet with cradle
- *Scanning limits.* Above iliac crest to below the perineum (below ischial tuberosities)
- *Other.* Urethrogram or MRI recommended; empty rectum (enema 1–2 hours prior to simulation), moderately full bladder

Target Volume(s)

Prostate bed:

- *CTV:*
  - Superior: 2 cm above pubic symphysis, at least posterior 2 cm of bladder should be included and area between bladder and rectum to anterior rectal wall
  - Inferior: top of penile bulb, or 1.5 cm below urethrogram beak
  - Lateral: medial edge of each obturator internus muscle
  - Anterior: posterior aspect of pelvis, above the pelvic symphysis, gradual reduction of the anterior bladder is made for at least 1 to 2 cm
  - Include any clips in the seminal vesicle bed, and seminal vesicle remnants
  - Posterior: anterior-most aspect of ano-rectum
- *PTV:* CTV + 0.8 to 1.5 cm in all dimensions
  - May decrease posterior border to 0.6 cm

Pelvis:

(See RTOG contouring atlas, www.rtog.org)

- *CTV:* obturator, presacral, external iliac, proximal internal iliac, and common iliac nodes to L5–S1 junction
  - 7-mm around iliac vessels, carving out bowel and bone
  - Obturator and presacral spaces to be included
  - Include prostate bed CTV
- *PTV:* CTV + 0.8 to 1.5 cm in all dimensions
  - May decrease posterior border to 0.6 cm

Treatment Planning

- ≥ 95% of PTV should receive prescribed dose
- Maximum dose heterogeneity in PTV is 7% (3DCRT) or 15% (IMRT)

Treatment Delivery

- *Technique.* 3DCRT/IMRT
- *Image-guidance.* At least one port film or pre-treatment alignment film per field or simulation verification radiograph

Organ(s) at Risk

- *Bladder.* $D_{50\%} \leq 65$ Gy, $D_{70\%} \leq 40$ Gy (bladder minus prostate bed CTV)
- *Rectum.* $D_{35\%} \leq 65$ Gy, $D_{55\%} \leq 40$ Gy
- *Femoral heads.* $D_{10\%} \leq 50$ Gy
- *Small bowel.* $V_{45Gy} \leq 150$ mL bowel space
- *Penile bulb.* No constraints, but record dose

Toxicity

Acute:

- Abdominal cramping, diarrhea, rectal urgency, proctitis, hematochezia
- Urinary frequency, urgency, dysuria, hematuria, infection, incontinence
- Radiation dermatitis, epilation, fatigue

Late:

- Diarrhea, rectal urgency, proctitis, hematochezia, intestinal obstruction
- Urinary frequency, urgency, dysuria, hematuria, incontinence
- Erectile dysfunction, secondary malignancy

Clinical Protocol Reference

RTOG 0534: a phase III trial of short-term androgen deprivation with pelvic lymph node or prostate bed only radiotherapy (SPPORT) in prostate cancer patients with rising PSA after radical prostatectomy.

19.6. LOW-RISK BLADDER

Therapeutic Considerations

- *Patient population.* T1 (grade 2–3), N0, transitional cell histology
- *Concurrent treatments.* Cisplatin
- *Alternative treatments.* Cystectomy

Dose Specification

- 61.2 Gy in 34 fractions (1.8 Gy/fraction)
- *Pelvic fields.* 41.4 Gy in 23 fractions (1.8 Gy/fraction) followed by
- *Boost.* 19.8 Gy in 11 fractions (1.8 Gy/fraction)

Simulation

- *Imaging.* CT simulation
- *Position.* Supine
- *Immobilization.* Leg immobilizer or cradle
- *Other.* Empty bladder and rectum
- Optional 30 mL dilute contrast in bladder

Target Volume(s)

Pelvis:

- *GTV.* Gross tumor
- *CTV.* GTV + bladder, prostate (men), prostatic urethra (men), lymph node regions (internal iliac, external iliac, and obturator vessels)
- *Field borders:*
  - *Superior.* S1–2 junction
  - *Inferior.* 1 cm below obturator foramen
- *Laterally.* 1.5 cm beyond bony pelvis
- *Posterior.* 3.0 cm posterior to CTV bladder
- *Anterior.* 1.0 cm anterior to pubic symphysis or 1.5 cm anterior to anterior tip of the bladder (whichever is most anterior)
- *Blocks:*
  - *Anterior/posterior fields:* shield medial border of femoral heads
  - *Lateral fields:* block anal canal posteriorly, inferiorly shield soft tissue anterior to pubic symphysis, superiorly to exclude small bowel and anterior rectus fascia (if anterior to external iliac chain)

Bladder:

- *GTV.* Gross tumor
- *CTV.* GTV + bladder
- *PTV.* CTV + 0.5 cm, except superiorly (margin = 1.5 cm)

Treatment Planning

- Applies to CTV pelvis and PTV bladder
- *Minimum dose.* 95% prescription dose, $D_{99\%}$ > 95% prescription dose
- D_{max}: < 107% prescription dose

Treatment Delivery

- *Technique.* 3DCRT: pelvis: four-field box
- *Image-guidance.* Not specified

Organ(s) at Risk

- *Femoral heads.* D_{max} < 45 Gy
- *Rectum.* D_{55Gy} < 50%

Toxicity

Acute:
- Urinary frequency, nocturia, hematuria
- Proctitis, rectal bleeding, hematochezia, nausea, vomiting
- Radiation dermatitis, alopecia, fatigue

Late:
- Urinary frequency, nocturia, hematuria, ureteral obstruction
- Rectal irritation, bowel obstruction or bleeding, rectal ulcers, fistulization
- Vaginal bleeding

Clinical Protocol Reference

RTOG 0926: a phase II protocol for patients with stage T1 bladder cancer to evaluate selective bladder preserving treatment by radiation therapy concurrent with cisplatin chemotherapy following a thorough transurethral surgical re-staging.

19.7. HIGH-RISK BLADDER

Therapeutic Considerations

- *Patient population.* Muscle-invasive bladder cancer post-transurethral surgery, stage T2–T4a, Nx/0/1, M0
- *Concurrent treatments.* Transurethral resection then chemotherapy with induction radiotherapy, cystectomy if ≥T1 and feasible, otherwise consolidation radiation with chemotherapy
- *Alternative treatments.* Cystectomy, radiation therapy, chemotherapy, or a combination of these, also can use low-risk bladder regimen (Section 20.6)

Dose Specification

Twice daily (BID) regimen (bladder sparing):
Induction:
- 20.8 Gy in 13 fractions (1.6 Gy/fraction, qam) to CTVpelvis plus:
- 19.5 Gy in 13 fractions (1.5 Gy/fraction, qpm [4–6 hours later]) first 5 days to CTVbladder, then CTVboost for 8 days
- Total to CTVboost is 40.3 Gy in 26 fractions

Consolidation:
- 24 Gy in 16 fractions (1.5 Gy/fraction, BID) × 8 days to CTVpelvis
- Total: 64.3 Gy in 42 fractions

Daily (OD) regimen (bladder sparing):
Induction:
- 20 Gy in 10 fractions (2 Gy/fraction) for first 10 days to CTVpelvis
- Then 8 Gy in four fractions (2 Gy/fraction) for 4 days to CTVbladder
- Then 12 Gy in six fractions (2 Gy/fraction) for 6 days to CTVboost
- Total to CTVboost is 40 Gy in 20 fractions

Consolidation:
- 24 Gy in 12 fractions (2 Gy/fraction) to CTVpelvis
- Total: 64 Gy in 32 fractions

Unresectable regimen:
- 39.6 Gy in 22 fractions (1.8 Gy/fraction) to CTVpelvis
- Then 14.4 Gy in eight fractions (2 Gy/fraction) for 4 days to CTVbladder
- Then 10.8 Gy in six fractions (2 Gy/fraction) for 6 days to CTVboost
- Total: 64.8 Gy in 36 fractions

Simulation

- *Imaging.* CT simulation
- *Position.* Supine
- *Immobilization.* Pelvic immobilization device
- *Other.* Empty bladder, optional bladder and rectal contrast, optional urinary catheter

Target Volume(s)

- *GTV.* Gross tumor
- *CTV pelvis: superior.* Mid-sacrum (anterior aspect of S2–3 junction)
  - Inferior: lower pole of obturator foramen
  - Lateral: 1.5 cm beyond bony pelvis
  - Anterior: anterior to bladder covering external iliac nodes
  - Posterior: at S1–S2 junction
  - Anterior–posterior (AP)/posterior–anterior (PA) field shielding: medial border of femoral heads
  - Lateral field shielding: soft tissue anterior to pubic symphysis, anal canal, superiorly exclude small bowel and anterior rectus fascia anteriorly
  - Ensure covering CTVbladder
- *CTV bladder.* GTV + whole bladder
- *CTV boost.* GTV
- *Field edge.* 2 to 2.5 cm beyond CTVs

Treatment Planning

- Dose prescribed to isocenter, or mid-plane if AP/PA fields used
- $D_{99\%} > 95\%$ of prescribed dose for each CTV
- Volume of any CTV to receive 107% of prescribed dose should be < 0.12 mL
- Minimum 4 hours between BID treatments

Treatment Delivery

- *Technique.* 3DCRT
- *Image-guidance.* Not specified

Organ(s) at Risk

- *Rectum.* $D_{50\%} < 30$ Gy, $D_{10\%} < 55$ Gy
- *Femoral heads.* $D_{20\%} < 50$ Gy

Toxicity

Acute:

- Urinary frequency, nocturia, hematuria, cystitis, ureteral obstruction
- Proctitis, hematochezia, mucous-like stools
- Dyspareunia, erythema, epilation, weight loss, fatigue

Late:

- Frequency, nocturia, hematuria, cystitis, ureteral obstruction
- Bowel obstruction, hematochezia, rectal ulcers, fistula, colitis
- Epilation/loss of pubic hair
- Ovarian failure, erectile dysfunction, sterility

Clinical Protocol References

RTOG 0712: a phase II randomized study for patients with muscle-invasive bladder cancer evaluating transurethral surgery and concomitant chemoradiation by either BID irradiation plus 5-fluorouracil and cisplatin or QD irradiation plus gemcitabine followed by selective bladder preservation and gemcitabine/cisplatin adjuvant chemotherapy.

RTOG 0524: a phase I/II trial of a combination of paclitaxel and trastuzumab with daily irradiation or paclitaxel alone with daily irradiation following transurethral surgery for non-cystectomy candidates with muscle-invasive bladder cancer.

19.8. STAGE I SEMINOMA

Therapeutic Considerations

- *Patient population.* Stage I seminomatous germ cell tumor of the testis, categorized as either "classical" or "anaplastic," pT1–3
- *Concurrent treatments.* None
- *Alternative treatments.* Active surveillance, carboplatin

Dose Specification

- 30 Gy in 15 fractions (2 Gy/fraction) or 20 Gy in 10 fractions (2 Gy/fraction)

Simulation

- *Position.* Supine
- *Immobilization.* Institutional standard
- *Other.* Planned with aid of an IV urogram to definite kidney position, scrotal shielding, unless CT simulation

Target Volume(s)

Para-aortic field:

- Anterior and posterior beams
- *Superior border.* T10–11 disc space
- *Inferior.* L5–S1 disc space
- *Ipsilateral margin.* Out to the renal hilum, otherwise transverse process
- *Contralateral margin.* Include transverse process in para-aortic area

Dogleg field (Figure 19.1)—if previous inguino-pelvic or scrotal surgery:

- *Superior.* T10–11 disc space
- *Inferior.* Mid-obturator foramen
- *Ipsilateral margin.* Renal hilum down to L5–51, then diagonally to the lateral edge of the acetabulum, then vertically down to the mid obturator level
- *Contralateral margin.* Inclusion on the transverse process down to L5–S1, then diagonally in parallel with the ipsilateral border, then vertically to the median border of the obturator foramen

Treatment Delivery

- *Technique.* EBRT
- *Image-guidance.* Target fields checked by verification port films

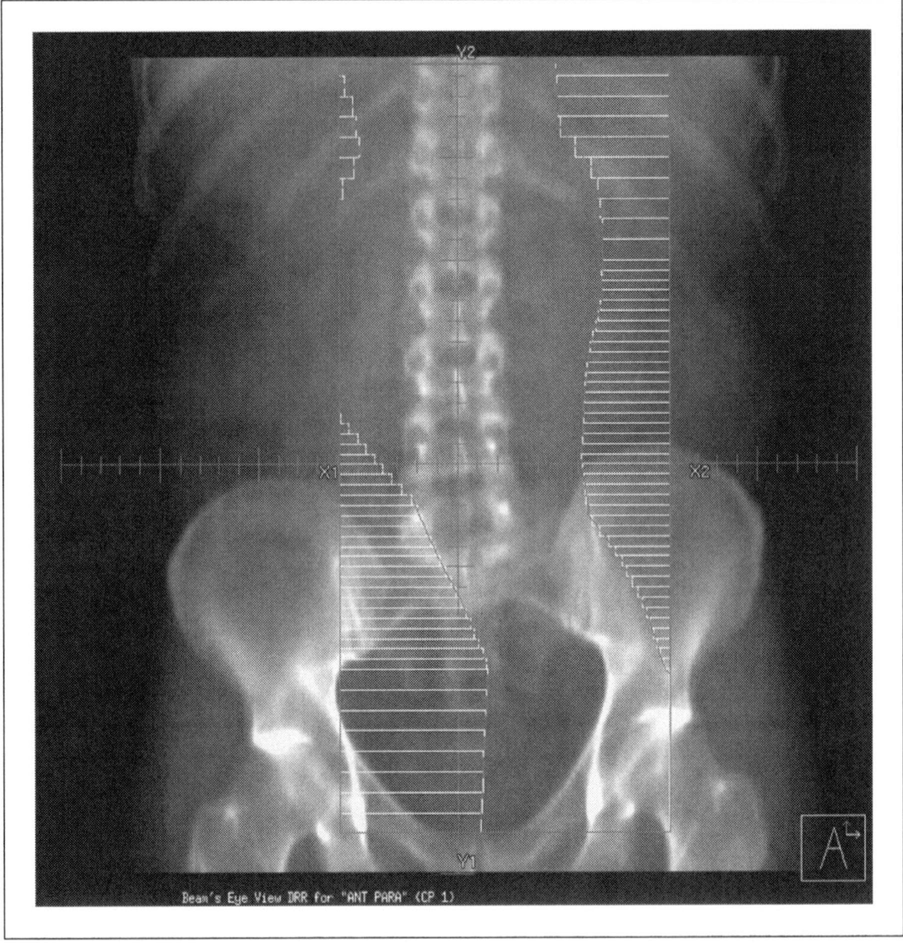

FIGURE 19.1 AP seminoma dogleg digitally reconstructed radiograph (DRR)

Organ(s) at Risk

- Kidney, dose constraints not specified

Toxicity

Acute:
- Nausea, vomiting, anorexia
- Diarrhea, dyspepsia, abdominal cramping
- Leukopenia
- Erythema, lethargy

Late:
- Decreased fertility
- Second malignancy

- Peptic ulcer disease
- Lymphedema, peripheral vascular disease

Clinical Protocol Reference

EORTC 30982: radiation therapy compared with chemotherapy in treating patients with stage I testicular cancer.

Chapter 20

Gynecological Treatment Planning

20.1. CERVIX

Therapeutic Considerations

- *Patient population.* Cervical cancer; FIGO stage IIB–IIIB or FIGO IB–IIA with pelvic node metastases and/or tumor size ≥ 5 cm
- *Concurrent treatments.* Weekly cisplatin

Dose Specification

- *Pelvic field.* 45 Gy in 25 fractions (1.8 Gy/fraction) plus
- *LDR brachytherapy.* 85 Gy (cumulative point A dose including external beam component) in two fractions 1 to 3 weeks apart

Or

- *HDR brachytherapy.* 30 Gy in five fractions
- May boost positive parametria to 60 Gy

Simulation

- *Imaging.* CT simulation preferred
- *Position.* Supine or prone
- *Immobilization.* Belly board (prone)
- *Scanning limits.* Not specified
- *Other.* Full bladder, small bowel contrast recommended, distal most aspect of cervico-vaginal disease marked with radio-opaque seeds or radio-opaque vaginal tampon, barium/radio-opaque device to localize rectum if conventional simulation

Target Volume(s)

Pelvic field:

- Anterior–posterior (AP)–posterior–anterior (PA) portals
  - Superior: L4/5 or 1 cm above the uterus (whichever is more superior)

- Inferior: below the obturator foramen or 3 cm below most distal vaginal disease (whichever is most inferior)
- Lateral: 2 cm lateral from bony pelvis
- Block: small bowel and femoral heads, but maintaining a 1-cm margin on the common iliac nodes, do not shield the obturator foramina (leave at least 1.5 cm)

- Lateral portals
  - Superior, anterior: as for AP–PA
  - Anterior: 5 mm anterior to symphysis pubis, and ≥ 1 cm anterior to common iliac nodes at L4–5
  - Posterior: entire bony sacrum. Ensure gross disease encompassed by ≥ 3-cm margins. In small volume disease, split posterior sacrum may be used (but maintain a 3- to 4-cm margin around cervical disease)
- Stage IIIA or IIIB with lower third vaginal involvement
  - AP–PA or four-field techniques acceptable
  - 2 cm around inguino-femoral vessels, to the lesser trochanter inferiorly. A 2-cm margin on the inferior extent of tumor is required

Parametrial boost:

- AP–PA fields with lateral borders identical to pelvic fields
- *Inferior.* Same as the pelvic field or brought up to the mid-obturator foramen
- *Superior.* 9 to 12 cm above the inferior border, tailor position from the radio-opaque markers and intracavitary films. Central blocking should measure at least 4.5 cm at midplane, and should be tailored to the position of the intracavitary system

Lymph node boost:

- At least 4 cm × 4 cm, and maintain a margin of 1 to 1.5 cm

LDR brachytherapy:

- Cesium intracavitary system in two applications
- Interstitial brachytherapy may be used to treat distal vaginal disease

HDR brachytherapy:

- Iridium-192
- Tandem and ovoids or tandem and ring systems
- Tandem and cylinder for lower third vaginal involvement

Treatment Planning

- Complete radiotherapy in ≤ 56 days
- *Pelvic field:*
  - Four-field technique with dose prescribed to isocenter
  - Maximum dose heterogeneity ≤ 5%
- *Parametrial and/or nodal boosts:*
  - AP–PA technique or CT-simulated multi-field plans are acceptable (ensure no overlap with brachytherapy)
  - If using a CT-based plan planning target volume (PTV) = gross tumor volume (GTV) + 1 cm
  - Boost dose: 60 Gy
  - Maximum dose heterogeneity: ≤ 5%
- *LDR brachytherapy:*
  - May be performed as soon as the fourth week of external beam radiotherapy

- Interval between two applications is 1 to 3 weeks
- Minimum cumulative dose to Point A (ICRU38): 85 Gy in two fractions
- Point A definition: 2 cm superior to cervical os along intrauterine tandem and 2 cm lateral in the plane of the intrauterine system

- *HDR brachytherapy:*
    - Can be performed as soon as week 2
    - One insertion per week, with no external beam radiotherapy on the same day
    - If most of the external beam radiotherapy is complete, then two insertions per week can be done to ensure completion of therapy within 56 days
    - Minimum dose to Point A (ICRU38): 30 Gy in five fractions
    - Recommend tandem and ring or ovoid system

Treatment Delivery

- *Technique.* Three-dimensional conformal radiation therapy (3DCRT)
- *Image-guidance.* Not specified

Organ(s) at Risk

- Total cumulative doses allowed for external beam radiation and LDR brachytherapy:
    - Small bowel: 60 Gy
    - Bladder: 80 Gy
    - Rectum: 70 Gy
    - Vaginal surface: 135 Gy
- HDR brachytherapy:
    - Bladder: ≤ 77% point A dose for each fraction
    - Rectum: ≤ 68% point A dose for each fraction

Toxicity

Acute:

- Fatigue, local epilation, erythema, decreased blood counts
- Diarrhea, proctitis
- Urinary frequency, dysuria

Late:

- Local skin changes and hair loss
- Vaginal narrowing, shortening, dyspareunia, induction of menopause, vaginal vault necrosis/fibrosis
- Rectal bleeding, loose stool, rectal ulcer, bowel obstruction
- Dysuria, urinary frequency, hematuria, ureteral obstruction

Clinical Protocol Reference

RTOG 0417: a phase II study of bevacizumab in combination with definitive radiotherapy and cisplatin chemotherapy in untreated patients with locally advanced cervical carcinoma.

20.2. POST-OPERATIVE CERVIX

Therapeutic Considerations

- *Patient population.* Clinical stage IA2, IB, IIA cervical cancer with any/all: positive pelvic nodes, positive parametrium, and/or positive para-aortic nodes. Complete resection, with negative post-operative CT and PET scans
- *Concurrent treatments.* Concurrent weekly cisplatin and external beam radiotherapy (with or without brachytherapy)
- *Alternative treatments.* Addition of adjuvant chemotherapy, surgery alone, adjuvant radiotherapy

Dose Specification

- 45 to 50.4 Gy in 25 to 28 fractions (1.8 Gy/fraction)
- ±20 to 25 Gy in one fraction (LDR brachytherapy) or 12 to 18 Gy in two to three fractions (HDR brachytherapy)

Simulation

- *Imaging.* CT simulation, slice thickness ≤ 3 mm (intensity-modulated radiation therapy [IMRT]) or ≤ 5 mm (3DCRT)
- *Position.* Supine
- *Immobilization.* Cradle that fixes upper body, trunk, and proximal legs
- Scanning limits:
  - *3DCRT.* At least L3 to mid-femur, if para-aortics being treated then superior border is T10
  - *IMRT.* T10 to below the perineum
- *Other.* full bladder radio-opaque marker at the vaginal cuff
  - IV contrast may be used to help define vessels
  - IMRT: requires a full bladder and empty bladder scans; which are used for planning

Target Volume(s)

3DCRT pelvic fields:

- AP–PA (anterior–posterior) field borders:
  - Superior: L4/5
  - Inferior: below the obturator foramen and at least 4 cm below the vaginal cuff
  - Lateral: 1 to 2 cm lateral to bony pelvis
  - Blocking: small bowel, femoral heads, but maintain a margin of at least 1 cm from common iliac vessels, do not shield the obturator foramina
- Lateral field borders:
  - Superior/inferior: same as AP–PA fields
  - Anterior: line through the pubic symphysis ≥ 1 cm anterior to the common iliac vessels at L4–5
  - Posterior: include S3–4

- Blocking: anterior small bowel if possible, but maintain a margin of ≥ 1 cm from common and external iliac vessels; blocking may split the L4–5 vertebral body to shield posterior soft tissue; may split the sacrum but maintain a margin on presacral nodes; posterior rectum may be blocked

3DCRT para-aortic fields:
(if positive common iliac or para-aortic nodes)
- AP–PA field borders:
  - Superior (only positive common iliac nodes): L1–2 interspace
  - Superior (positive para-aortic nodes): T11–12 interspace
  - Inferior: top of pelvic field
  - Lateral border: transverse processes
  - Blocking: shield kidneys, bowels
- Lateral field borders:
  - Superior/inferior: same as AP–PA fields
  - Anterior: at least 2 cm anterior to the vertebral body and/or 1 cm anterior to the para-aortic nodal region
  - Posterior: at least 1 cm posterior to the para-aortic nodal region and/or 1 to 1.5 cm of the vertebral body
  - Blocking: block small bowel and kidneys

IMRT:
(as per the RTOG contouring atlas, www.rtog.org)
- *CTVnodal.* Internal iliacs, hypogastric, obturator, external iliac, common iliac and presacral lymph node, and soft tissue down S3
  - Common iliac vessels +7 mm (excluding muscle, bone, small bowel)
  - 1 to 2 cm of tissue anterior to S1–3 (presacral lymph nodes, uterosacral ligaments)
  - External iliac contours should stop at the level of the femoral head (+7 mm, excluding muscle, bone, small bowel)
  - Obturator nodes: inferiorly to upper 1/3 of the obturator fossa
  - Superior limit: 7 mm below L4–5
  - If common iliacs are positive: superior limit is 7 mm below L2
  - If para-aortics are positive: superior limit is 7 mm below T12
- *CTVvagina.* Include vagina, paravaginal soft tissues on both the full and the empty bladder scans
  - Inferior limit: upper 1/3 of the pubic symphysis, or based on the tumor location, ensure ≥ 3 cm vagina covered
  - Lateral: obturator muscle
- *ITV vagina.* CTVvagina (empty bladder) + CTVvagina (full bladder)
- *PTV.* CTVnodal + ITVvagina + 7 mm

Brachytherapy:
- Vaginal cuff only
- No more than 2/3 of the vagina should be included in the treatment volume
- May use colpostats/ovoids or cylinders
- May use LDR or HDR brachytherapy

Treatment Planning

- *3DCRT:*
  - D_{min} ≥ 96% of prescription dose
  - D_{max} ≤ 107% of prescription dose

- *IMRT:*
  - PTVvagina, PTVnodes: dose prescribed to cover 97% of PTV
  - D_{min} > 93% of prescription dose
  - D_{max} < 110% of prescription dose
- *LDR brachytherapy:*
  - To start within 7 days of completion of external beam radiation
  - 25 Gy in one fraction (if external beam is 50.4 Gy in 28 fractions)
  - 20 Gy in one fraction (if external beam is 45 Gy in 25 fractions)
  - Dose prescribed to the vaginal surface
- *HDR brachytherapy:*
  - To start within 7 days of completion of external beam radiation
  - 12 Gy in two fractions (if external beam is 50.4 Gy in 28 fractions)
  - 18 Gy in three fractions (if external beam is 45 Gy in 25 fractions)
  - Dose prescribed to the vaginal surface

Treatment Delivery

- *Technique.* IMRT/3DCRT
- *Image-guidance.* Port film verification for all fields at least every 5 days
  - Treated with full bladder

Organ(s) at Risk

- *Kidneys (each).* $D_{66\%} \leq 18$ Gy
- *Spinal cord.* $D_{max} \leq 45$ Gy
- *Bladder.* $D_{35\%} < 45$ Gy
- *Bowel.* $D_{30\%} < 40$ Gy
- *Rectum.* $D_{60\%} < 45$ Gy

Toxicity

Acute:

- Urinary frequency, dysuria
- Diarrhea, nausea, vomiting, proctitis
- Local epilation, skin erythema, decreased blood counts

Late:

- Dysuria, hematuria
- Chronic malabsorption, rectal ulcer, rectal bleeding or stricture, bowel obstruction
- Shortening of the vagina, dyspareunia, vaginal vault necrosis or fistula, vaginal dryness
- If para-aortics are treated: long-term kidney damage, myelitis

Clinical Protocol Reference

RTOG 0724, GOG-0724: phase III randomized study of concurrent chemotherapy and pelvic radiation therapy with or without adjuvant chemotherapy in high-risk patients with early stage cervical carcinoma following radical hysterectomy.

20.3. POST-OPERATIVE ENDOMETRIUM

Therapeutic Considerations

- *Patient population.* Stage IA (with myometrial invasion) grade 3 with lymphovascular space involvement–LVSI, stage 1B grade 3, stage II, stage IIIA or C, stage IIIB if parametrial invasion only, stage IA (with myometrial invasion) or IB or stage II or stage III with serous or clear cell histology
- *Concurrent treatments.* Cisplatin with radiotherapy followed by four cycles of carboplatin and paclitaxel

Dose Specification

- 48.6 Gy in 27 fractions (1.8 Gy/fraction)
  - 45 Gy in 25 fractions and 50.4 Gy in 28 fractions allowed
- Brachytherapy (for cervical involvement)

Simulation

- *Imaging.* CT simulation
- *Position.* supine or prone
  - Prone: use of belly-board recommended
- *Other.* Full bladder recommended

Target Volume(s)

3DCRT:

- *Pelvic field:*
  - AP–PA portals (Figures 20.1 and 20.2)
    - Superior: L4/5 or 1 cm above the uterus (whichever is more superior)
    - Inferior: below the obturator foramen or 3 cm below most distal vaginal disease (whichever is most inferior)
    - Lateral: 2 cm lateral to pelvic brim
    - Block: small bowel and femoral heads, but maintaining a 1-cm margin on the common iliac nodes, do not shield the obturator foramina (leave at least 1.5 cm)
  - Lateral portals
    - Superior, anterior: as for AP, PA
    - Anterior: 5 mm anterior to symphysis pubis, and at least 1 cm anterior to common iliac nodes at L4–5
    - Posterior: entire bony sacrum. Ensure gross disease encompassed by at least 3-cm margins. In small volume disease, a line through the posterior sacrum may be used (but maintain a 3- to 4-cm margin around cervical disease)

IMRT:

- As per the RTOG contouring atlas (www.rtog.org)
- Planned with a full bladder and empty bladder CT
- Clinical target volume (CTV): proximal ½ vagina, parametrial tissues, internal, external, and distal common iliac lymph node regions to the upper S1 level

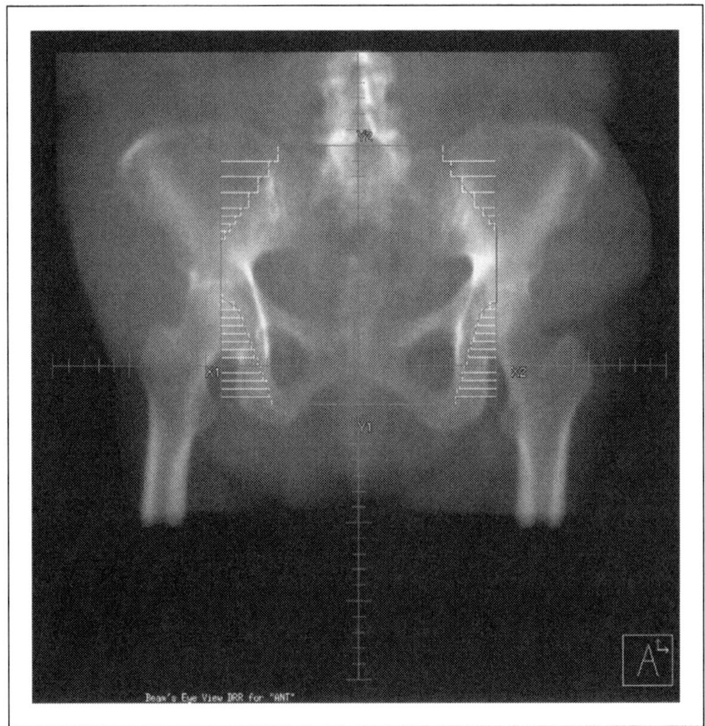

FIGURE 20.1 AP female pelvis endometrium

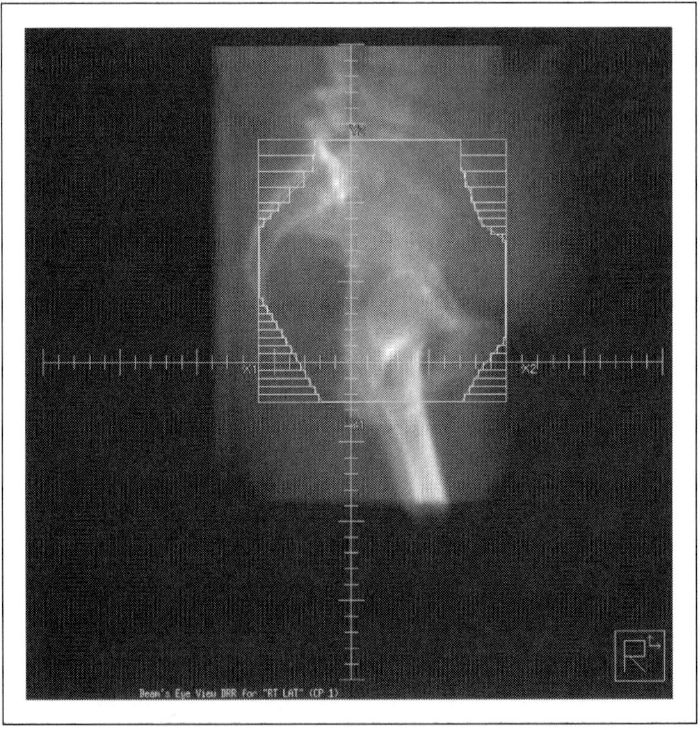

FIGURE 20.2 Right lateral female pelvis endometrium

- CTVnodes: internal iliac, external iliac, common iliac vessels, hypogastric, and obturator lymph nodes:
  - Iliac nodes: Start 7 mm below L4/5 and stop and the top of the femoral heads. Contour vessels with a 7-mm margin
  - Exclude muscle, bowel, bone
  - If the cervix is involved: add presacral lymph nodes (1–2 cm anterior to S1–3)
  - If external or internal iliac node involvement, common iliac lymph node regions included to aortic bifurcation (vessel + 7 mm)
  - If common iliac node involvement, peri-aortic lymph node region should be included to at least 2 cm above highest involved lymph node (vessel + involved nodes + 7 mm)
- CTV (full bladder): proximal half of vagina, parametrial tissues on the full bladder scan
- CTV (empty bladder): proximal half of vagina, parametrial tissues on the empty bladder scan
- Internal target volume (ITV): CTV (full bladder) + CTV (empty bladder)
- PTV: CTVnodes + 7 mm, ITV + 7 mm (except lateral margin which should extend to obturator muscle)
  - Ensure at least 3 cm of vagina or at least 1 cm of obturator foramen is covered.

Vaginal brachytherapy:
- Ovoids or vaginal cylinder, active length 2 to 3 cm

Treatment Planning

Pelvic field:
- Prescription dose shall encompass ≥ 97% of PTV
- ≤ 20% of PTV will receive > 110% of prescription dose
- ≤ 1% of the volume outside the PTV will receive > 110% of prescription dose
- ≤ 1% of PTV will receive < 93% of prescribed dose

Brachytherapy—if cervical involvement:
- Start on the last 1 to 2 weeks of radiotherapy, with no external beam radiotherapy on same day or week after completion of radiotherapy
- *HDR.* 10 Gy in two fractions with fractions at least 3 days apart
- *LDR.* 14 Gy in one fraction
- Prescribe dose to 5 mm from ovoids or vaginal cylinder

Complete total course of treatment within 50 days

Treatment Delivery

- *Technique.* IMRT or 3DCRT
- *Image-guidance.* Portal imaging at least day 1 and after 1 week of treatment

Organ(s) at Risk

- Total cumulative doses for external beam radiotherapy and brachytherapy
  - Rectum: D_{max} (to 2 mL) ≤ 75 Gy
  - Bladder: D_{max} (to 2 mL) ≤ 90 Gy

- External beam radiotherapy
  - Bladder: $D_{35\%} \leq 45$ Gy
  - Femoral head: $D_{15\%} \leq 30$ Gy
  - Rectum: $D_{60\%} \leq 30$ Gy
  - Small bowel: $D_{30\%} \leq 40$ Gy

Toxicity

Acute:
- Diarrhea, abdominal cramping, rectal bleeding
- Dysuria, hematuria
- Vaginal dryness

Late:
- Diarrhea, abdominal cramping, bowel obstruction, fistula, rectal ulcer
- Hematuria
- Vaginal shortening, dyspareunia, vaginal vault necrosis, fistula
- Pedal edema

Clinical Protocol Reference

PORTEC-3, EN7: randomized phase III trial comparing concurrent chemoradiation and adjuvant chemotherapy with pelvic radiation alone in high risk and advanced stage endometrial carcinoma.

Chapter 21

Sarcoma Treatment Planning

21.1. PREOPERATIVE EXTREMITY SARCOMA

Therapeutic Considerations

- *Patient population.* Primary soft tissue sarcoma of the extremity excluding hands and feet
- *Concurrent treatments.* Radiation with or without chemotherapy followed by surgery and radiotherapy boost if surgical margins are positive
- *Alternative treatments.* Upfront surgery followed by radiation, surgery alone, radiation followed by surgery with or without chemotherapy

Dose Specification

- *50 Gy in 25 fractions (2 Gy/fraction).* If receiving neoadjuvant and/or adjuvant chemotherapy or no chemotherapy
- *44 Gy in 22 fractions (2 Gy/fraction).* If concurrent or interdigitated chemotherapy
- *Boost (positive surgical margins).* 16 Gy in eight fractions (2 Gy/fraction) for external beam radiation therapy

Simulation

- *Imaging.* CT simulation
- *Position.* Depends on tumor location
- *Immobilization.* Alpha cradle, thermoplastic casts, or other method for stability
- *Other.* MRI fusion recommended

Target Volume(s)

- *GTV.* Gross tumor defined by MRI T1 plus contrast images
- CTV for intermediate-to-high grade tumors ≥ 8 cm:

  - GTV + edema (defined by MRI T2 images) + 3 cm in longitudinal directions (proximal and distal)
  - Field can be shortened to the end of a compartment
  - *Radial margin.* 1.5 cm, include any tumor not confined by an intact fascial barrier, bone, or skin surface
- CTV for remaining tumors:
  - GTV + suspicious edema (defined by MRI T2 images) + 2 cm in longitudinal directions (proximal and distal)
  - Field can be shortened to the end of a compartment
  - Radial margin: 1 cm, including any tumor not confined by an intact fascial barrier, bone, or skin surface
- *Planning target volume (PTV).* CTV + 5 mm

Treatment Planning

- 100% isodose line to cover ≥ 95% of PTV
- ≥ 99% of PTV should receive > 97% of prescribed dose
- ≤ 20% of PTV to receive ≥ 110% of prescription dose

Post-operative boost:
- Positive tumor margin or residual tumor + 1-cm margin
  - To be given 2 weeks following surgery or after adequate wound healing
  - May be external beam, brachytherapy, or intraoperative
  - External beam: 16 Gy in eight fractions (2 Gy/fraction)
  - LDR brachytherapy: 16 Gy at ≤ 80 cGy/hour
  - HDR brachytherapy: 13.6 Gy in four fractions (3.4 Gy/fraction) twice daily
  - Intraoperative (electron or HDR brachytherapy): 10 to 12.5 Gy

Treatment Delivery

- *Technique.* 3DCRT/IMRT
- *Image-guidance.* Daily imaging using one of:
  - Orthogonal 2D kV and MV electronic portal imaging device images
  - Linac mounted kV and MV cone-beam CT
  - Linac mounted MV CT images

Organ(s) at Risk

- Avoid treating full circumference of an extremity
- Avoid treating anus, vulva, scrotum, lung
- Avoid treating full dose to skin
- *Anus.* $D_{50\%} < 30$ Gy
- *Vulva.* $D_{50\%} < 30$ Gy
- *Testis.* $D_{50\%} < 3$ Gy (if patient prefers to reserve fertility)
- *Lungs.* $V_{20Gy} < 20\%$

- *Femoral head/neck.* $D_{5\%} < 60$ Gy
- *Joints.* $D_{50\%} < 50$ Gy (shoulder, elbow, knee)
- *Kidney.* $D_{50\%} < 14$ Gy
- *Longitudinal strip of skin or subcutaneous tissue.* $D_{50\%} < 20$ Gy
- *Weight-bearing bone.* $D_{50\%} < 50$ Gy

Toxicity

Acute:

- Erythema, desquamation, fatigue, reduced blood counts
- Diarrhea (if pelvis is treated)
- Slow healing

Late:

- Skin changes and fibrosis, pain, edema
- Increased risk of fracture
- Bowel stricture, perforation
- *If heart treated.* Dizziness, weakness, dyspnea, coronary artery disease, arrhythmia
- *If lung treated.* Pneumonitis, fibrosis, cough, dyspnea
- *If liver or stomach treated.* Fatigue, altered digestion, pain, bloating, constipation, nausea, and vomiting
- Radionecrosis of the spinal cord

Clinical Protocol Reference

RTOG 0630: a phase II trial of image-guided preoperative radiotherapy for primary soft tissue sarcomas of the extremity.

Chapter 22
Lymphoma

22.1. LYMPHOMA PLANNING

Therapeutic Considerations

- *Patient population.* Lymphoma

Classic Hodgkin's lymphoma (HL):
- Favorable, stage I/II:
  - ABVD chemotherapy for two cycles or consider Stanford V and
  - IFRT (20 Gy in 10 fractions)
- Unfavorable, stage I/II:
  - Chemotherapy for four cycles and
  - IFRT (30 Gy in 20 fractions)
- Advanced stage:
  - Chemotherapy for six to eight cycles and
  - IFRT (30 Gy in 20 fractions, with consideration of boost to additional 5 to 10 Gy for residual disease)

Nodular lymphocyte predominant HL:
- Stage I–IIA:
  - Consider chemotherapy
  - IFRT (30 Gy in 20 fractions), consider boost to 5 to 10 Gy for residual disease
- Stage III/IV A or B:
  - Chemotherapy, and
  - IFRT (30 Gy in 20 fractions), consider boost to 5 to 10 Gy for residual disease

Indolent non-Hodgkin's lymphoma:
- *IFRT.* 25 to 40 Gy with conventional fractionation (1.8 to 2 Gy/fraction), or consider chemotherapy if extensive

Aggressive non-Hodgkin's lymphoma (NHL):
- Chemotherapy and IFRT
- *Limited stage IFRT.* 30 to 36 Gy
- *Advanced stage.* Consider IFRT for bulky or residual disease
- *Primary bone.* 40 Gy in 20 fractions, consider boost of 5 to 6 Gy to primary site

Simulation

- *Imaging.* Conventional or computed tomography (CT) simulation
- *Fields.* Anterior–posterior (AP)/posterior–anterior (PA)
- *Other.* Consider pre- and post-chemotherapy positron emission tomography (PET)

Clarifications:

- Give radiotherapy to initially involved pre-chemotherapy sites and volume
    - Exceptions: transverse diameter of the mediastinum and para-aortic lymph nodes, for which the post-chemotherapy volume is used
- Supraclavicular (SCL) lymph nodes are considered part of the cervical chain

Cervical and SCL region:

- Simulation:
    - Imaging: conventional or CT simulation
    - Position: supine, neck hyper-extended (mandible in line with mastoid process), arms at sides
    - Immobilization: as per institutional guidelines
- Borders (Figure 22.1):
    - Superior: 1 to 2 cm above the lower tip of the mastoid process and mid-point through the chin
    - Inferior: 2 cm below the bottom of the clavicle
    - Lateral: include the medial 2/3 of the clavicle or to the coracoid process

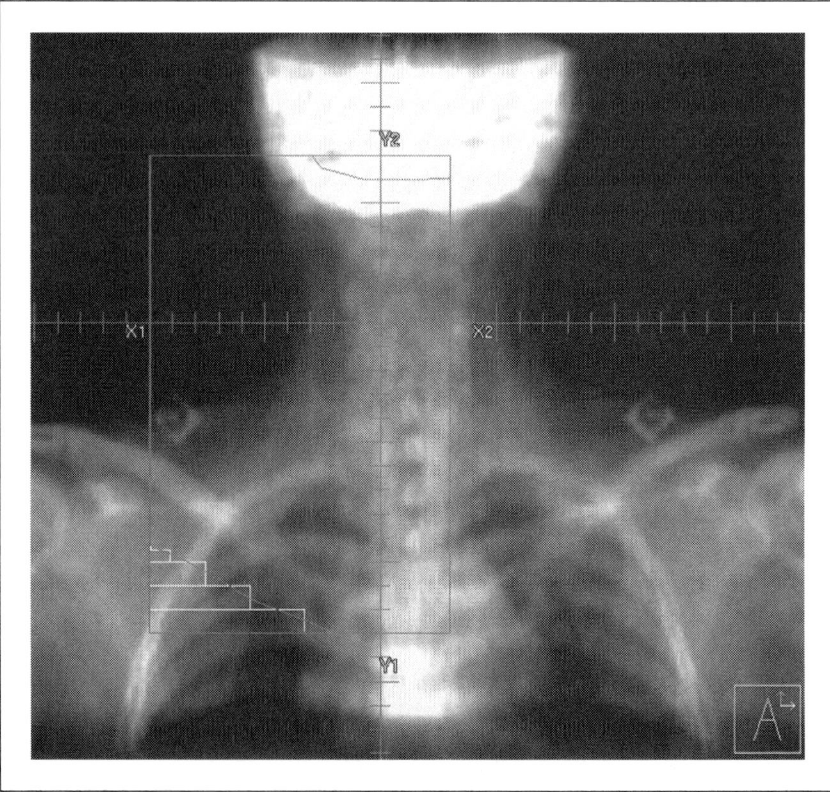

FIGURE 22.1 AP cervical and supraclavicular lymphoma

- Medial (for unilateral involvement):
  - SCL nodes not involved: ipsilateral transverse processes, unless medial nodes are close to the vertebral bodies (then include entire vertebral body)
  - SCL involved: contralateral transverse processes (for stage I patients, the larynx and vertebral bodies above the larynx can be blocked if there are no medial cervical nodes)
- Blocks:
  - Posterior cervical cord block if the cord dose exceeds 40 Gy
  - Larynx block: unless nodes were present at that location (2 × 3 cm block on AP field only at approximately C5–6)
  - Oral cavity: include 1 cm of mandible
  - Lung: start 2 cm from vertebral body, stay 1.5 cm below clavicle to chest wall, then 2 cm below clavicle to cover infraclavicular nodes

Mediastinum/hilum:

- Simulation:
  - Imaging: conventional or CT simulation
  - Position: supine, arms up (axillary involvement) otherwise arms akimbo or at sides
  - Immobilization: alpha cradle or similar device
- Borders (Figure 22.2):
  - Superior: C5/6 interspace
    - If SCL involved: top of larynx (consider coverage of ipsilateral cervical nodes)

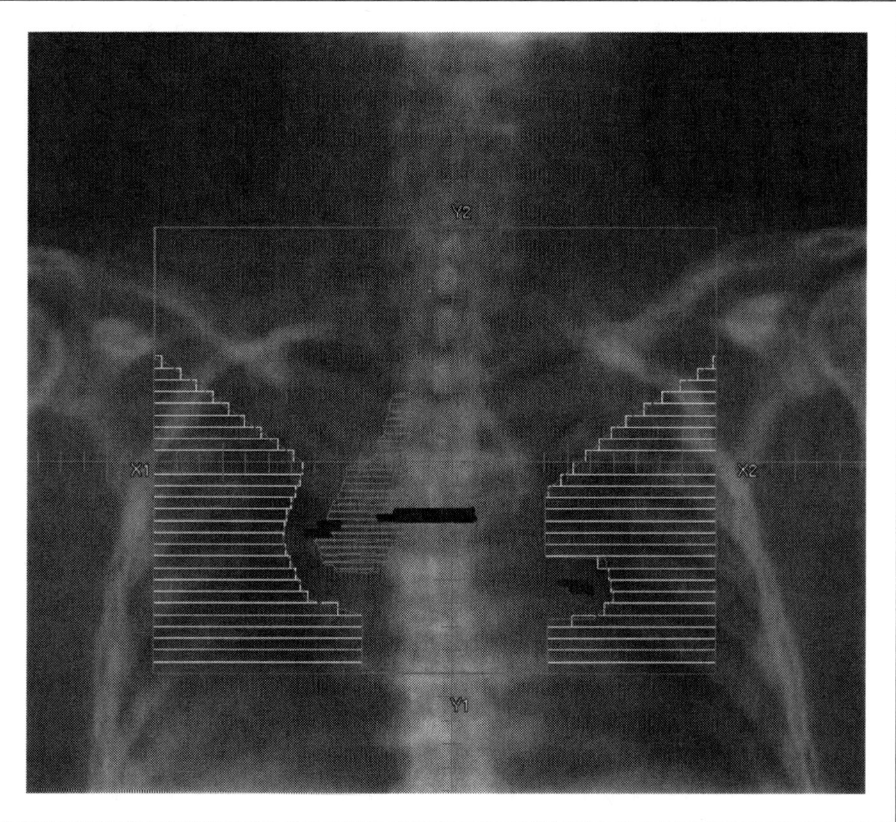

FIGURE 22.2 AP mediastinum lymphoma

- Inferior: 5 cm below the carina or 2 cm below the pre-chemotherapy tumor volume, whichever is more inferior
- Lateral: open field to coracoid process or 2/3 of clavicle
- Hilar margin: 1 cm, unless initially involved (then use 1.5-cm margin)
- Blocks:
  - Lung: start 1.5 cm from vertebral body, 1 cm around hila, 1.5 cm inferior to clavicle until reaching chest wall, then 2 cm inferior to clavicle
  - Ensure 1.5 cm border on any residual disease
  - Mediastinal field should have ≥ 8 cm width

Axillary:

- Simulation:
  - Imaging: conventional or CT simulation
  - Position: supine, arms up, or akimbo
  - Immobilization: breast board (arms up), or alpha cradle/similar device
- Borders (Figure 22.3):
  - Superior: C5/6 interspace
  - Inferior: tip of scapula or 2 cm below the lowest axillary node, whichever is more inferior
  - Lateral: lateral edge of the surgical neck of the humerus or flash axilla
  - Medial: ipsilateral cervical transverse processes
    - Include to entire vertebrae if SCL involved

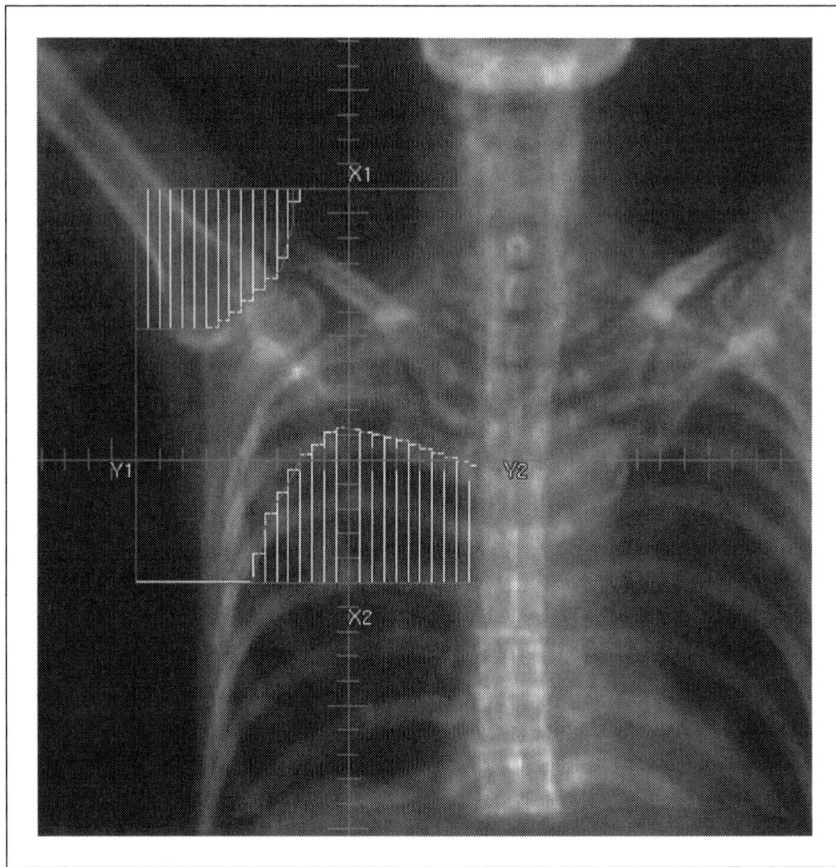

FIGURE 22.3 AP axillary lymphoma

- Blocks:
  - Humerus: medial border is the glenoid, leaving approximately 1 cm medial and inferior aspect of the humeral head, block the humeral shaft
  - Lung: 1.5 cm below the clavicle to chest wall, 1 cm of lung along the lateral chest wall; where two meet, round the corner following the inferior aspect of the fifth rib

Para-aortics:

- Simulation:
  - Imaging: conventional or CT simulation
  - Position: supine, arms at sides
  - Immobilization: alpha cradle or similar device
- Borders (Figure 22.4):
  - Superior: top of T11 or 2 cm above the pre-chemotherapy volume, whichever is more superior
  - If the para-aortics are not involved, may decrease to L1
  - Inferior: bottom of L4 or 2 cm below the pre-chemotherapy volume, whichever is more inferior
  - Lateral: edge of the transverse processes + 2 cm, or 2 cm from post-chemotherapy residual disease
- Blocks:
  - Contour kidneys for possible block if needed

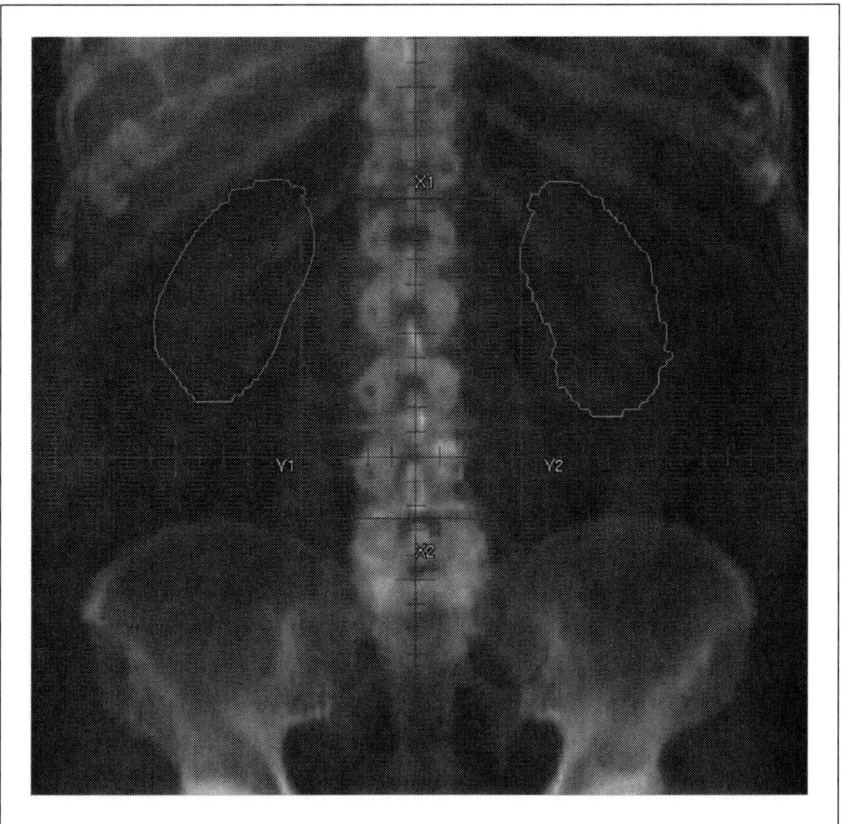

FIGURE 22.4 AP para-aortic lymphoma

Spleen:

- Simulation:
  - Imaging: CT simulation
  - Position: supine, arms at sides
  - Immobilization: alpha cradle or similar device
- Borders:
  - Post-chemotherapy volume + 1.5-cm margin
    - Contour left kidney for possible block

Iliacs:

- Simulation:
  - Imaging: conventional or CT simulation
  - Position: supine, arms at sides
  - Immobilization: alpha cradle or similar device
- Borders (Figure 22.5):
  - Superior: L4/5 interspace
  - Inferior: top of pubic symphysis
  - Lateral: greater trochanter or anterior superior iliac spine (ASIS) or 2 cm lateral to pre-chemotherapy involved nodes, whichever is more lateral
  - Medial: edge of the transverse processes + 2 cm, or 2 cm from post-chemotherapy residual disease

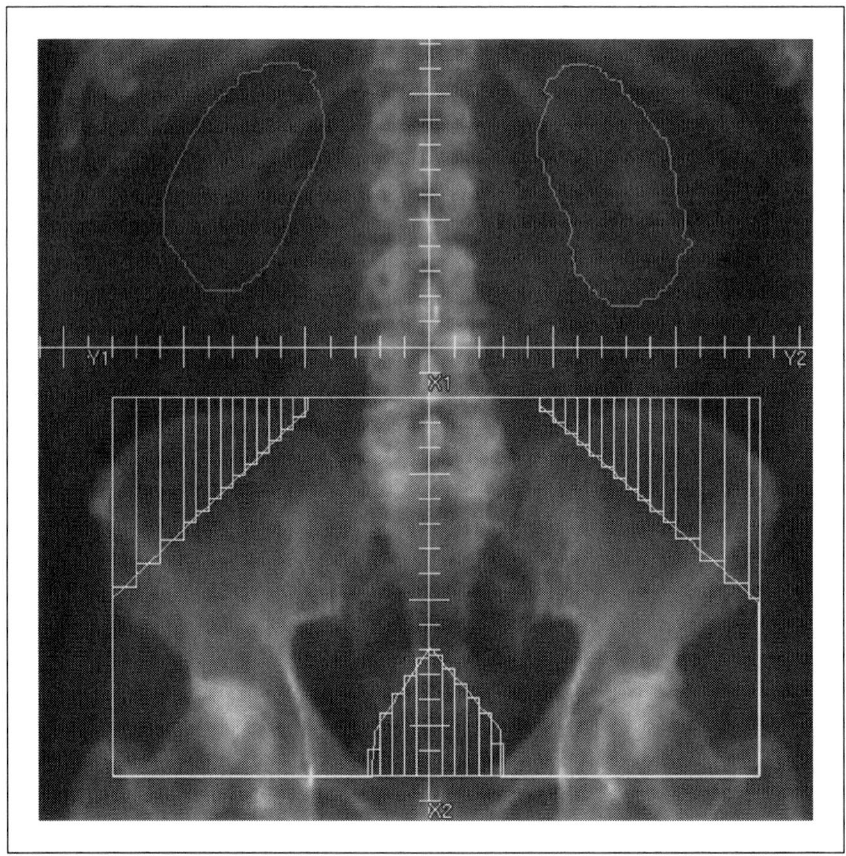

FIGURE 22.5 AP iliacs lymphoma

- Blocks:
  - Lateral dogleg: edge of the transverse processes + 2 cm until L4/5 interspace, then diagonal to ASIS
  - Medial dogleg if treating contralateral iliacs: continue 2 cm from edge of transverse processes until bottom of SI joint, then diagonal to top of pelvic brim in line with medial border of obturator foramen
  - Medial dogleg if not treating contralateral iliacs: same as above, but start diagonal at the top of the SI joint to the medial border of the obturator foramen

Inguinal/femoral:

- Simulation:
  - Imaging: conventional or CT simulation
  - Position: supine, arms at sides
  - Immobilization: alpha cradle or similar device
- Borders (Figure 22.6):
  - Superior: mid-sacroiliac joint
  - Inferior: 5 cm below lesser trochanter of 2 cm below disease, whichever is most inferior
  - Lateral: greater trochanter or 2 cm lateral to pre-chemotherapy involved nodes, whichever is more lateral
  - Medial: medial border of obturator foramen or 2 cm from pre-chemotherapy nodes, whichever is more medial
    - Or pubic symphysis with block for groin/vulva (1.5-cm margin on residual disease or medial border of obturator foramen to pelvic brim then diagonal to medial border)

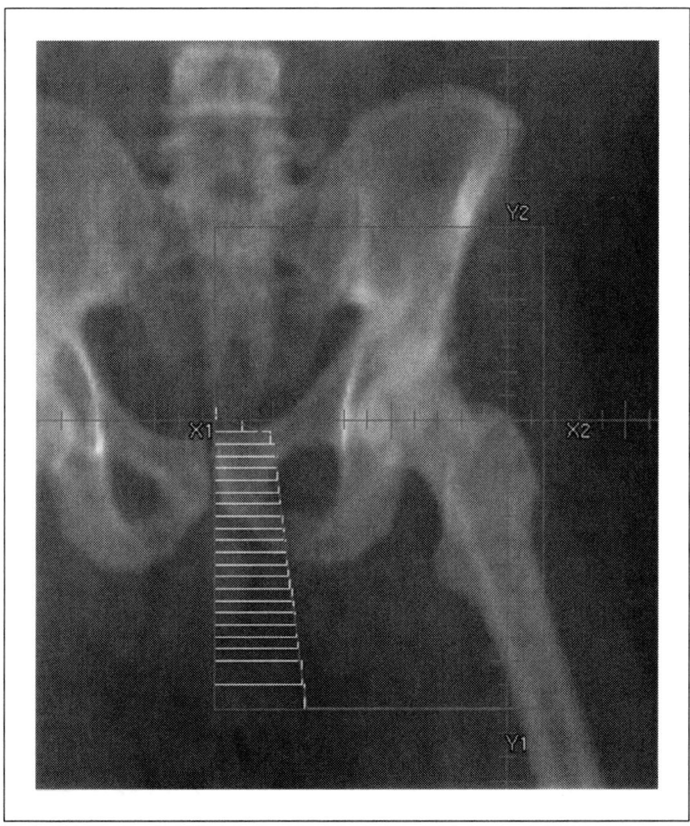

FIGURE 22.6 AP inguinal/femoral lymphoma

Clinical Protocol References

Sheplan LJ, Macklis RM. Lymphoma and myeloma radiotherapy. In: Videtic GM, Vassil AD, eds. *Handbook of Treatment Planning in Radiation Oncology*. New York: Demos Medical Publishing, 2011:157–169.

Engert A. Reduced treatment intensity in patients with early-stage Hodgkin's lymphoma. *NEJM* 2010;363:640–652.

Noordijk EM. First results of the EORTC-GELA H9 randomized trials: the H9-F9 comparing 3 radiation dose levels) and H9-U trial (comparing 3 chemotherapy schemes) in patients with favorable or unfavorable early stage Hodgkin's lymphoma (HL). *JCO* 2005;23(16s):6505.

Yahalom J, Mauch P. The involved field is back: issues in delineating the radiation field in Hodgkin's disease. *Ann Oncol* 2002;13(suppl 1):79–83.

Chapter 23

Skin Cancer Treatment Planning

23.1. SKIN PLANNING

Therapeutic Considerations

- *Patient population.* BCC or SCC of the skin
- *Concurrent treatments.* Consideration of surgery prior to radiotherapy
- *Alternative treatments.* Surgery, cryotherapy, curettage, topical chemotherapy, photodynamic therapy

Basal cell carcinoma:

- Low-risk
  - Curettage and electrodessication: non-hair-bearing area
  - Excision with 4-mm margin
  - Radiotherapy for nonsurgical candidate
  - If superficial can consider topical chemotherapy, photodynamic therapy, or cryotherapy
- High-risk
  - Excision with 10-mm margin
  - Radiotherapy for nonsurgical candidate, substantial perineural invasion
- Postoperative positive or close margins
  - Re-excision
  - Radiotherapy

SCC:

- Local, low-risk
  - Curettage and electrodessication: non-hair-bearing area
  - Excision with 4- to 6-mm margin
  - Radiotherapy for nonsurgical candidate
- Local, high-risk
  - Excision with 10-mm margin
  - Radiotherapy for nonsurgical candidate, substantial perineural invasion
- Positive regional adenopathy, with primary on trunk and extremities (operable)
  - Lymph node dissection then consider radiotherapy (especially if multiple positive nodes or extensive extracapsular extension)

- Positive regional adenopathy, with primary on trunk and extremities (inoperable)
  - Radiotherapy, consider concurrent chemotherapy
- Positive regional adenopathy of the head and neck
  - One positive node, ≤ 3 cm, no extracapsular extension: radiotherapy or observe
  - ≥ two positive nodes or one node, > 3 cm, and no extracapsular extension: radiotherapy
  - Extracapsular extension: radiotherapy, consider concurrent chemotherapy
  - Incompletely excised: radiotherapy, consider concurrent chemotherapy

Simulation

- *Imaging.* Conventional or computed tomography (CT) simulation
- *Fields.* Anterior–posterior (AP)/posterior–anterior (PA)
- *Other.* Consider pre- and post-chemotherapy positron emission tomography for lymph node positive disease

Treatment Planning

- Dose fractionation schedules (see Table 23.1)
- Smaller margins can be used for orthovoltage or if near a critical structure
- Bolus necessary when using electrons to achieve adequate surface dose
- Electron beam doses are specified at 90% of D_{max}
- Orthovoltage are specified at D_{max} (skin surface) and is used for superficial tumor < 5 mm in depth

Treatment Delivery and Image-Guidance

- *Technique.* Superficial, orthovoltage, electrons, three-dimensional conformal radiation therapy, intensity-modulated radiation therapy

Scalp:

- Simulation
  - Imaging: CT simulation or mark-up
  - Position: depends on lesion location and treatment modality used
  - Immobilization: depends on lesion location and treatment modality used
- Beam set-up
  - Direct appositional field (superficial, orthovoltage, electrons)
  - Variable if photons, usually tangential
- Shielding
  - Lead shielding on skin to mark field border for superficial or orthovoltage
- Considerations
  - Depth and location of tumor will determine modality used

Eyelid:

- Simulation
  - Imaging: mark-up
  - Position: supine
  - Immobilization: none for superficial or orthovoltage
- Beam set-up
  - Direct appositional field

TABLE 23.1 Skin Cancer Dose Fractionation Recommendations

Primary Tumor		
Tumor Diameter	Margins	Dose and Fractionation
< 2 cm	1–1.5 cm	64 Gy in 32 fractions
		55 Gy in 20–30 fractions
		50 Gy in 15–20 fractions
		35 Gy in 5 fractions
≥ 2 cm	1.5–2 cm	64–66 Gy in 32–33 fractions
		60 Gy in 30–34 fractions
		55 Gy in 20–30 fractions
Postoperative		60–66 Gy in 30–33 fractions
		50 Gy in 20 fractions
		40 Gy in 15 fractions
		36 Gy in 12 fractions
Cosmesis not important		40 Gy in 10 fractions
		30 Gy in 5 fractions
		18–20 Gy in 1 fraction
Regional disease—after lymph node dissection (using shrinking field technique)		
Head and neck, extracapsular extension (ECE)		60–66 Gy in 30–33 fractions
Head and neck, no ECE		56 Gy in 28 fractions
Axilla or groin, ECE		60 Gy in 30 fractions
Axilla or groin, no ECE		54 Gy in 27 fractions
Regional disease—no lymph node dissection (using shrinking field technique)		
Clinically negative but at risk for subclinical disease		50 Gy in 25 fractions (2 Gy/fraction)
Head and neck adenopathy		66–70 Gy in 33–35 fractions
Axilla or groin adenopathy		66 Gy in 33 fractions

- Shielding
  - Lead eye shielding on eye
  - Lead shielding on skin to mark field border
- Considerations
  - Ophthalmic anesthetic drops applied prior to insertion of eye shield
  - Suggest protracted fractionation for cosmetic and functional results
  - Attempt to shield the lacrimal gland (if feasible)

Canthus of eye:

- Simulation
  - Imaging: mark-up
  - Position: supine
  - Immobilization: none for superficial or orthovoltage

- Beam set-up
  - Direct appositional field
- Shielding
  - Lead eye shielding on eye
  - Lead shielding on skin to mark field border
- Considerations
  - Ophthalmic anesthetic drops applied prior to insertion of eye shield
  - Respect natural boundaries (if on lower eyelid, not going to spread to upper eyelid)
  - Suggest protracted fractionation for cosmetic and functional results
  - Attempt to shield the lacrimal drainage system (if feasible)

Ear (pinna):
- Simulation
  - Imaging: mark-up, simulation in select cases
  - Position: lateral decubitus
  - Immobilization: none
- Beam set-up
  - Direct appositional field
  - Consider: electrons (or orthovoltage), photons in select cases
- Shielding
  - Lead shielding behind ear (depending on location of tumor and beam used)
- Considerations
  - Wax or wet gauze in and behind ear to bring perpendicular to scalp

Nasolabial fold/nasal ala:
- Simulation
  - Imaging: CT simulation if unsure of infiltration depth
  - Immobilization: thermoplastic mask with nose cut out
- Beam set-up
  - Direct appositional field for orthovoltage or electrons
  - Consider: orthovoltage, electrons (or photons)
- Shielding
  - Lead coated in wax in nose
  - Lead shielding on skin to mark field border for orthovoltage
- Considerations
  - Include nasolabial fold for nasal ala lesions
  - Can use wax bolus on irregular surfaces for homogeneity if using electrons

Tip of nose:
- Simulation
  - Imaging: CT simulation or mark-up
  - Position: supine
  - Immobilization: thermoplastic mask
- Beam set-up
  - Pair of opposed lateral fields, half beam block sup (protect eyes) and post (protect maxillary sinuses) for photons
  - Direct appositional field for superficial or orthovoltage
- Borders (for photon treatment)
  - Sup: bridge of nose
  - Inf: 1 cm below inferior aspect of nose
  - Post: most lateral part of nose that will allow beam to clear cheek
  - Ant: 1 cm above tip of nose or gross disease

- Considerations (for photon treatment)
  - Wax bolus from bridge of nose to 1 cm inferior to most inferior portion of nose; build up 1 cm above and beyond nose laterally

Lip:
- Simulation
  - Imaging: CT simulation or mark-up
  - Position: supine
  - Immobilization: thermoplastic mask
- Beam set-up
  - Direct appositional field
  - Consider: orthovoltage, electrons, or external beam depending on tumor depth
  - Interstitial brachytherapy implant in select cases
- Shielding
  - Lead shield behind lip to shield teeth and mandible
  - Lead shielding on skin to mark field border (orthovoltage)

Toxicity:

Acute:
- Skin erythema, dry and wet desquamation

Late:
- Skin atrophy, telangiectasia, hyper- or hypo-pigmentation
- Local epilation, decreased sebaceous and sweat gland function
- Subcutaneous fibrosis

Clinical Protocol References

NCCN Clinical Practice Guidelines in Oncology: Basal cell and squamous cell skin cancers. Version 1.2012.

Principles and practice of radiation oncology. Chapter 30: Skin Cancer. 5th Edition. Halperin, Perez, Brady, eds. Philadelphia, PA: Lippincott Williams & Wilkins, 2008:694–695, 700.

23.2. POSTOPERATIVE HIGH-RISK SKIN

Therapeutic Considerations

- *Patient population.* High-risk nodal disease or advanced primary disease from a SCC of the skin in the head and the neck
- *Concurrent treatments.* None
- *Alternative treatments.* Consideration of concurrent chemotherapy, re-excision, observation

High-risk nodal disease:
- Intraparotid nodal disease
- Cervical nodal disease within the drainage basin of a synchronous or previously (≤ 2 years) resected index lesion within the corresponding nodal drainage basin and exclusion of a mucosal primary
- For cervical nodal disease to be eligible there must be ≥ one of the following:
  - ≥ 2 nodes involved
  - Largest node ≥ 3 cm
  - Extracapsular extension

Advanced primary disease:
- T3–4 primary disease (cartilage, skeletal, muscle, bone involvement or > 4 cm or in transit metastases)

Dose Specification

- 60 to 66 Gy in 30 to 33 fractions (2 Gy/fraction)

Simulation

- *Imaging.* CT simulation, slice thickness ≤ 5 mm
- *Position.* Supine
- *Immobilization.* Thermoplastic mask or vacuum formed mask
- *Other.* Wire all surgical scars
  - Suggest use of an intraoral stent or tongue depressor
  - For an appositional electron field, an open neck technique is recommended
  - For posterior vertex of the scalp or suboccipital nodes requiring irradiation, the patient may be positioned prone

Target Volume(s)

- *CTV1.* Site of resected gross disease, surgical bed/scar
  - First echelon of clinically uninvolved nodes
- *CTV2.* Site of resected gross disease, surgical bed/scar
- *CTV3.* Site of resected gross disease
- *PTV1.* CTV1 + ≥ 0.5 cm
- *PTV2.* CTV2 + ≥ 0.5 cm
- *PTV3.* CTV3 + ≥ 0.5 cm

Treatment Planning

- *PTV1.* 50 Gy in 25 fractions (2 Gy/fraction)
- *PTV2.* 54 Gy in 27 fractions (2 Gy/fraction)
- *PTV3.* 60 to 66 Gy in 30 to 33 fractions (2 Gy/fraction)
- *For electrons.* The dose is specified to the depth of the 90% isodose line
- *Dose homogeneity.* Minimum 95% prescribed dose
  - Maximum 107% prescribed dose
  - Where there is a photon/electron match, a small volume hotspot of $\leq$ 120% is permissible
- *Advanced local disease, N0.* Bolus to achieve full tumor dose on skin at primary site
  - Where elective nodal dissection is performed and no disease is detected, this is considered part of the surgical bed/scar (bolus of this scar is optional)
  - Elective nodal irradiation may be omitted where it is technically difficult or the toxicity is high
- High-risk nodal disease or advanced disease with low-risk nodal disease
  - For positive intraparotid or upper cervical nodal metastases the ipsilateral lower neck and supraclavicular region are considered the first echelon of nodes (part of CTV1)
  - When nodal metastases occur > 12 months following treatment of the index cutaneous lesion and there is no evidence of local recurrence, treatment of the primary and intervening lymphatics is optional
  - When high-risk nodal metastases occur $\leq$ 12 months after treatment of the index lesion, suggest inclusion of the primary site and intervening dermal lymphatic as part of PTV1–3 (treated to 60–66 Gy)

Treatment Delivery and Image-Guidance

- *Technique.* Appositional electron field or photons
- *Image-guidance.* Day 1 portal film/image for each photon beam
  - Weekly portal film/image for each photon beam
  - For electrons: simulation field, photograph, or digitally reconstructed radiograph available as a reference image

Organ(s) at Risk

- *Spinal cord.* $D_{max} \leq 45$ Gy
- *Brainstem.* $D_{max} \leq 54$ Gy
- *Optic chiasm.* $D_{max} \leq 54$ Gy

Toxicity

Acute:

- Skin erythema, desquamation
- Loss of taste, dysphagia, dry mouth
- Alopecia, weight loss, lethargy

Late:

- Thinning of the skin, skin fibrosis, alopecia
- Hearing loss, dry mouth
- Osteoradionecrosis of the mandible, nerve damage, cataracts

Clinical Protocol Reference

TROG 0501 (POST study): post-operative concurrent chemo-radiotherapy versus post-operative radiotherapy in high-risk cutaneous squamous cell carcinoma of the head and neck.

Suggested Readings

Andriole GL, Crawford ED, Grubb RL 3rd, PLCO Project Team. Prostate cancer screening in the randomized Prostate, Lung, Colorectal, and Ovarian Cancer Screening Trial: mortality results after 13 years of follow-up. *J Natl Cancer Inst.* 2012;104(2):125–132.

Aune D, Lau R, Chan DS, et al. Nonlinear reduction in risk for colorectal cancer by fruit and vegetable intake based on meta-analysis of prospective studies. *Gastroenterology.* 2011;141(1):106–118.

Boffetta P, Couto E, Wichmann J, et al. Fruit and vegetable intake and overall cancer risk in the European Prospective Investigation into Cancer and Nutrition (EPIC). *J Natl Cancer Inst.* 2010;102(8):529–537.

Booth CM, Li G, Zhang-Salomons J, Mackillop WJ. The impact of socioeconomic status on stage of cancer at diagnosis and survival: a population-based study in Ontario, Canada. *Cancer.* 2010;116(17):4160–4167.

Buys SS, Partridge E, Black A, PLCO Project Team. Effect of screening on ovarian cancer mortality: the Prostate, Lung, Colorectal and Ovarian (PLCO) Cancer Screening Randomized Controlled Trial. *JAMA.* 2011;305(22):2295–2303.

Chen WY, Rosner B, Hankinson SE, Colditz GA, Willett WC. Moderate alcohol consumption during adult life, drinking patterns, and breast cancer risk. *JAMA.* 2011;306(17):1884–1890.

Dalton-Griffin L, Kellam P. Infectious causes of cancer and their detection. *J Biol.* 2009;8(7):67.

Danaei G, Vander Hoorn S, Lopez AD, Murray CJ, Ezzati M; Comparative Risk Assessment collaborating group (Cancers). Causes of cancer in the world: comparative risk assessment of nine behavioural and environmental risk factors. *Lancet.* 2005;366(9499):1784–1793.

Davis JS, Wu X. Current state and future challenges of chemoprevention. *Discov Med.* 2012;13(72):385–390.

DeVita VT, Lawrence TS, Rosenberg SA. *DeVita, Hellman, and Rosenberg's Cancer: Principles and Practice of Oncology.* 9th ed. Philadelphia, PA: Wolters Kluwer Health/Lippincott Williams & Wilkins; 2011: p. xlvii.

Edge SB, American Joint Committee on Cancer. *AJCC Cancer Staging Manual.* 7th ed. New York, NY; London: Springer; 2010: p. xiv.

Edge SB, Compton CC. The American Joint Committee on Cancer: the 7th edition of the AJCC cancer staging manual and the future of TNM. *Ann Surg Oncol.* 2010;17(6):1471–1474.

Eheman C, Henley SJ, Ballard-Barbash R, et al. Annual Report to the Nation on the status of cancer, 1975–2008, featuring cancers associated with excess weight and lack of sufficient physical activity. *Cancer.* 2012;118(9):2338–2366.

Engert A, Plütschow A, Eich HT, et al. Reduced treatment intensity in patients with early-stage Hodgkin's lymphoma. *N Engl J Med.* 2010;363(7):640–652.

Gaspar LE, Scott C, Murray K, Curran W. Validation of the RTOG recursive partitioning analysis (RPA) classification for brain metastases. *Int J Radiat Oncol Biol Phys.* 2000;47(4):1001–1006.

Gomez D, Cahlon O, Mechalakos J, Lee N. An investigation of intensity-modulated radiation therapy versus conventional two-dimensional and 3D-conformal radiation therapy for early stage larynx cancer. *Radiat Oncol.* 2010;5:74.

Goossens MC, De Grève J. Individual cancer risk as a function of current age and risk profile. *Eur J Cancer Prev.* 2010;19(6):485–495.

Greene KL, Albertsen PC, Babaian RJ, et al. Prostate specific antigen best practice statement: 2009 update. *J Urol.* 2009;182(5):2232–2241.

Grégoire V, Eisbruch A, Hamoir M, Levendag P. Proposal for the delineation of the nodal CTV in the node-positive and the post-operative neck. *Radiother Oncol.* 2006;79(1):15–20.

Guillem JG, Berchuck A, Moley JF, et al. Role of surgery in cancer prevention. In VT DeVita, TS Lawrence, SA Rosenberg, eds. *DeVita, Hellman, and Rosenberg's Cancer: Principles & Practice of Oncology.* Philadelphia, PA: Wolters Kluwer Health/Lippincott Williams & Wilkins; 2011: p. xlvii.

Guyatt G, Rennie D. *Users' Guides to the Medical Literature: Essentials of Evidence-Based Clinical Practice.* Chicago, IL: AMA Press; 2002: p. xxxi.

Hall EJ, Giaccia AJ. *Radiobiology for the Radiologist.* 6th ed. Philadelphia, PA: Lippincott Williams & Wilkins; 2006: p. ix.

Hanahan D, Weinberg RA. The hallmarks of cancer. *Cell.* 2000;100(1):57–70.

Hartman M, Loy EY, Ku CS, Chia KS. Molecular epidemiology and its current clinical use in cancer management. *Lancet Oncol.* 2010;11(4):383–390.

Hinz EK, Kudesia R, Rolston R, Caputo TA, Worley MJ Jr. Physician knowledge of and adherence to the revised breast cancer screening guidelines by the United States Preventive Services Task Force. *Am J Obstet Gynecol.* 2011;205(3):201.e1–201.e5.

ICRU. *Prescribing, Recording and Reporting Photon Beam Therapy. Report 50*; 1993: Bethesda, MD.

ICRU. *Prescribing, Recording and Reporting Photon Beam Therapy (Supplement to report 50). Report 62*; 1999: Bethesda, MD.

Kane MA. Preventing cancer with vaccines: progress in the global control of cancer. *Cancer Prev Res (Phila).* 2012;5(1):24–29.

Kumar V, Cotran RS, Robbins SL. *Robbins Basic Pathology.* 7th ed. Philadelphia, PA: Saunders; 2003: p. xii.

Lichtenstein P, Holm NV, Verkasalo PK, et al. Environmental and heritable factors in the causation of cancer–analyses of cohorts of twins from Sweden, Denmark, and Finland. *N Engl J Med.* 2000;343(2):78–85.

Lutz S, Lo SS, Chow E, Sahgal A, Hoskin P. Radiotherapy for metastatic bone disease: current standards and future prospectus. *Expert Rev Anticancer Ther.* 2010;10(5):683–695.

Menon U, Kalsi J, Jacobs I. The UKCTOCS experience–reasons for hope? *Int J Gynecol Cancer.* 2012;22(Suppl 1):S18–20.

Moyer VA, on behalf of the U.S. Preventive Services Task Force*. Menopausal Hormone Therapy for the Primary Prevention of Chronic Conditions: U.S. Preventive Services Task Force Recommendation Statement. *Ann Intern Med.* 2012.

Nelson HD, Tyne K, Naik A, Bougatsos C, Chan BK, Humphrey L, U.S. Preventive Services Task Force. Screening for breast cancer: an update for the U.S. Preventive Services Task Force. *Ann Intern Med.* 2009;151(10):727–37, W237.

Oster S, Penn L, Stambolic V. Oncogenes and tumor suppressor genes. In I Tannock, ed. *The Basic Science of Oncology.* New York, NY:McGraw-Hill, Medical Pub. Division;2005: p. x.

Parkin DM. The global health burden of infection-associated cancers in the year 2002. *Int J Cancer.* 2006;118(12):3030–3044.

QUANTEC. *Quantitative Analysis of Normal Tissue Effects in Clinic (QUANTEC).* IJROBP. 2010;76(3):S1-S160.

Rex DK, Johnson DA, Anderson JC, Schoenfeld PS, Burke CA, Inadomi JM; American College of Gastroenterology. American College of Gastroenterology guidelines for colorectal cancer screening 2009 [corrected]. *Am J Gastroenterol.* 2009;104(3):739–750.

Rodrigues G, Macbeth F, Burmeister B, et al. Consensus statement on palliative lung radiotherapy: third international consensus workshop on palliative radiotherapy and symptom control. *Clin Lung Cancer.* 2012;13(1):1–5.

Rubin P, Hansen, JT. *TNM Staging Atlas.* Philadelphia, PA: Lippincott Williams & Wilkins; 2008: xii.

Saslow D, Solomon D, Lawson HW, et al.; American Cancer Society; American Society for Colposcopy and Cervical Pathology; American Society for Clinical Pathology. American Cancer Society, American Society for Colposcopy and Cervical Pathology, and American Society for Clinical Pathology screening guidelines for the prevention and early detection of cervical cancer. *Am J Clin Pathol.* 2012;137(4):516–542.

Schröder FH, Hugosson J, Roobol MJ, et al. ERSPC Investigators. Screening and prostate-cancer mortality in a randomized European study. *N Engl J Med.* 2009;360(13):1320–1328.

Schulz KF, Altman DG, Moher D; CONSORT Group. CONSORT 2010 Statement: updated guidelines for reporting parallel group randomised trials. *BMC Med.* 2010;8:18.

Sheplan L, Macklis R. Lymphoma and myeloma radiotherapy. In A Vassil and GM Videtic, eds. *Handbook of treatment planning in radiation oncology.* Demos Medical Publishing; 2011: p. 157–169.

Solan MJ, Brady LW. Skin cancer. In EC Halperin, CA Perez, LW Brady, eds. *Perez and Brady's Principles and Practice of Radiation Oncology.* Philadelphia, PA:Wolters Kluwer/Lippincott Williams & Wilkins; 2008: p. xxxii.

Sperduto PW, Chao ST, Sneed PK, et al. Diagnosis-specific prognostic factors, indexes, and treatment outcomes for patients with newly diagnosed brain metastases: a multi-institutional analysis of 4,259 patients. *Int J Radiat Oncol Biol Phys.* 2010;77(3):655–661.

Stewart BW. Priorities for cancer prevention: lifestyle choices versus unavoidable exposures. *Lancet Oncol.* 2012;13(3):e126–e133.

Tannock I. *The Basic Science of Oncology.* 4th ed. New York, NY: McGraw-Hill, Medical Pub. Division. 2005, p. x, 555.

Tepper, J.E. and L.L. Gunderson, Radiation treatment parameters in the adjuvant postoperative therapy of gastric cancer. *Semin Radiat Oncol,* 2002. 12(2): p. 187–95.

Therasse P, Arbuck SG, Eisenhauer EA, et al. New guidelines to evaluate the response to treatment in solid tumors. European Organization for Research and Treatment of Cancer, National Cancer Institute of the United States, National Cancer Institute of Canada. *J Natl Cancer Inst.* 2000;92(3):205–216.

Tonelli M, Connor Gorber S, Joffres M, et al. Recommendations on screening for breast cancer in average-risk women aged 40–74 years. *CMAJ,* 2011;183(17):1991–2001.

UPSTF. Screening for breast cancer: U.S. Preventive Services Task Force recommendation statement. *Ann Intern Med,* 2009;151(10):716–26, W-236.

Vassil A, Videtic GM. (eds.) Palliative radiotherapy. In *Handbook of Treatment Planning in Radiation Oncology.* Demos Medical Publishing; 2011: p. 215–217.

Vengalil S, O'Sullivan JM, Parker CC. Use of radionuclides in metastatic prostate cancer: pain relief and beyond. *Curr Opin Support Palliat Care,* 2012:6(3), 310–5.

Weitzel JN, Blazer KR, Macdonald DJ, et al. Genetics, genomics, and cancer risk assessment: State of the Art and Future Directions in the Era of Personalized Medicine. *CA Cancer J Clin,* 2011.

Yahalom J, Mauch P. The involved field is back: issues in delineating the radiation field in Hodgkin's disease. *Ann Oncol,* 2002;13(Suppl 1):79–83.

Index

Note: Page numbers followed by "*f*" and "*t*" denote figures and tables, respectively.